Hematology Board Review

Hematology Board Review
Blueprint Study Guide and Q&A

Second Edition

Editors

Rami N. Khoriaty, MD
Associate Professor
Department of Internal Medicine, Division of Hematology/Oncology
University of Michigan Medical School
Ann Arbor, Michigan

Morgan Jones, MD, PhD
Clinical Professor
Department of Internal Medicine, Division of Hematology/Oncology
University of Michigan Medical School
Ann Arbor, Michigan

Francis P. Worden, MD
Professor of Medicine
Director of the Hematology/Oncology Fellowship Program
University of Michigan Medical School
Ann Arbor, Michigan

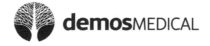

Springer Publishing Company, LLC
www.springerpub.com
connect.springerpub.com

Acquisitions Editor: David D'Addona
Compositor: Exeter Premedia
ISBN: 978-0-8261-8802-1
ebook ISBN: 978-0-8261-8803-8
DOI: 10.1891/9780826188038

23 24 25 26 / 5 4 3 2 1

Medicine is an ever-changing science. Research and clinical experience are continually expanding our knowledge, in particular our understanding of proper treatment and drug therapy. The authors, editors, and publisher have made every effort to ensure that all information in this book is in accordance with the state of knowledge at the time of production of the book. Nevertheless, the authors, editors, and publisher are not responsible for any errors or omissions or for any consequence from application of the information in this book and make no warranty, expressed or implied, with respect to the content of this publication. Every reader should examine carefully the package inserts accompanying each drug and should carefully check whether the dosage schedules therein or the contraindications stated by the manufacturer differ from the statements made in this book. Such examination is particularly important with drugs that are either rarely used or have been newly released on the market. The publisher has no responsibility for the persistence or accuracy of URLs for external or third-party Internet websites referred to in this publication and does not guarantee that any content on such websites is, or will remain, accurate or appropriate.

Library of Congress Cataloging-in-Publication Data

Names: Khoriaty, Rami N., editor. | Jones, Morgan, MD, PhD, editor. |
  Worden, Francis P., editor.
Title: Hematology board review : blueprint study guide and Q&A / Rami N.
  Khoriaty, Morgan Jones, Francis P. Worden.
Description: Second edition. | New York : Springer Publishing, [2024] |
  Includes bibliographical references and index.
Identifiers: LCCN 2023039332 (print) | LCCN 2023039333 (ebook) | ISBN
  9780826188021 (paperback) | ISBN 9780826188038 (ebook)
Subjects: MESH: Hematologic Diseases | Hematology--methods | Examination
  Questions
Classification: LCC RC636 (print) | LCC RC636 (ebook) | NLM WH 18.2 |
  DDC 616.1/50076--dc23/eng/20231023
LC record available at https://lccn.loc.gov/2023039332
LC ebook record available at https://lccn.loc.gov/2023039333

Contact sales@springerpub.com to receive discount rates on bulk purchases.

Publisher's Note: New and used products purchased from third-party sellers are not guaranteed for quality, authenticity, or access to any included digital components.

Printed in the United States of America by Gasch Printing.

Contents

Contributors

Asra Z. Ahmed, MD, Division of Hematology/Oncology, Department of Internal Medicine, University of Michigan, Ann Arbor, Michigan

Emily Bellile, MS, Senior Statistician, Cancer Data Science, School of Public Health, University of Michigan, Ann Arbor, Michigan

Dale L. Bixby, MD, PhD, Clinical Professor, Division of Hematology/Oncology, University of Michigan, Ann Arbor, Michigan

Patrick Burke, MD, Associate Professor of Internal Medicine, Division of Hematology/Oncology, Department of Medicine, University of Michigan, Ann Arbor, Michigan

Erica Campagnaro, MD, Clinical Associate Professor, Rogel Cancer Center, Department of Medicine, University of Michigan, Ann Arbor, Michigan

Shannon A. Carty, MD, Assistant Professor of Internal Medicine, Division of Hematology/Oncology, Department of Internal Medicine, University of Michigan, Ann Arbor, Michigan

Jason C. Chen, MD, Clinical Assistant Professor, Department of Medicine, University of Michigan, Ann Arbor, Michigan

Mark Y. Chiang, MD, PhD, Associate Professor of Internal Medicine, University of Michigan, Ann Arbor, Michigan

Laura Cooling, MD, MS, Professor, Department of Pathology, Associate Director, Transfusion Medicine, Director, Immunohematology Reference Laboratory and Cellular Therapy Laboratory, University of Michigan Hospitals, Ann Arbor, Michigan

Charles E. Foucar, MD, Assistant Professor, Division of Hematology/Oncology, University of New Mexico, Albuquerque, New Mexico

Marcus Geer, MD, Fellow, Department of Internal Medicine, Division of Hematology/Oncology, University of Michigan, Ann Arbor, Michigan

Monalisa Ghosh, MD, Clinical Associate Professor, Department of Internal Medicine, Division of Hematology/Oncology, University of Michigan, Ann Arbor, Michigan

Jennifer E. Girard, MD, Department of Internal Medicine, Division of Hematology/ Oncology, University of Michigan, Ann Arbor, Michigan

Morgan Jones, MD, PhD, Clinical Instructor, Department of Internal Medicine, Division of Hematology/Oncology, University of Michigan Medical School, Ann Arbor, Michigan

Yasmin H. Karimi, MD, Clinical Assistant Professor, Department of Internal Medicine, Division of Hematology/Oncology, University of Michigan, Ann Arbor, Michigan

Rami N. Khoriaty, MD, Associate Professor, Department of Internal Medicine, Division of Hematology/Oncology, University of Michigan Medical School, Ann Arbor, Michigan

Darren King, MD, Assistant Professor of Internal Medicine, Division of Hematology/ Oncology, Department of Medicine, University of Michigan, Ann Arbor, Michigan

Richard King, MD, Physician, TriHealth Cancer Institute, Cincinnati, Ohio

Erin M. Kropp, MD, PhD, Fellow, Department of Internal Medicine, Division of Hematology/Oncology, University of Michigan, Ann Arbor, Michigan

Thomas F. Michniacki, MD, Clinical Assistant Professor, Division of Pediatric Hematology/Oncology, Department of Pediatrics, University of Michigan, Ann Arbor, Michigan

Kristen Pettit, MD, Clinical Associate Professor, Division of Hematology/Oncology, Department of Medicine, University of Michigan, Ann Arbor, Michigan

Matthew J. Pianko, MD, Clinical Assistant Professor, Department of Internal Medicine, Division of Hematology/Oncology, Rogel Cancer Center, University of Michigan, Ann Arbor, Michigan

Samuel B. Reynolds, MD, Fellow, Department of Internal Medicine, Division of Hematology/Oncology, University of Michigan, Ann Arbor, Michigan

Mary Mansour Riwes, DO, Division of Hematology/Oncology, Department of Internal Medicine, University of Michigan, Ann Arbor, Michigan

Dahlia Sano, MD, Assistant Professor, Department of Internal Medicine, Hematology/Oncology, Rogel Cancer Center, University of Michigan, Ann Arbor, Michigan

Jordan K. Schaefer, MD, Department of Internal Medicine, Division of Hematology/ Oncology, University of Michigan, Ann Arbor, Michigan

Lauren Shevell, MD, Department of Internal Medicine, Division of Hematology/ Oncology, University of Michigan, Ann Arbor, Michigan

Sharon A. Singh, MD, Associate Professor, Department of Pediatrics, Division of Pediatric Hematology/Oncology, University of Michigan, Ann Arbor, Michigan

Suman L. Sood, MD, Department of Internal Medicine, Division of Hematology/Oncology, University of Michigan, Ann Arbor, Michigan

Christopher T. Su, MD, MPH, Clinical Fellow, Division of Hematology/Oncology, University of Michigan, Ann Arbor, Michigan

Radhika Takiar, MD, Fellow, Division of Hematology/Oncology, Department of Internal Medicine, University of Michigan, Ann Arbor, Michigan

Jane Tolkinen, DO, Fellow, Hematology/Medical Oncology, Trinity Health, Ann Arbor, Michigan

Kelly J. Walkovich, MD, Clinical Associate Professor, Division of Pediatric Hematology/Oncology, Department of Pediatrics, University of Michigan, Ann Arbor, Michigan

Jonathan Weiss, MD, Division of Hematology/Oncology, Department of Internal Medicine, Rogel Cancer Center, Michigan Medicine, Ann Arbor, Michigan

Ryan Wilcox, MD, PhD, Division of Hematology/Oncology, Department of Internal Medicine, Rogel Cancer Center, Michigan Medicine, Ann Arbor, Michigan

Victoria Wytiaz, MD, Hematology/Oncology Fellow, Department of Internal Medicine, Division of Hematology/Oncology, University of Michigan, Ann Arbor, Michigan

James Yoon, MD, Fellow, Division of Hematology/Oncology, Department of Medicine, University of Michigan, Ann Arbor, Michigan

Preface

Preparation for board examinations can be a daunting and overwhelming process for many. As trainees, we are often busy with research projects, manuscripts, and a large clinical volume, making it difficult to find time to study for the examinations. As practicing physicians, we find it hard to keep up with material needed for board recertification.

Questions on the board examinations are drawn from well-established, validated medical literature and widely accepted clinical guidelines. With this said, the University of Michigan Hematology and Oncology Fellowship Program has designed this board review book to serve as an excellent resource for individuals preparing for their hematology boards as well as for hematologists or oncologists needing a refresher in practice or in preparation for maintenance of certification (MOC). This book is not intended to be an all-encompassing review; rather, it is intended to help summarize important facts that one might need to know for the board examination or MOC. We created each chapter to cover all topics listed by the American Board of Internal Medicine (ABIM) that one should know for the hematology board examination.

In this book, we provide up-to-date information, including well-established treatment regimens for a variety of blood disorders, iron disorders, bone marrow failure syndromes, platelet and megakaryocytic disorders, hemostasis, thrombosis, and hematologic malignancies, as well as indications, risks, and complications for transfusion medicine and hematopoietic cell transplantation (HCT).

Importantly, we have engaged our fellows and faculty to develop *Hematology Board Review, Second Edition*. Each chapter was written by a fellow and edited by an expert faculty member or an ancillary staff clinician at the University of Michigan. The book is similarly formatted to the *Oncology Board Review, Third Edition*, with several questions, answers, and rationales provided at the end of each chapter so that individuals preparing for the boards will be able to assess their readiness for all key topics they will find on the actual exam.

Our goal is to help our readers summarize and solidify many important clinical facts and to help them build confidence in their exam preparation. We hope that fellows, practicing hematologists, and practicing medical oncologists preparing for their certification or recertification find the *Hematology Board Review, Second Edition*, a useful tool.

Finally, we dedicate this book to Michelle Reinhold for her continued devotion and immeasurable service to the University of Michigan Hematology/Oncology Fellowship Program as program coordinator.

Rami N. Khoriaty, MD
Morgan Jones, MD, PhD
Francis P. Worden, MD

Stem Cell Biology and Hematopoiesis

1

Erin M. Kropp and Morgan Jones

1. How many blood cells are produced every day?
- Humans produce approximately 300 to 500 billion blood cells per day.

2. What is hematopoiesis?
- Hematopoiesis is the process by which blood cells are produced.
- Hematopoietic stem cells (HSCs) differentiate into the various cellular components of blood.
- In adults, hematopoiesis occurs primarily in the bone marrow of the pelvis, ribs, vertebrae, sternum, and skull.

3. What are HSCs?
- HSCs are defined by their ability to self-renew and give rise to all mature blood cell types.
- HSCs can differentiate into lineage-committed precursors, which can then differentiate into erythrocytes, lymphocytes, platelets, neutrophils, eosinophils, basophils, natural killer cells, dendritic cells, and monocytes.
- HSCs represent 1 in 10,000 to 20,000 cells in the bone marrow.

4. What is the difference between HSCs and hematopoietic progenitor cells (HPCs)?
- HSCs are the pluripotent undifferentiated cells that can replenish the whole blood system, HPCs are those that are more committed toward a specific lineage.

TABLE 1.1

Hematopoietic Stem Cell (HSC)	Hematopoietic Progenitor Cell (HPC)
Undifferentiated and has the ability to self-renew	Progressively lose self-renewal capacity
Pluripotent: can replenish the entire blood system	Oligopotent: can replenish lineage-specific cells
Usually in quiescent state (G0 phase)	More proliferative
Can undergo unlimited cell divisions	Limited cell divisions

5. How do HSCs differentiate into mature blood cells?
- Hematopoietic growth factors (erythropoietin [EPO], thrombopoietin, and granulocyte colony-stimulating factor [G-CSF]), nutrients, and the bone marrow microenvironment are all essential for the regulation of differentiation and normal blood production.

- Signaling through transcription factors and growth factors regulates HSC differentiation and self-renewal.
  - Specific driver mutations in these transcription factors, such as GATA2, RUNX1, Ikaros, CEBPA, and PAX5, are pathogenic in malignant hematologic diseases such as leukemia and lymphoma.
- Growth factors not only are essential for maintaining HSCs and regulating differentiation, but can also be utilized clinically.

TABLE 1.2 ■ Summary of Hematopoietic Growth Factor Production and Target Cells

Growth Factor	Source of Production	Target Cells
EPO	Renal peritubular cells	Erythroid progenitors
TPO	Liver, kidney	Stem cells
G-CSF	Marrow stromal cells	Megakaryocyte progenitors
GM-CSF	Marrow stromal cells	Granulocytes
M-CSF	Marrow stromal cells	Granulocytes, macrophages
SCF (C-kit ligand)	Marrow stromal cells	Monocyte progenitors
Cytokines (interleukins)	Marrow stromal cells	Stem cells
Chemokines	Marrow stromal cells	Multipotent precursor cells of myeloid and lymphoid lineage

EPO, erythropoietin; G-CSF, granulocyte colony-stimulating factor; GM-CSF, granulocyte/macrophage colony-stimulating factor; M-CSF, macrophage colony-stimulating factor; SCF, stem cell factor; TPO, thrombopoietin.

- Recombinant EPO-stimulating agents, such as darbepoetin and epoetin, are used in anemia of chronic kidney disease and myelodysplastic syndromes (MDS).
- G-CSF and granulocyte/macrophage colony-stimulating factor (GM-CSF) are used in chemotherapy-induced neutropenia.
- G-CSF is used in stem cell collection prior to stem cell transplant.
- Thrombopoietin mimetics are used in idiopathic thrombocytopenia purpura, aplastic anemia, and prior to procedures/surgeries in patients with liver cirrhosis.

6. What is the purpose and process of a bone marrow examination?
- Bone marrow examination is used to diagnose and characterize disorders affecting the bone marrow and to assess hematopoiesis.
- The bone marrow is assessed for cellularity, cell morphology, and cell maturation. More specialized testing such as flow cytometry, cytogenetic analysis, and molecular testing can be performed on bone marrow specimens.
- Bone marrow examination consists of bone marrow biopsy (trephine biopsy) and aspiration.
- Bone marrow is usually taken from the posterior iliac spine using a Jamshidi™ needle.
- A bone marrow examination should include analysis of the following:
  - Percent cellularity: an estimate of expected cellularity which can be calculated by subtracting the patient's age from 100
  - Myeloid:erythroid ratio: normally 2–4:1
  - Myeloid and erythroid maturation

■ Stages of myeloid maturation: myeloblast → promyelocyte → myelocyte → metamyelocyte → band cell → mature myeloid cell (basophil, neutrophil, eosinophil)

■ Stages of erythroid maturation: proerythroblast → basophilic erythroblast → polychromatophilic erythroblast → orthochromatic erythroblast → polychromatic erythrocyte (reticulocyte) → erythrocyte

● Dysplasia in the erythroid and myeloid elements and megakaryocytes

■ Evidence of erythroid dysplasia: nuclear cytoplasmic dyssynchrony and the presence of multinucleated erythroid precursors

■ Evidence of myeloid dysplasia: hyper- or hyposegmented neutrophils or hypogranular neutrophils

■ Findings of megakaryocytic dysplasia: micro-megakaryocytes and hypolobated megakaryocytes

● Characterization of lymphocytes, lymphoid aggregates, megakaryocytes, and plasma cells to identify abnormal populations

● Determination of iron stores by iron staining and assessment for "ringed sideroblasts"

● Other findings might include infiltration by carcinoma, bacterial infections, fungal infections, intracellular yeast, or hemophagocytosis

7. How are HSCs identified?

■ HSCs can be identified and selected by analyzing characteristic surface markers using flow cytometry.

■ Most HSCs express the cell surface marker CD34, which is a marker of immaturity.

■ The most common cell surface marker phenotype of HSCs are CD34+, CD38–, CD45RA–, CD90+.

8. Where are HSCs located?

TABLE 1.3 ■ Origin of Hematopoiesis During Development

Hematopoietic Organ	Timeline
Yolk sac	3–5 weeks of gestation until about 3 months
AGM	4–6 weeks of gestation
Liver and spleen	Starts at about 2 months until 6 months of gestation
Bone marrow	Starts around 4 months and continues onward into postnatal life

AGM, aorta-gonad-mesonephros.

9. What is the stem cell niche?

■ The bone marrow is composed of fat, other stromal cell populations, hematopoietic cells, and vascular sinuses. Mature cells can exit the bone marrow through thin-walled sinusoids lined by endothelial cells. The bone marrow stem cell niche is located near the perivascular space, which is close to the endosteal surface.

- HSCs have complex interactions with osteoblasts, neurons, macrophages, reticular cells, endothelial cells, mesenchymal cells, and adipocytes, among other cells. These interactions all contribute to hematopoiesis.

10. How is HSC localization regulated?

- HSCs can leave the bone marrow, circulate through the systemic vasculature, and then either enter other organs or return through the circulation to the bone marrow.
- Adhesions and chemokines interact with cell surface receptors on HSCs to promote cellular homing.
- Areas of high chemokine expression attract HSCs. Such areas include sites of constitutive chemokine production (bone marrow, secondary lymph organs, and sites of inflammation).
- Two important subfamilies of chemokines are the CXC and CC.
  - CXC: important for neutrophil migration and activation
  - CC: important for monocyte and lymphocyte homing
- The interaction between CXCL12 (also known as SDF-1α) and CXCR4 is particularly important in HSC homing and homeostasis in the marrow.
  - CXCL12 is produced by reticular cells of the bone, sinus endothelial cells, and cells in the perivascular space.
  - CXCR4 is expressed on HSCs, mature blood cells, and endothelial cells.
  - G-CSF mobilizes stem cells through decreased chemokine and adhesion interactions.
  - Stem cells can be mobilized using the drug plerixafor, which is an inhibitor of CXCR4.
- CXCL12-mediated HSC homing through the marrow sinusoid endothelial cells occurs via two main mechanisms:
  - Integrin binding: $\alpha4\beta1$ integrin (also known as very-late antigen [VLA] 4) on HSCs binds to Vascular cell adehsion molecule 1 (VCAM-1) on the marrow venous sinus endothelial cells. Other integrins also play supporting roles.
  - Selectin ligands: P-selectin glycoprotein ligand-1 (PSGL-1) expressed on HSCs binds to P-selectin expressed on endothelial cells. Similarly, L-selectin and E-selectin ligands expressed on HSCs bind to E-selectin on marrow venous sinus endothelial cells.

11. How are HSCs and other cells from the bone marrow released into the circulation?

- HSCs pass through a series of steps to leave the bone marrow.
  - Detach from the niche, at least in part due to proteolytic cleavage
  - Travel between adventitial cells
  - Attach to endothelial cells of the marrow sinusoidal network at adhesion proteins, such as VCAM-1, Intercellular adhesion molecule 1 (ICAM-1), E-selectin, and P-selectin
- Several factors promote the release of HSC into the bloodstream.
  - G-CSF
    - Likely has a direct impact on the CXCR4–CXCL12 interaction and may trigger neutrophil-mediated proteolysis of adhesion molecules
    - Takes several days for maximal effect
  - Plerixafor
    - Small molecule antagonist of CXCR4
    - Rapidly mobilizes HSCs for peripheral blood collection for transplant and is thus used when rapid mobilization is needed

- Alpha-4 integrin binding blockade
  - Disrupts VLA-4 activity
  - Causes HSC mobilization

12. What can HSCs be used for?

- HSCs can be transplanted between individuals for a variety of therapeutic uses.
- HSCs are able to traffic into and out of the bone marrow niche. They are able to engraft in the recipient's bone marrow.
- G-CSF is used to stimulate HSC mobilization from the bone marrow niche into the peripheral blood where they can be collected to be used for HSC transplantation.
- In clinical practice, isolation of 100% pure stem cells is not necessary for bone marrow transplantation. It is possible to safely use only CD34+ purified grafts for stem cell transplant.
- HSC transplantation can be utilized for the following therapeutic indications:
  - Bone marrow failure or genetic disorders that cause bone marrow failure
  - Malignant disease (mostly hematologic malignancies): for reconstitution of hematopoiesis following high doses of chemotherapy and/or radiation
  - Gene therapy for various genetic disorders including X-linked severe combined immunodeficiency (X-SCID), chronic granulomatous disease, or Wiskott–Aldrich syndrome: normal gene copies can be inserted into genetically defective stem cells

QUESTIONS

1. **What is the immunophenotype for human hematopoietic stem cells (HSCs)?**
   A. Lin− CD34+, CD38+, CD45RA−
   B. Lin+, CD34−, CD38+, CD45RA−
   C. Lin−, CD34+, CD38−, CD45RA+
   D. Lin+, CD34+, CD38+, CD45RA+
   E. None of the above

2. **Genetic alterations in which of these transcription factors that are important in hematopoiesis has NOT been implicated in human leukemia?**
   A. CEBPA
   B. RUNX1
   C. GATA1
   D. Pax5
   E. None of the above

3. **Embryonic hematopoietic activity is first found in which of these areas in the developing human embryo?**
   A. The neural crest
   B. The notochord
   C. The aorta-gonad-mesonephros
   D. The embryonic ectoderm
   E. The embryonic endoderm

4. A person undergoes stem cell mobilization with granulocyte colony-stimulating factor (G-CSF). The absolute CD34+ cell count is checked during peripheral blood cell collection and is found to be 1.5×10^6 CD34+ cells per kilogram. The decision is made to add plerixafor (AMD3100) to increase the yield. This agent works primarily through:

A. Disruption of the very-late antigen 4 (VLA-4) activity
B. Antagonism of CXCR4
C. Impact on CXCR4–CXCL12 interaction and possible triggering of neutrophil-mediated proteolysis of adhesion molecules

5. Which of the following is NOT a location where hematopoietic stem cells can be found during NORMAL human hematopoietic development?

A. The bone marrow
B. The liver
C. The aorta-gonad-mesonephros
D. The kidney

ANSWERS

1. **A. Lin− CD34+, CD38+, CD45RA−.** Current evidence suggests that HSC are Lin−, CD34+, CD38+, CD45RA−. HSCs used for transplant are taken from a pool of CD34+ cells. CD34 is a marker of immaturity.

2. **E. None of the above.** CEBPA, RUNX1, GATA1, and Pax5 are all implicated in human leukemia. In addition, SCL/TAL1, MLL, LMO2, PU.1, and E2A have all been implicated in human leukemia.

3. **C. The aorta-gonad-mesonephros.** Although the earliest primitive hematopoiesis occurs in the embryonic yolk sac, the first embryonic hematopoiesis is detected in the mesoderm, specifically in the area around the ventral wall of the dorsal aorta. This is detected at 4 to 5 weeks of gestation.

4. **B. Antagonism of CXCR4.** Plerixafor (AMD3100) is a small molecule that acts as an antagonist on CXCR4 and can be used to increase the yield when G-CSF alone results in a suboptimal number of CD34+ cells in the collection. Alpha-4 integrin binding blockade disrupts VLA-4 binding. G-CSF has numerous effects on the bone marrow environment and is thought to cause stem cell mobilization through effects on CXCR4–CXCL12 interaction and stimulation of neutrophil-mediated proteolysis of adhesion molecules.

5. **D. The kidney.** The bone marrow, liver, and aorta-gonad-mesonephros are all areas where hematopoietic stem cells can be found at different developmental timepoints. Although the kidney serves as a site of hematopoietic stem cell development in fish, it is not an organ where hematopoietic stem cells are found in humans.

Red Blood Cell Production Disorders

Erin M. Kropp and Asra Ahmed

Background

1. What are the mechanisms of normal erythropoiesis?

- The typical life span of a red blood cell (RBC) is 120 days; steady-state erythropoiesis replaces approximately 1% of RBCs daily.
- For erythropoiesis, cells are derived from common myeloid progenitors which become progressively more committed to erythroid cells. Maturation occurs through the accumulation of hemoglobin (Hgb) and enucleation.
- Reticulocytes represent the final stage of development as cells acquire biconcave shape.
- Erythropoietin is essential for erythroid progenitor cell survival and induces transcription factor expression that prompts differentiation.

2. What are the main features of anemia induced by an RBC production disorder (hypoproliferative anemia)?

- Inadequate erythropoiesis relative to the degree of anemia
- Established by calculating reticulocyte count or reticulocyte index
  - Reticulocyte index = reticulocyte % × (hematocrit [HCT]/45) × (1/maturation time): <2 (or absolute reticulocyte count <100,000/microL) indicates hypoproliferative anemia.

3. What are the common signs and symptoms of anemia?

- Depends on the degree of anemia and the time over which it develops
- Fatigue and decreased exercise tolerance
- Pallor
- Systolic murmur on examination
- Dyspnea
- Weakness
- Headache
- Angina

4. **What are the systemic causes of hypoproliferative anemia?**

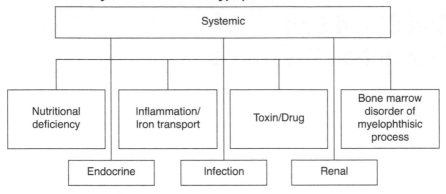

FIGURE 2.1 ■ Systemic causes of hypoproliferative anemia.

Nutritional Deficiencies

IRON DEFICIENCY

1. **What is the role of iron in RBC production?**
   - Iron is required for Hgb synthesis, which facilitates the transport and delivery of oxygen by RBCs.

2. **What are the key steps in iron absorption?**
   - Iron is absorbed in the duodenum and upper jejunum.
   - Iron exit from small intestinal cells and from macrophages into the circulation is mediated by ferroportin.

3. **How is iron distributed in the body?**
   - Iron binds to protein and is primarily distributed intracellularly. In the body, it is bound to Hgb in erythrocytes, myoglobin in myocytes, and ferritin in macrophages and hepatocytes, and is utilized by the bone marrow for Hgb synthesis in erythropoiesis.
   - A minority of the total body iron is in circulation, which binds to transferrin for transport to cells.

4. **How is iron regulated within the body?**
   - Iron levels are tightly regulated to prevent iron overload but also ensure adequate intracellular iron stores for Hgb production.
   - When iron stores are adequate, hepcidin is produced, which degrades ferroportin to decrease intestinal absorption.
   - In iron deficiency, ferroportin and transferrin levels increase and facilitate iron absorption and transport into cells.
     - Soluble transferrin receptor, a cleaved portion of the cellular transferrin receptor on erythroid precursors, is released into the circulation and its level is increased in iron deficiency.
   - In the setting of inflammation or infection, cellular iron export is reduced, resulting in increased intracellular iron in both enterocytes of the small bowel (leading to reduced iron absorption from the diet) and macrophages. This results in reduced circulating iron.

5. What are the common risk factors for iron deficiency?
- Decreased intake
  - Limited iron accessibility in diet is the most common risk factor for iron deficiency worldwide.
- Decreased absorption
  - Inflammatory gastrointestinal disease or bariatric surgery
  - Decreased gastric acidity
  - Phytates, tannins, and calcium from diet
- Increased blood loss
  - Clinical or subclinical gastrointestinal blood loss
  - Menses/menorrhagia
  - Frequent blood donation
- Increased demands
  - Pregnancy and lactation

6. What are the signs and symptoms of iron deficiency?
- Restless legs syndrome
- Pica
- Cheilosis or koilonychia on exam
- Delayed growth or development in children

7. What are the diagnostic criteria for iron deficiency anemia?
- Microcytic anemia (mean corpuscular volume [MCV] <80): present in moderate to severe iron deficiency anemia but may not be present in mild iron deficiency
- Low serum iron and low transferrin saturation (typically <20%)
- Increased total iron binding capacity (TIBC) and increased serum transferrin
- Low ferritin: <12 to 15 ng/mL (99% specific, 57% sensitive), <30 ng/mL (92% specific, 98% sensitive)
  - Ferritin is an acute phase reactant so it may be falsely normal or elevated with acute inflammation. In these settings, reticulocyte Hgb concentration, soluble transferrin receptor index (ratio of soluble transferrin receptor and ferritin), and bone marrow iron stains can help.
- Soluble transferrin receptor increases with iron deficiency and can be used to differentiate iron deficiency from anemia of chronic disease (ACD).
- Decreased iron staining of the bone marrow aspirate smear is considered the gold standard for diagnosis, but it is typically not required.
- Mentzer index is MCV/RBC, which differentiates iron deficiency from thalassemia: >13 iron deficiency is likely, <13 thalassemia is more likely.

8. What is the treatment for iron deficiency anemia?
- Transfusion of RBCs if the patient is severely symptomatic or has evidence of end-organ damage
- Iron replacement dose based on the calculated iron deficit (mg) = body weight × (14 − Hgb) × (2.145) + 500

9. How is iron supplemented?
- Oral or intravenous (IV) iron can be used depending on the underlying cause of iron deficiency, availability, cost, and the patient's compliance and ability to tolerate oral iron.
  - Intramuscular (IM) iron repletion is another option, but is not commonly used as it is painful.

- Oral preparations include ferrous fumarate, ferrous gluconate, ferrous sulfate, ferrous succinate, ferric citrate, ferrous ascorbate, and polysaccharide iron complex. Dose is dependent on patient age and estimated iron deficit, but typically is ~200 mg of elemental iron every other day; ferrous sulfate is the cheapest and is well-absorbed. Coated preparations should not be used as >90% of iron is absorbed in the duodenum.
  - Recent data suggest every other day dosing may increase the efficacy of absorption as more frequent dosing leads to upregulation of hepcidin and thus decreases absorption.
  - Vitamin C may help with absorption, but Hgb response is comparable with oral iron supplementation alone.
  - Treatment failure may be from poor adherence secondary to intolerance (constipation, abdominal pain, bloating), impaired absorption from diet (milk, caffeine, phytates), or unrecognized malabsorption disorder.
- IV preparations may be used with oral intolerance, malabsorption, or severe iron deficiency. Formulations include iron sucrose, low molecular weight iron dextran, ferric derisomaltose, ferumoxytol, ferric gluconate, and ferric carboxymaltose. Each can cause hypotension and hypersensitivity reactions. The exact risk of hypersensitivity reactions is unknown and likely underreported, but is estimated at <1%.
  - Low molecular weight iron dextran, ferric carboxymaltose, ferumoxytol, and ferric derisomaltose can be given as a single dose. Low molecular weight iron dextran requires a test dose as it has been associated with higher risk of severe anaphylaxis (<0.1%).

FOLATE DEFICIENCY

1. What is the role of folic acid in erythropoiesis?
- Cofactor for methyl and formyl transferases
  - Methyl donor for conversion of homocysteine to methionine, required for DNA synthesis
- Folate required during erythroblast proliferation and differentiation

2. How are folic acid levels regulated?
- Stored in the liver, enterohepatic recirculation is important for redistribution to the body.
- It is absorbed in the small intestine, mostly the jejunum.
- Stores are adequate for 2 to 4 months.

3. What are specific risk factors for deficiency?
- Decreased nutritional intake
- Decreased absorption
  - Inflammatory gastrointestinal disease or bariatric surgery
- Excessive loss
  - External biliary drainage
- Increased demands
  - Cell turnover in hemolysis or psoriasis
  - Pregnancy
- Altered metabolism
  - Drugs that affect folate metabolism

4. **What symptoms or signs are indicative of folate deficiency?**
   - Glossitis
   - Weight loss
   - Neural tube defects or low birth weight in pregnancy

5. **What are the diagnostic features of folate deficiency?**
   - Macrocytic, megaloblastic anemia, hypersegmented neutrophils (>5% neutrophils with five lobes or one with six lobes), and thrombocytopenia may be present.
   - Serum folate level below 2 ng/mL is diagnostic.
   - Serum folate values between 2 and 4 ng/mL are equivocal and can be further worked up with methylmalonic acid and homocysteine levels. Normal methylmalonic acid and elevated homocysteine are indicative of folate deficiency.

6. **What is the treatment for folate deficiency?**
   - Treatment is 1 to 5 mg of oral folic acid daily for 2 to 4 months. Plasma folate levels are corrected immediately and normal erythropoiesis is restored. Repletion of folate stores requires several weeks of therapy or can be indefinite if ongoing losses or a reversible cause cannot be identified.
   - IV folic acid can be given in those unable to receive oral replacement or those with extensive small bowel resections or pathology.

VITAMIN B$_{12}$ DEFICIENCY

1. **What is the role of vitamin B$_{12}$ erythropoiesis?**
   - Essential cofactor for methyltransferases
     - Converts homocysteine to methionine, required for DNA synthesis
     - Converts methylmalonyl CoA (MMA) to succinyl CoA
   - Required during erythroblast proliferation and differentiation

2. **How is vitamin B$_{12}$ absorbed?**
   - Intrinsic factor (IF) is produced by the parietal cells in the stomach and binds to vitamin B$_{12}$; the complex of IF–vitamin B$_{12}$ is absorbed in the ileum.
   - Transcobalamin transports vitamin B$_{12}$ to the tissues.
   - Vitamin B$_{12}$ is stored in the liver. Stores can usually support levels for 3 years.

3. **What are specific risk factors?**
   - Decreased nutritional intake
     - Vegan diet (vitamin B$_{12}$ is present in meat, liver, fish, and eggs)
   - Decreased absorption
     - Inflammatory gastrointestinal disease
     - Terminal ileal resection
     - IF deficiency
       - Pernicious anemia (autoantibody against parietal cell or against IF)
       - Gastrectomy
     - Atrophic gastritis (lack of acid leads to decreased absorption)
     - Competition of vitamin B$_{12}$ with pathogens
       - Small bowel bacterial overgrowth syndrome
       - *Diphyllobothrium latum* infection

4. **What signs and symptoms can be indicative of vitamin B$_{12}$ deficiency?**
   - Glossitis
   - Neurologic symptoms
     - Peripheral neuropathy
     - Dorsal column abnormalities: ataxia and loss of vibration sense
     - Subacute degeneration of the spinal cord, optic atrophy, and psychiatric disorders

5. **What are the diagnostic criteria for vitamin B$_{12}$ deficiency?**
   - Macrocytic anemia (MCV >100), hypersegmented neutrophils (>5% neutrophils with five lobes or one with six lobes), and thrombocytopenia may also be present.
   - Serum vitamin B$_{12}$ less than 200 pg/mL is diagnostic.
   - Serum vitamin B$_{12}$ between 200 and 300 pg/mL is equivocal.
     - Elevated methylmalonic acid and elevated homocysteine are diagnostic of vitamin B$_{12}$ deficiency in this situation.
   - Pernicious anemia may be identified by testing for autoantibodies to IF.

6. **What is the treatment for vitamin B$_{12}$ deficiency?**
   - Recent studies suggest high-dose oral vitamin B$_{12}$ (1,000–2,000 mcg daily) is equivalent to parenteral supplementation.
     - High-dose vitamin B$_{12}$ can be absorbed in an IF independent mechanism and has been shown to be equally effective in pernicious anemia.
   - IM supplementation with 1,000 mcg (IM or subcutaneous) once per week for 4 weeks followed by 1,000 mcg per month can be used in individuals with symptomatic anemia or neuropsychiatric symptoms, those with altered gastrointestinal anatomy, or if oral compliance is a concern.
   - Response: Neutrophil hypersegmentation improves in 1 to 2 weeks, Hgb normalizes in 5 to 6 weeks, and MCV normalizes in 10 weeks.

COPPER DEFICIENCY

1. **How are copper levels regulated?**
   - Absorbed in the stomach and proximal duodenum
   - Majority stored in hepatocytes

2. **What are specific risk factors for deficiency?**
   - Decreased nutritional intake
     - Parenteral nutrition without copper supplement
   - Decreased absorption
     - High zinc intake, often through denture adhesive; competes for copper absorption
     - Gastric bypass surgery or celiac disease

3. **What are the clinical and lab features of copper deficiency?**
   - Myelopathy or myeloneuropathy may occur.
     - Gait disorders with ataxia or spasticity
     - Peripheral neuropathy
   - Leukopenia or thrombocytopenia may be present.
   - Anemia could be microcytic or macrocytic.
   - Bone marrow may show myelodysplastic changes with ringed sideroblasts, erythroid hyperplasia, or cytoplasmic vacuoles in erythroid and myeloid precursors.

4. **What are the diagnostic criteria for copper deficiency?**
   - Patient has decreased serum copper or ceruloplasmin.
   - Decreased 24-hour urinary copper excretion is less sensitive.
   - Concurrent vitamin B_{12} and folate should be ruled out.

5. **What is the treatment for copper deficiency?**
   - Mild to moderate: 2 mg/day
   - Severe: 2 to 4 mg/day IV, then 3 to 8 mg daily PO until levels normalize
   - Anemia typically reverses within 8 weeks

COMBINED DEFICIENCIES

1. **What are the common causes?**
   - Decreased intake
     - Nutrition access
     - Nutritional disorders such as anorexia nervosa
   - Decreased absorption
     - Inflammatory bowel disease
     - Altered gastrointestinal anatomy (gastrectomy, gastric bypass surgery)
     - Celiac sprue

2. **What if folate and vitamin B_{12} are both deficient?**
   - Vitamin B_{12} replacement should precede folate supplementation.
   - Treatment with folic acid alone can mask B_{12} deficiency and may exacerbate neurologic disease from vitamin B_{12} deficiency.

3. **What is the typical presentation in anorexia?**
   - Often presents with multiple vitamin deficiencies
   - Bone marrow biopsy with gelatinous transformation; may be reversible with adequate intake

Iron Transport Deficiency

1. **What is the etiology of iron transport deficiency?**
   - Exceedingly rare; mutation in *TMPRSS6,* which regulates hepcidin production

2. **What are the diagnostics?**
   - Microcytic anemia with very low transferrin saturation and low ferritin
   - Hepcidin levels inappropriately high
   - Genetic testing

3. **What is the treatment?**
   - Typically refractory to PO iron supplementation; IV iron preparation recommended

Anemia of Chronic Disease/Inflammation

ETIOLOGY AND RISK FACTORS

1. **How is ACD defined?**
   - Hypoproliferative anemia due to limited iron availability caused by systemic inflammatory conditions

■ Can occur with chronic disease that leads to prolonged inflammatory state, but can also be observed in conditions with acute inflammation, such as an infection

2. **What is the etiology of anemia of chronic disease or inflammation?**
   ■ Cytokine-mediated effects
     ● Increase hepcidin production
     ● Stimulate iron uptake in macrophages
     ● Decrease erythropoietin production and blunted response to erythropoietin
     ● Increase apoptosis in RBC precursors in the bone marrow
     ● Shorten RBC survival in circulation
   ■ Increased hepcidin levels, which lead to decreased iron release from the liver and impaired iron absorption, which restricts iron availability for erythropoiesis

3. **What are the common underlying diseases associated with ACD?**
   ■ Infections (acute infections, HIV, etc.)
   ■ Autoimmune diseases
   ■ Malignancy
   ■ Inflammatory bowel disease
   ■ Heart failure
   ■ Diabetes
   ■ Chronic kidney disease
   ■ Chronic obstructive pulmonary disease (COPD)

DIAGNOSTIC WORKUP/CRITERIA

1. **What are the most common presenting signs/symptoms?**
   ■ Many patients present with a mild normocytic, normochromic anemia. In ~25% of cases, the anemia is microcytic.
   ■ Red cell distribution width is nonspecific and can be normal to increased.
   ■ Mean corpuscular hemoglobin (MHC) is normal to low.
   ■ Peripheral smear may be normal or show signs of an underlying inflammatory condition (toxic granulation, left shift, etc.).

2. **How is the diagnosis of ACD made?**
   ■ The diagnosis is suspected when the following are present:
     ● Ferritin is normal or high.
     ● Serum iron and TIBC are low.
     ● Transferrin saturation may be normal or low.
     ● Hepcidin levels are elevated.
     ● Soluble transferrin receptor is normal. Soluble transferrin to ferritin index can be used to differentiate between ACD and iron deficiency anemia. Soluble transferrin receptor (mg/L) divided by ferritin (mcg/L): <1 suggests ACD and >2 suggests iron deficiency anemia.

TREATMENT

1. **What is the preferred treatment for ACD?**
   ■ The primary treatment is correction of the underlying disorder.

2. What are additional treatment options?
- Use of erythropoietin-stimulating agents (ESAs) if the patient is symptomatic and has not responded to treatment of the underlying disorder; erythropoietin decreases hepcidin and thus it immediately releases iron from the stores, permitting productive erythropoiesis
- Red cell transfusions
- Supplemental iron to achieve transferrin saturation of ≥20% and serum ferritin ≥100 ng/mL

Renal Disease

1. What is the etiology of anemia of chronic kidney disease?
- Decreased production of erythropoietin in the peritubular cells of the kidneys
- May be multifactorial with ACD or iron deficiency
- Increased risk with declining glomerular filtration rate (GFR)

2. How is the diagnosis made?
- Erythropoietin levels are normal to mildly elevated but are inappropriate for the degree of anemia.

3. What is the treatment?
- Dosing should be adjusted to the lowest dose required to achieve an Hgb goal of 10 g/dL. The starting dose of ESA with epoetin is 50 to 100 units/kg three times weekly or darbepoetin 0.45 or 0.75 mcg/kg every 1 or 2 weeks, respectively, for patients on dialysis. Dose and frequency of administration are adjusted based on Hgb response.
- Iron should be monitored at least every 3 months as deficiency can be induced with ESA administration.

4. What precautions or contraindications exist for ESA therapy?
- There is increased risk of thrombosis, stroke, myocardial infarction, heart failure, and hypertension. Risk of complications increases with higher Hgb goals (>11 g/dL).
- In patients with active malignancy (excluding myeloid), it may be associated with tumor progression or recurrence.
- ESAs may induce iron deficiency anemia as iron stores get mobilized.

Systemic Effects on Bone Marrow

BONE MARROW TOXINS

1. What drugs or toxins can induce hypoproliferative anemia?
- Alcohol
- Chemotherapy
- Toxic chemicals: benzene or solvents
- Medications associated with aplastic anemia

INFECTION

1. What infections can induce hypoproliferative anemia?

- Parvovirus B19: infects erythroid progenitor cells; mechanisms unclear but can cause direct cytotoxicity in erythroid progenitors; more prominent effect in patients with chronic hemolytic conditions who have a baseline higher percentage of reticulocytes
- Epstein–Barr virus (EBV), HIV, and hepatitis

ENDOCRINE

1. What endocrine disorders are associated with hypoproliferative anemia?

- Hypothyroidism
- Primary adrenal insufficiency
- Hypogonadism

Bone Marrow Process

1. What bone marrow processes result in hypoproliferative anemia?

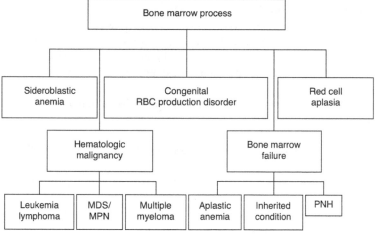

FIGURE 2.2 ■ Etiologies in the bone marrow that can cause hypoproliferative anemia.
MDS, myelodysplastic syndrome; MPN, myeloproliferative neoplasm; PNH, paroxysmal nocturnal hemoglobinuria; RBC, red blood cell.

Red Cell Aplasia

ETIOLOGY AND RISK FACTORS

1. What are the causes of pure red cell aplasia?

- Idiopathic: most common cause
- Thymoma
- Congenital form: Diamond–Blackfan syndrome

- Large granular lymphocyte leukemia
- Drugs including phenytoin, isoniazid, valproic acid, chloramphenicol, azathioprine, and mycophenolate
- T-cell and B-cell lymphoproliferative disorders (chronic lymphocytic leukemia, [CLL] etc.)
- ABO incompatible hematopoietic cell transplant
- Infection including parvovirus B19, mumps, hepatitis, EBV, and HIV
- Anti erythropoietin antibody-mediated red cell aplasia from subcutaneous erythropoietin administration, which is exceedingly rare with newer erythropoietin preparations

DIAGNOSTIC WORKUP/CRITERIA

1. **What is the diagnostic workup?**
   - Reticulocyte count markedly decreased (often <10,000/microL)
   - Bone marrow aspiration and biopsy
   - CT or MRI of the chest to rule out thymoma
   - Viral studies (parvovirus B19, HIV, EBV, etc.), medication history, and detailed malignancy workup as indicated

2. **What are the diagnostic criteria?**
   - An absolute reticulocyte count <10,000/microL or 0.5%
   - Normal white blood cell and platelet counts
   - Few or no erythroid precursors in the bone marrow, but normal white cell and platelet precursors

TREATMENT

1. **What is the initial management for red cell aplasia?**
   - Treat the underlying cause if identified or remove the offending drug.
   - Transfusion of packed red blood cells (prbc) are offered for symptomatic anemia.
   - Intravenous immunoglobulin (IVIG) is used to treat red cell aplasia induced by parvovirus B19.
   - Malignancy-induced red cell aplasia should be treated according to disease-specific guidelines.
   - A short period of observation is reasonable for idiopathic red cell aplasia since some cases will spontaneously remit (10%–15% of cases). If it does not resolve, glucocorticoids, cyclosporine A, or glucocorticoids and cyclosporine A are reasonable initial treatments. There have been no randomized trials comparing these treatments.
   - Patients with recurrent or refractory disease can be treated with IVIG, cyclophosphamide, azathioprine, rituximab, sirolimus, alemtuzumab, or daclizumab. Hematopoietic stem cell transplantation may be considered in select refractory cases.

Sideroblastic Anemia

ETIOLOGY AND RISK FACTORS

1. **What is the cause of sideroblastic anemia?**
   - Sideroblastic anemias are due to inherited or acquired abnormalities in heme synthesis and mitochondrial function.

- The specific mitochondrial pathways that are typically affected include heme synthesis, iron–sulfur cluster production, and mitochondrial protein synthesis.

2. **What are the common congenital and acquired causes of sideroblastic anemia?**
   - Congenital
     - X-linked, X-linked with ataxia
     - Glutaredoxin 5 deficiency
     - Erythropoietic protoporphyria
     - Mitochondrial defects
     - Pearson marrow-pancreas syndrome
     - Thiamine-responsive megaloblastic anemia
   - Acquired
     - Clonal acquired sideroblastic anemias—myeloid neoplasms with ring sideroblasts–will be discussed in the myelodysplastic syndrome (MDS) Chapter 14
     - Alcoholism (the most common cause)
     - Drugs including isoniazid, chloramphenicol, and linezolid
     - Copper deficiency
     - Lead poisoning

SIGNS AND SYMPTOMS

1. **What are the signs or symptoms that can indicate sideroblastic anemia?**
   - Hepatosplenomegaly
   - Congenital forms: often present with microcytic or normocytic anemia
   - Acquired forms: often present with normocytic or macrocytic anemia

DIAGNOSTIC WORKUP/CRITERIA

1. **What is the diagnostic workup when sideroblastic anemia is suspected?**
   - Complete blood count (CBC) and blood smear
   - Iron studies
   - Erythrocyte folate level
   - Plasma copper and ceruloplasmin levels
   - Lead level
   - Bone marrow aspirate and biopsy
   - Genetic testing or medication history

2. **What are the diagnostic criteria?**
   - Ring sideroblasts on the bone marrow aspirate smear: erythroblasts with iron-loaded mitochondria; appear as a ring of blue granules surrounding the nucleus with Prussian blue staining
   - Genetic testing if applicable

PROGNOSTIC FACTORS

1. **What is the prognosis for sideroblastic anemia?**
   - Patients with acquired sideroblastic anemia who have a reversible cause typically have no long-term sequelae of the disease.
   - Thrombocytosis is a good prognostic sign.
   - Transfusion dependence is a poor prognostic sign.

2. **What are the major causes of death in sideroblastic anemia?**
   - Secondary hemochromatosis: organ failure
   - Leukemia

TREATMENT

1. **What is the treatment for congenital sideroblastic anemia?**
   - In patients with nonsyndromic forms, treatment is aimed at relieving the symptoms of anemia and preventing organ damage from iron overload. Periodic transfusions are appropriate to treat symptomatic anemia, but they should be minimized to prevent iron overload.
   - In patients with syndromic forms, treatment is dictated by other features of the disease and symptom management.
   - Patients should be referred for genetic evaluation and counseling.
   - Thiamine-responsive sideroblastic anemia is treated with thiamine.

2. **What is the treatment for acquired sideroblastic anemia?**
   - Remove the offending drug toxin. For isoniazid-induced sideroblastic anemia, vitamin B_6 can be given while continuing the drug.
   - In copper deficiency, remove excessive zinc and/or administer copper replacement.

Congenital Dyserythropoietic Anemias

1. **What is congenital dyserythropoietic anemia (CDA)?**
   - CDAs are heritable conditions characterized by inefficient erythropoiesis and abnormal erythroblasts findings in the bone marrow, including increased percentage of binucleated erythroblasts.
   - These are heterogeneous conditions with three main subtypes: CDA types I, II, and III.
     - CDA type II is the most common subtype.
   - They can share features of ineffective hematopoiesis with iron overload and varying degrees of hemolysis.
   - They are initially classified by morphologic features on bone marrow biopsy, and now can be diagnosed with genetic testing.

2. **How is CDA diagnosed?**
   - Family history
   - Genetic testing
   - Bone marrow biopsy

CONGENITAL DYSERYTHROPOIETIC ANEMIA TYPE I

1. **What are the common presenting features of type I CDA?**
   - Patients present with mild to severe anemia, often with macrocytosis.
   - Hepatomegaly, splenomegaly, and cholelithiasis are common.
   - Dysmorphic skeletal features may be present, typically affecting the hands and feet. Less common are small stature, almond-shaped blue eyes, hypertelorism, and micrognathia.

- Bone marrow with shows internuclear chromatin bridges between nuclei in erythroblasts. Nuclei have a spongy appearance under electron microscopy due to vacuoles in the heterochromatin.

2. **What is the etiology of type I CDA?**
   - It is caused by mutations in codanin-1 (*CDAN1*) or in CDAN1 interacting nuclease 1 (*CDIN1*, previously known as *C15orf41*), which have roles in DNA repair and chromatin reassembly. Type I CDA is autosomal recessive.

3. **What is the treatment for type I CDA?**
   - Red cell transfusions may be necessary; iron chelation should be instituted when the ferritin level exceeds 500 to 1,000 mcg/L.
   - Folic acid should be given if hemolysis is present.
   - Interferon alpha is effective in most patients with type I CDA.
   - Splenectomy may be effective for anemia but carries risk of morbidity and mortality.
   - Stem cell transplantation has been used in few patients and should be considered in severe disease.
   - Osteoporosis is present in almost 90% of cases and should be screened for and treated if identified.

CONGENITAL DYSERYTHROPOIETIC ANEMIA TYPE II

1. **What are the common presenting features of type II CDA?**
   - Normocytic anemia varies from mild to severe; jaundice and splenomegaly are associated with hemolytic anemia.
   - Moderate to marked anisocytosis, poikilocytosis, anisochromia, and contracted spherocytes are present in the peripheral blood.
   - More than 10% of bi- and multinucleated red cell precursors is a morphologic hallmark. Electron microscopy shows a double plasma membrane appearance. Pseudo-Gaucher macrophages may be present in bone marrow. Positive acidified serum lysis (tests susceptibility to hemolysis) is present in majority of cases.

2. **What is the etiology of type II CDA?**
   - Due to mutations in the *SEC23B* gene, a component of the coat protein complex II (COPII), responsible for the biogenesis of endoplasmic reticulum-derived vesicles; also known by its acronym HEMPAS (hereditary erythroblastic multinuclearity associated with a positive acidified serum lysis test); autosomal recessive

3. **What is the treatment for type II CDA?**
   - Red cell transfusions may be necessary; iron chelation should be instituted when the ferritin level exceeds 500 to 1,000 mcg/L.
   - Folic acid supplementation should be given if hemolysis is present.
   - Splenectomy is less effective in type II CDA but should be considered in severely anemic or symptomatic patients with splenomegaly.
   - Stem cell transplantation has been used in few patients and should be considered in severe disease.

CONGENITAL DYSERYTHROPOIETIC ANEMIA TYPE III

1. **What are the common presenting features of type III CDA?**
   - Most patients are asymptomatic with mild to moderate normocytic anemia, mild jaundice, and commonly cholelithiasis.

- Intravascular hemolysis is common.
- Some macrocytes may be extremely large. The marrow has marked erythroid hyperplasia, with large multinucleate erythroblasts with big lobulated nuclei, and giant multinucleate erythroblasts.

2. **What is the etiology of type III CDA?**
   - Autosomal dominant; mutations in the *KIF23* gene encoding mitotic kinesin-like protein 1 (MKLP1), critical for cytokinesis
   - Rare autosomal recessive form of the disease resulting from mutations in *RACGAP1*, which encodes the partner of MKLP1 in the centralspindlin complex that is critical for cytokinesis

3. **What is the treatment for type III CDA?**
   - Type III CDA generally does not require treatment. Folic acid supplementation should be given if hemolysis is present.

QUESTIONS

1. **A 68-year-old male with a history of alcoholism and poor nutrition presents with several months of shortness of breath and fatigue. Physical examination is unremarkable. Laboratory values include the following:**

Laboratory Evaluation for Patient in Question 1

Laboratory Test	Patient's Value	Reference Range
White blood cell count	4×10^9/L	$4–10 \times 10^9$/L
Hemoglobin	6 g/dL	13–16 g/dL
MCV	116 fL	80–100 fL
Platelet count	180×10^9/L	$150–400 \times 10^9$/L
Reticulocyte count	1.0%	0.7%–2.07%
Ferritin	110 ng/mL	35–150 ng/mL
TIBC	243 mcg/dL	240–450 mcg/dL
Transferrin saturation	13%	20%–50%
Vitamin B12	220 pg/mL	(211–911 pg/mL)
Folate	3 ng/mL	(≥3 ng/mL)
Methylmalonic acid	2.8 mcg/dL	(0–4.7 mcg/dL)
Homocysteine	77 micromol/L	(<11 µmol/L)

MCV, mean corpuscular volume; TIBC, total iron binding capacity.

Which of the following most likely accounts for the patient's anemia?
A. Folate deficiency
B. B_{12} deficiency
C. Erythropoietin deficiency
D. Iron deficiency

2. **A 49-year-old female is evaluated in the clinic for progressive dyspnea on exertion, pallor, and fatigue. She has a history of congestive heart failure, diabetes mellitus, and latent tuberculosis for which she is taking isoniazid. Her laboratory data are as follows:**

Laboratory Evaluation for Patient in Question 2

Laboratory Test	Patient's Value	Reference Range
White blood cell count	$3.8 \times 10^9/L$	$4-10 \times 10^9/L$
Hemoglobin	8.2 g/dL	13–16 g/dL
MCV	102 fL	80–100 fL
Platelet count	$310 \times 10^9/L$	$150-400 \times 10^9/L$
Ferritin	72 ng/mL	35–150 ng/mL
TIBC	273 mcg/dL	240–450 mcg/dL
Transferrin saturation	27%	20%–50%
Vitamin B12	240 pg/mL	211–911 pg/mL
Folate	5 ng/mL	≥3 ng/mL

MCV, mean corpuscular volume; TIBC, total iron binding capacity.

A bone marrow biopsy reveals ringed sideroblasts. What is the appropriate next step in the care of this patient?
A. Refer for genetic testing.
B. Stop isoniazid.
C. Start vitamin B_6.
D. Start vitamin B_{12}.

3. **A 31-year-old male presents to the clinic with progressive anemia. He has a history of Crohn's disease and previously underwent resection of his ileum and proximal colon. Laboratory studies are notable for the following:**

Laboratory Evaluation for Patient in Question 3

Laboratory Test	Patient's Value	Reference Range
White blood cell count	$4.1 \times 10^9/L$	$4-10 \times 10^9/L$
Hemoglobin	9 g/dL	13–16 g/dL
MCV	102 fL	80–100 fL
Platelet count	$211 \times 10^9/L$	$150-400 \times 10^9/L$
Ferritin	30 ng/mL	35–150 ng/mL
TIBC	440 mcg/dL	240–450 mcg/dL
Transferrin saturation	18%	20%–50%
Vitamin B12	180 pg/mL	211–911 pg/mL
Folate	2.8 ng/mL	≥3 ng/mL

MCV, mean corpuscular volume; TIBC, total iron binding capacity.

Oral supplementation should be avoided with which vitamin?
A. Iron
B. Vitamin B$_{12}$
C. Folic acid
D. Copper

4. **A 61-year-old male with a history of chronic kidney disease (CKD) stage 2 and polymyalgia rheumatica presents for evaluation of anemia. He is not currently taking medications. He reports fatigue, proximal weakness, and mild shortness of breath on exertion. Physical exam is notable for mild proximal weakness. Laboratory studies are notable for hemoglobin of 8.3 (13–16 g/dL), mean corpuscular volume 78 (80–100 fL), ferritin 195 (35–150 ng/mL), total iron binding capacity 230 mcg/dL (240–450 mcg/dL), transferrin saturation 14% (20%–50%), folate 7 (>3 ng/mL), and erythropoietin 30 mU/mL (2.5–18.5 mU/mL). What is the most likely diagnosis and appropriate initial treatment?**
A. Iron-deficient anemia; oral iron supplementation
B. Iron-deficient anemia; intravenous iron supplementation
C. Anemia of chronic disease; treatment of polymyalgia rheumatica
D. Anemia of chronic disease; initiate darbepoetin
E. Beta-thalassemia; observation

5. **A 54-year-old female with a history of chronic kidney disease (CKD) stage 5 presents to the clinic for evaluation of anemia. She has exertional shortness of breath and fatigue but denies any bleeding source. Physical exam is positive for elevated jugular venous pressure (JVP), pedal edema, and bibasilar crackles in the lung.**

Laboratory Evaluation for Patient in Question 5

Laboratory Test	Patient's Value	Reference Range
White blood cell count	5.0 × 10^9/L	4–10 × 10^9/L
Hemoglobin	8.0 g/dL	13–16 g/dL
MCV	84 fL	80–100 fL
Platelet count	280 × 10^9/L	150–400 × 10^9/L
Ferritin	72 ng/mL	35–150 ng/mL
TIBC	220 mcg/dL	240–450 mcg/dL
Transferrin saturation	17%	20%–50%
Erythropoietin	20 mU/mL	2.6–18.5 mU/mL

MCV, mean corpuscular volume; TIBC, total iron binding capacity.

What is the best treatment option for this patient?
A. No active intervention
B. Darbepoetin
C. Oral iron supplementation
D. Combined darbepoetin and intravenous iron supplementation

6. A 45-year-old female with a sickle cell disease presents with acute-onset dyspnea at rest and light headedness with standing for the last 2 days. She works as a kindergarten teacher and developed a facial rash with fatigue about 1 week prior. Orthostatic vitals are positive and systolic murmur is noted on physical exam. Her laboratory studies are notable for white blood cells (WBC) of 6 (4–10 × 10^9/L), hemoglobin 5.2 (13–16 g/dL), platelet 304 (150–450 × 10^9/L), and absolute reticulocyte count 10,000. At baseline, her hemoglobin is 8 to 9 g/dL and reticulocyte count 4.5%. Chest x-ray is without focal consolidation. What is the best initial management?
   A. Transfusion of packed red blood cells
   B. Intravenous immunoglobulin (IVIG) 2 g/kg over 5 days
   C. Glucocorticoids
   D. Treatment of acute chest syndrome
   E. Observation

7. A 25-month-old female presents with jaundice and is found to have anemia. She is referred to hematology for further evaluation. Her mother notes a history of syndactyly at birth requiring surgical intervention. Laboratory studies are notable for hemoglobin of 8.0 (13–16 g/dL), mean corpuscular volume (MCV) 100.5 (80–100 fL), lactate dehydrogenase (LDH) 410 (50–180 U/L), haptoglobin undetectable, and indirect bilirubin 3.2 (0.2–0.6 mg/dL). Bone marrow biopsy shows abnormal erythroblasts with "spongy" nuclei and internuclear chromatin bridges. Mutation in what gene most likely led to this presentation?
   A. *KIF23*
   B. *SEC23B*
   C. *CDAN1*
   D. Glutaredoxin 5

8. A 20-year-old man is referred to a hematologist because he was found to have anemia (hemoglobin of 10.5 with normal mean corpuscular volume of 86) with normal white blood cell and platelet counts. Workup demonstrated normal B$_{12}$, folate, thyroid stimulating hormone (TSH), liver tests, and renal function. Iron studies showed an elevated transferrin saturation (TSAT) at 65% and a ferritin of 600. The patient has no known inflammatory or chronic disorders. A full review of systems was negative. *HFE* mutation analysis was negative. Lactate dehydrogenase (LDH) was elevated at 280, haptoglobin was low, and retic production index was 0.9%. Direct antiglobulin test (DAT) was negative, as was paroxysmal nocturnal hemoglobinuria (PNH) flow cytometry. Peripheral smear showed no increased spherocytes or schistocytes. Bone marrow analysis demonstrated expansion of the erythroid lineage with increased percentage of binucleated erythroblasts at 25%. The myeloid and megakaryocytic lineages were normal. Cytogenetics was 46,[XY]. What test result is not consistent with a diagnosis of congenital dyserythropoietic anemia (CDA) type II?
   A. Internuclear chromatic bridging
   B. Homozygous or compound heterozygous mutations in *SEC23B*
   C. Positive acidified serum lysis test
   D. Double membrane appearance on erythroid cells by transmission electron microscopy

9. A 70-year-old man is referred to a hematology clinic for neutropenia (absolute neutrophil count [ANC] 0.9) and mild anemia (hemoglobin 11). The platelet count is normal. Iron studies, TSH, vitamin B_{12}, and folate acid levels are normal. Lactate dehydrogenase (LDH) and haptoglobin are normal. Peripheral blood flow cytometry does not show evidence of clonal disease. The patient has not had gastrointestinal (GI) surgeries. Testing for HIV, Epstein–Barr virus (EBV), cytomegalovirus (CMV), and hepatitis viruses is negative. Abdominal ultrasound shows normal liver findings and no splenomegaly. Bone marrow biopsy showed normocellular marrow and presence of ringed sideroblasts and cytoplasmic vacuoles in myeloid and erythroid cells. Cytogenetics and next-generation sequencing for mutations in myeloid genes in the bone marrow are negative. Which of the following is correct?
   A. The patient may have copper deficiency.
   B. The patient may have zinc deficiency.
   C. The patient has B_{12} deficiency despite adequate vitamin B_{12} levels, as suggested by the cytoplasmic vacuoles in myeloid and erythroid cells.
   D. The patient most likely has Fanconi anemia.

ANSWERS

1. **A. Folate deficiency.** The patient presents with macrocytic anemia and an equivocal serum folate level. When the folate is between 2 and 4 ng/mL, methylmalonic acid and homocysteine levels are used to differentiate between vitamin B_{12} and folic acid deficiency. An elevated homocysteine level and a normal methylmalonic acid are consistent with folic acid deficiency. Poor nutrition with lack of vegetables, compounded by moderate alcohol interference with folate metabolism, is a risk factor for folate deficiency. However, it is seen in those drinking only hard liquor and wine (no folate content). The patient also has functional iron deficiency (transferrin saturation <20%); however, this does not explain the patient's macrocytic anemia.

2. **C. Start vitamin B_6.** This patient has sideroblastic anemia, which is likely acquired from the isoniazid that she is taking for latent tuberculosis. Isoniazid-induced sideroblastic anemia is unique in that you can continue treatment and supplement with vitamin B_6.

3. **B. Vitamin B_{12}.** Intrinsic factor complex is absorbed in the ileum. The remaining nutrients are absorbed higher in the small intestine and may be adequately supplemented orally. Vitamin B_{12} should be provided parenterally in the setting of ileal resection, symptomatic B_{12} deficient anemia, or failure of PO supplementation.

4. **C. Anemia of chronic disease; treatment of polymyalgia rheumatica.** His laboratory values are consistent with low iron levels, low total iron binding capacity, and elevated ferritin suggestive of anemia of chronic disease. His symptoms are concerning for recurrence of polymyalgia rheumatica. Treatment of anemia of chronic disease/inflammation should focus on reversal of the underlying etiology, although erythropoietin, transfusion, and iron supplementation may be considered as alternatives if primary therapy fails or the underlying etiology is not readily reversed.

5. **D. Combined darbepoetin and intravenous iron supplementation.** Even though the erythropoietin level is above the normal range, it is relatively low for the level of anemia. Supplementation of iron deficiency is recommended prior to initiation of erythropoietin-stimulating agent (transferrin saturation <20%). The goal of therapy is to keep hemoglobin (Hb) between 10 and 12 g/dL.

6. **A. Transfusion of packed red blood cells.** The patient presents with symptomatic severe anemia and transfusion should be considered for initial treatment. This patient's presentation is consistent with parvovirus B19; diagnostic testing and IVIG would be the appropriate subsequent steps to treat her viral-induced red cell aplasia. Glucocorticoids may be utilized as first-line therapy for some types of red cell aplasia but are not first line for parvovirus B19 infection. Her imaging is not consistent with acute chest syndrome and observation is not appropriate given her current anemia and underlying etiology.

7. **C. *CDAN1*.** The clinical scenario is most consistent with congenital dyserythropoietic anemia (CDA) type I and can be confirmed with genetic testing. CDA type I can be differentiated from other types by presence of skeletal anomalies, spongy nuclear appearance, and bridging nuclei on bone marrow biopsy. Patients who require transfusions should be monitored for iron overload and osteoporosis and receive folate supplementation if hemolysis is present. Other therapies such as interferon alpha or hematocrit may be considered in certain scenarios, although risks of morbidity and mortality must be weighed with the severity of the disease.

8. **A. Internuclear chromatic bridging.** CDA type II is an autosomal recessive disease resulting from mutations in *SEC23B*. Characteristic test findings include hemolysis with lack of appropriate increase in retic count, increased percentage of binucleated erythroblasts in the bone marrow, positive acidified serum lysis test, and double membrane appearance on erythroid cells by transmission electron microscopy. Internuclear chromatic bridging is a characteristic of CDA type I, not of CDA type II.

9. **A. The patient may have copper deficiency.** Ringed sideroblasts and cytoplasmic vacuoles in myeloid and erythroid cells are characteristic findings of copper deficiency in the right clinical setting and therefore a copper level should be obtained.

Red Blood Cell Destruction Disorders

3

Jane Tolkinen and Mark Y. Chiang

Warm Antibody Hemolytic Anemia

EPIDEMIOLOGY

1. **What is the incidence of warm antibody hemolytic anemia (WAHA)?**
   - The incidence of WAHA is 1 to 3 cases per 100,000 persons. Peak incidence is in the seventh decade, likely due to the increased incidence of lymphoproliferative diseases within this age group.

ETIOLOGY AND RISK FACTORS

1. **What is the pathophysiology of WAHA?**
   - WAHA is caused by autoantibodies against common red blood cell (RBC) antigens leading to eventual RBC destruction. The autoantibodies are almost always of the immunoglobulin G (IgG) subtype, but can be rarely mediated by Immunoglobulin A (IgA) or immunoglobulin M (IgM); (which are almost always seen in cold agglutinin disease [CAD]). The IgG panagglutinating antibodies optimally bind RBCs at 37°C. These antibodies do not cause lysis or agglutination of RBCs.
   - RBCs are cleared extravascularly through the reticuloendothelial system. IgG-coated RBCs bind to Fc receptor expressing splenic macrophages resulting in partial phagocytosis, producing spherocytes. Hepatic macrophages have receptors for C3 and can phagocytose RBCs with complement on their surface. *The presence of spherocytes in the peripheral blood is a defining feature of WAHA.*
   - Although rare, in severe cases intravascular hemolysis can be seen.

2. **What are the secondary causes of WAHA?**
   - Lymphoproliferative disorders, including chronic lymphocytic leukemia (CLL), monoclonal gammopathies, and Hodgkin and non-Hodgkin lymphoma
   - Autoimmune diseases, particularly systemic lupus erythematosus (SLE)
   - Drug-induced, including cephalosporins, penicillin derivatives, and nonsteroidal anti-inflammatory drugs (NSAIDs)
   - Chronic inflammatory conditions, including ulcerative colitis
   - Nonlymphoid neoplasia, including ovarian cancer

SIGNS AND SYMPTOMS

1. **What are the clinical features of WAHA?**
   - Onset can be insidious or rapid.
   - Patients may present with pallor, icterus, and symptoms of anemia.

2. **What are the laboratory features of WAHA?**
   - Normocytic or macrocytic anemia (due to compensatory reticulocytosis)
   - Signs of extravascular hemolysis, including reduced haptoglobin, increased lactate dehydrogenase (LDH), and increased unconjugated hyperbilirubinemia
   - Direct antiglobulin test (DAT; direct Coombs test) is positive for IgG, C3, or both in 90% to 95% of cases
   - Hemoglobinuria: a feature of intravascular hemolysis and is rare in WAHA

3. **What is the direct Coombs test and what are its limitations?**
   - Anti-IgG/anti-C3 serum is added to the patient's washed RBCs. If the patient's RBCs are coated with IgG or complement, agglutination will be observed, resulting in a positive DAT.
   - Most commercial reagents require a density of >150 molecules of IgG or C3/RBC to produce a positive DAT.
   - The standard DAT will not detect IgA- or IgG4-mediated antibodies.
   - The strength of DAT generally correlates with the severity of hemolysis, but a positive test does not always indicate hemolysis. Weakly positive DAT occurs in 1 in 10,000 healthy donors and 5% to 10% of hospitalized patients without hemolysis, which is usually caused by complement.

4. **What is DAT-negative WAHA?**
   - Immune mediated hemolysis with a negative DAT, which occurs in <5% of WAHA.
   - If the DAT is negative but there is high suspicion for WAHA, additional testing such as ELISA, radiolabeled anti-immunoglobulin, or IgA-specific assays should be tested.
   - Management and treatment responses are similar in DAT-positive and DAT-negative patients.

5. **What are the proposed mechanisms of DAT-negative WAHA?**
   - Low titers of autoantibodies and/or C3. The density of IgG or C3 on the RBC is below the detection threshold of the commercially available Coombs reagent.
   - Low-affinity IgG antibodies. These antibodies dissociate from the RBC surface during the DAT washing process.
   - Non-IgG antibodies, usually IgA antibodies or rarely IgM. The Coombs reagent used for initial screening has antibodies against only IgG and complement C3.

DIAGNOSTIC CRITERIA

1. **What is the differential diagnosis for DAT-negative hemolytic anemia?**
   - Hereditary spherocytosis (HS): HS is a *nonimmune* form of spherocytic hemolytic anemia which usually manifests at a younger age, but mild cases may not produce clinically significant anemia until later in life. Most patients will report family history of anemia.
   - Wilson disease: The oxidative damage of hemoglobin by copper leads to hemolytic anemia, and the cells appear contracted with small irregular projections representing Heinz bodies.
   - Acute hemolysis due to toxins such as lecithinase C produced by clostridium perfringens: Typically patients would have evidence of sepsis.
   - Zieve syndrome: This is due to recent heavy alcohol intake, accompanied by fatty liver, hyperlipidemia, and hemolytic anemia.

- Paroxysmal nocturnal hemoglobinuria (PNH) is a nonspherocytic hemolytic anemia.
- Delayed transfusion reactions

2. **What are the indications for red cell transfusion in WAHA and what are the specific considerations?**
   - In general, transfusion is safe in patients with WAHA and should not be withheld because a completely compatible donor cannot be found. However, transfusion should be limited to the minimum amount of blood necessary to prevent hemodynamic compromise and end-organ damage. *A dropping hemoglobin in the setting of reticulocytopenia is life-threatening and transfusion should not be delayed.*
   - Identification of a compatible donor is rare as nearly all antibodies in WAHA are panagglutinins (e.g., they bind to all donor RBCs), but the blood bank will provide the least incompatible blood for transfusions (i.e., the blood that gives the weakest reaction in crossmatch testing).
   - It is very important to identify the patient's ABO type to find either ABO-identical or ABO-compatible blood to avoid a concurrent hemolytic transfusion reaction. The risk of transfusion reaction with ABO and RhD-matched blood is nearly zero in patients who have not been previously sensitized to foreign antigens and <10% for patients with a history of pregnancy or prior RBC transfusion.
   - The presence of coexisting alloantibodies should be excluded. This process is accomplished by using the patient's red cells to absorb all of the autoantibody. If residual antibody is found after absorption, it can be tested for specificity so that donor RBCs expressing the particular alloantigen can be avoided.

TREATMENT

1. **What is the treatment for WAHA?**
   - All anemic patients should be started on folic acid.
   - If applicable, treat the underlying condition and/or remove the offending drug.
   - Corticosteroids are first-line therapy. Initial dose is typically prednisone 1 mg/kg/day. Steroids alone will result in sustained response in 60% to 70% of patients, but 50% of responders will relapse within 1 year, often during steroid taper or discontinuation. The addition of rituximab to initial corticosteroids leads to an improvement in relapse-free survival.
   - Once disease remission is obtained, steroids can be tapered at a rate of 10 to 20 mg/week until the patient reaches daily prednisone dose of 20 mg. Then slower tapers of 5 to 10 mg/week are recommended due to high risk of relapse.
   - As long as the dose of prednisone is ≥20 mg/day, patients should receive prophylactic *Pneumocystis jirovecii* pneumonia (PCP) therapy.
   - The goal of treatment is amelioration of symptoms and transfusion independence. *These goals can be achieved despite persistence of a positive DAT. Therefore, DAT negativity is not essential for successful treatment.*

2. **What are the indications for second-line treatment?**
   - Need for prednisone dose of more than 0.1 mg/kg per day or 0.15 mg/kg every other day
   - Fall in hemoglobin to less than 10 gm% with ongoing hemolysis (the acceptable hemoglobin concentration depends on the functional capacity of the patient)
   - Steroid intolerance

3. **What are the second-line treatment options in WAHA?**
   - Rituximab: 375 mg/m^2 or even lower doses, such as 100 mg/m^2, given weekly for four doses. When given as monotherapy, the overall response rate is between 70% and 90%, but about 50% of patients relapse, with a mean duration of response of 20 months.
   - Splenectomy: response rate of 60% to 90%, but about 30% of patients will have an early relapse (within 1–2 months of surgery). Prolonged remissions are observed in approximately 40% to 50% of patients. Patients who relapse after splenectomy often respond to low-dose glucocorticoids. Splenectomy is associated with an increased thrombosis and infection risk. Patients should be vaccinated against encapsulated organisms at least 14 days prior to splenectomy (pneumococcus, *Haemophilus influenzae* type B, and meningococcus).
   - IVIG: total of 2 g/kg given in two or five daily doses. Response is transient and IVIG should only be used as a temporizing measure.
   - **Immunomodulatory agents** including azathioprine, cyclophosphamide, cyclosporine, mycophenolate mofetil, and danazol. A common feature of these second-line treatments is a delayed response. Therefore, if tolerated, treatment should be continued for 3 to 4 months before considering it a failure in the unresponsive patient.

Cold Agglutinin Disease

EPIDEMIOLOGY

1. **What is the epidemiology of cold agglutinin disease (CAD)?**
   - CAD has a prevalence of ~14 per million people. It occurs in the older population, with a median age at diagnosis of 72 years.
   - The median overall survival is 10.6 years after diagnosis.

2. **What is the pathophysiology of CAD?**
   - Cold reactive autoantibodies bind optimally to RBCs at temperatures <37°C. The agglutinins in primary CAD are monoclonal autoantibodies, almost exclusively IgM isotype, directed against the carbohydrate antigen I/i on RBCs. Due to the large size of the pentameric configuration of IgM, cold agglutinins can span the distance of multiple RBCs to cause direct agglutination.
   - RBC agglutination occurs optimally at 0°C to 5°C, and agglutination in vivo leads to blood flow impediment. This results in vascular symptoms, predominately acrocyanosis affecting exposed areas, including the nose, ears, hands, and fingers.
   - IgM antibodies can activate complement on the surface of RBCs. This leads to extravascular hemolysis due to phagocytosis by reticuloendothelial cells (particularly those in the liver) that have receptors for activation and degradation products of complement C3. The activation of complement occurs at higher temperatures of 20°C to 25°C, and once complement C3 is covalently bound to the RBCs hemolysis occurs independent of whether or not the agglutinin is still bound to the RBCs. There are no reticuloendothelial receptors for IgM. Complement activation can cause direct (intravascular) lysis of red cells, but it is uncommon for clinically significant intravascular hemolysis to occur due to the presence of complement activation inhibitors in the plasma and on RBC surface.

- The highest temperature at which the agglutinin reacts is called its thermal amplitude. The higher the thermal amplitude, the more likely the disease will be symptomatic, as complement activation is initiated at 20°C to 25°C and is optimal at 37°C.

SIGNS AND SYMPTOMS

1. What are the clinical features of CAD?
- Patients present with chronic mild to moderate hemolysis with acute episodes of cold-induced hemolysis.
- Vascular manifestations include acrocyanosis and Raynaud's phenomenon. These processes occur due to agglutination of red cells in the microvasculature of areas of the body that are exposed to cold.

DIAGNOSTIC CRITERIA

1. What are the laboratory features of CAD?
- In addition to features of extravascular hemolysis, the mean corpuscular volume (MCV) and mean corpuscular hemoglobin concentration (MCHC) may be falsely elevated due to clumping of RBCs.
- Similarly, the blood smear exhibits RBC autoagglutination at room temperature. This can be prevented by processing blood at 37°C prior to slide preparation.
- DAT is positive for C3. The IgM antibody is not detected because the DAT reagent does not contain anti-IgM.
- A cold agglutinin titer >1:64 is needed for diagnosis, but a titer of 1:512 is generally considered clinically significant. In addition, the thermal amplitude should be determined for the cold agglutinin.
- Serum protein electrophoresis usually reveals a monoclonal IgM protein.
- Flow cytometry often shows monoclonal B-cells.
- Low complement levels are due to chronic consumption, but some of the complement proteins are acute phase reactants, and during stress their levels can increase, thereby exacerbating hemolysis.
- Bone marrow shows erythroid hyperplasia and may show lymphoplasmacytic aggregates, which can be clonal.

2. What are the secondary causes of CAD?
- Autoimmune disease
- Lymphoma/CLL
- Postinfectious, particularly *Mycoplasma pneumoniae* (anti-I) and infectious mononucleosis (anti-i); antibodies are polyclonal and self-limiting
- *All patients with CAD should undergo a bone marrow biopsy and imaging studies to investigate for an underlying lymphoproliferative neoplasm.*

TREATMENT

1. How do you treat CAD?
- Avoiding cold, such as washing hands in warm water, prewarming of IV infusions, wearing warm clothing, or moving to a warmer climate, may be sufficient for patients with mild disease.
- Often anemia is mild and does not require treatment. Treatment is indicated in symptomatic anemia with disabling vascular symptoms or transfusion-dependent hemolytic anemia.

- In secondary CAD, treat the underlying cause.
- *Splenectomy and corticosteroids are rarely effective in the treatment of CAD.*
- If the degree of anemia warrants blood transfusion, washed *RBCs* (washing removes complement component from contaminating plasma) infused through an in-line blood warmer should be given.
- As IgM can easily be removed from plasma, if the cold agglutinin needs to be removed urgently as in critically ill patients or in preparation for surgical procedures such as cardiothoracic bypass surgery, plasma exchange with albumin replacement can be used, but the benefits are transient.
- If the patient requires surgery, the operating room and the patient should be kept warm.
- In patients with chronic symptomatic hemolysis, rituximab 375 mg/m^2 weekly for 4 weeks results in a 50% response rate. If patients relapse after a durable response, rituximab at the same dose can be repeated.
- Rituximab with fludarabine achieves higher (70%) and longer responses (median 66 months) compared with rituximab monotherapy, but with increased rates of infection and neutropenia.
- Rituximab with bendamustine is also effective with 71% response rate, including 40% complete response (CR) with a median observed response duration of 32 months, and is better tolerated than rituximab-fludarabine.
- Sutimlimab, which is a humanized anti-C1s antibody, was approved by the FDA in 2022 for treatment of CAD. Given its rapid effect, it is useful for rapid increases in hemoglobin, similar to plasmapheresis, as a temporizing measure prior to definitive treatment with B-cell-targeted therapies.
- Second-line agents include IVIG, bortezomib (proteasome inhibitor), and daratumumab (anti-CD38 antibody).

Drug-Induced Hemolytic Anemia

1. **What are the basic mechanisms of drug-induced immune hemolytic anemia?**
   - **Hapten or drug adsorption mechanism**
     - This mechanism applies to drugs that bind firmly to proteins on the RBC membrane and is classically described with penicillin-induced hemolytic anemia.
     - Affected patients have usually received high doses of penicillin (10–30 × 10^6 units per day for 7–10 days or more), but other medications, including cephalosporins, semisynthetic penicillins, and tetracyclines, have been implicated.
     - IgG antibody is directed against epitopes of the drug. The antibodies bind to drug-coated RBCs and induce a positive IgG DAT. This mechanism produces extravascular hemolysis mainly through sequestration by splenic macrophages.
     - Indirect Coombs test performed with antibody from the sera or eluate from the red cell surface is *only positive when tested against penicillin-coated red cells*.
     - Hemolytic anemia typically occurs 7 to 10 days after the drug is started and abates a few days to weeks after drug discontinuation.
   - **Ternary or immune complex mechanism**
     - The drug-dependent antibody binds to a neoantigen that is formed by the interaction between the drug and a red cell membrane constituent. Drugs in this group exhibit only weak direct binding to RBC membranes, and even small doses of the drug are capable of triggering hemolysis.

- Antibodies are either IgG or IgM and activate complement on the RBC surface and can lead to *severe intravascular hemolysis*. Extravascular hemolysis is mediated by phagocytosis of the opsonized red cell by macrophages.
- The DAT is usually positive for C3 only because the loosely bound immunoglobulins are washed off during lab processing of the sample being tested.
- The indirect Coombs test to detect the drug-induced antibody is *positive only if the drug is added to all steps of the reaction.*
- Quinidine is the prototypic example of this type of drug-induced WAHA, but other drugs, including cephalosporins, have been implicated.

- **Autoantibody mechanism**
  - The most commonly implicated drug is alpha-methyldopa, an antihypertensive that is rarely used in the United States.
  - The clinical picture is characterized by IgG-mediated extravascular hemolysis similar to primary autoimmune hemolytic anemia.
  - The indirect Coombs test is positive from the eluate or the serum in the absence of the drug.
  - Autoimmune processes induced by methyldopa occur about 3 to 6 months after drug initiation.
  - Patients with CLL treated with fludarabine, cladribine, and pentostatin can also develop autoimmune hemolytic anemia.

Paroxysmal Nocturnal Hemoglobinuria

EPIDEMIOLOGY

1. **What is the epidemiology of PNH?**
   - The estimated prevalence is ~2 to 4 cases per million population, classifying PNH as an ultra-orphan disease.
   - The most common age of onset is in the 30s, with equal sex distribution.

ETIOLOGY AND RISK FACTORS

1. **What is the etiology and pathogenesis of PNH?**
   - Glycosylphosphatidylinositol (GPI) anchored proteins are absent due to somatic mutation in the *PIGA* gene located on the X chromosome. Males and females are affected equally because somatic cells use only one X chromosome. Males only have one X chromosome and in females the second X chromosome is inactivated.
   - As the mutations occur in multipotent hematopoietic stem cells (HSCs), all hematopoietic lineages (erythrocytes, platelets, granulocytes, monocytes, and lymphocytes) derived from the mutant clone are deficient in all GPI anchored proteins.
   - PNH can arise de novo or in the setting of underlying bone marrow failure (BMF) disorder (such as aplastic anemia and myelodysplastic syndromes [MDS]).
   - PNH is an acquired clonal disorder. Patients can have more than one *PIGA*-mutant clone with discrete mutations among the clones, but usually one clone is dominant.
   - CD55 and CD59 are GPI anchored proteins that are important in protecting the red cells from the steady-state, low-grade activation of the alternative pathway

of complement (APC). CD55, also known as decay acceleration factor (DAF), functions to prevent extravascular hemolysis by inhibiting C3 convertases and accelerating their decay. CD59, also known as membrane inhibitor of reactive lysis (MIRL), functions to prevent intravascular hemolysis by inhibiting C9 incorporation to form the membrane attack complex (MAC).

- The mechanisms that account for the clonal selection and clonal expansion of the *PIGA*-mutant HSCs are incompletely understood, with different hypotheses attributing clonal selection to a survival advantage for the GPI-negative cells in the setting of immune-mediated attack on the bone marrow (particularly aplastic anemia) and clonal expansion due to mutations in genes other than *PIGA* that provide a growth/survival advantage.
- Unlike other acquired clonal processes, PNH does not lead to replacement of normal hematopoiesis. Therefore, PNH is a clonal disease but not a malignant disease.
- BMF in PNH is not due to the PNH clone but by autoimmune destruction of HSCs by the T-cells, hence the close association of PNH with aplastic anemia and immune-mediated MDS. The *PIGA*-mutant HSCs survive the immune attack due to deficiency of one or more GPI-anchored proteins. The exact survival mechanism of the *PIGA*-mutant, GPI anchored protein-deficient HSC in the setting of immune attack is speculative.

SIGNS AND SYMPTOMS

1. **What are the clinical features of PNH?**
   - Anemia
     - Non sperocytic hemolytic anemia which is characterized by high LDH, low haptoglobin and a negative DAT. Although PNH is complement-mediated, the DAT is negative because PNH RBCs are destroyed rapidly in the vasculature. Reticulocytosis is present but may be lower than expected for the degree of anemia because of an element of BMF with PNH.
     - Acute hemolysis can be triggered by infection, surgery, immunizations, pregnancy, or any inflammatory condition.
     - Features of intravascular hemolysis (often with markedly elevated LDH).
     - Iron deficiency due to persistent hemoglobinuria.
     - Nocturnal hemoglobinuria (noticed in the morning) is a presenting symptom in only 25% of patients.
   - Thrombosis
     - Venous thrombosis occurs more than arterial thrombosis.
     - Unusual site thrombosis including hepatic veins causing hepatic veins causing Budd–Chiari syndrome, and the mesenteric, cerebral, and dermal veins.
     - The etiology of thrombophilia in PNH is incompletely understood and has been attributed to a variety of mechanisms, including intravascular hemolysis and platelet activation by complement.
     - Thrombosis can occur in any patient with PNH, but those with >50% WBC PNH clone are at the highest risk. Thrombosis is the most common cause of mortality in patients with PNH.
   - Smooth muscle dystonia
     - The intravascular hemolysis of PNH red cells releases free hemoglobin. This free hemoglobin is normally bound by haptoglobin and hemopexin, but once

- No concomitant BMF syndrome
- PNH clone >40% (often greater than 90%)

TREATMENT

1. When should patients with PNH be treated?
- Clinically significant hemolytic anemia
- Symptoms attributed to hemolysis
- Thrombotic event
- In asymptomatic patients, watchful waiting may be appropriate and patients with PNH clones <10% rarely require clinical intervention.

2. How is PNH treated?
- Eculizumab is a humanized mAB that binds to complement C5 and prevents its conversion to C5b, thereby blocking the formation of the cytolytic MAC.
- Treatment with eculizumab reduces intravascular hemolysis, reduces transfusion requirements, and ameliorates constitutional symptoms.
- Side effects of eculizumab include temporary headaches due to increased nitric oxide levels and increased risk of *Neisseria* sepsis. Patients should be prevaccinated for *Neisseria meningitidis* and revaccinated every 3 to 5 years.
- Eculizumab does not stop extravascular hemolysis and therefore patients will have persistently elevated reticulocyte count.
- Eculizumab does not treat BMF and ultimately does not address the underlying cause of PNH. It therefore must be administered indefinitely.
- Ravulizumab, another anti-C5 mAB, is FDA-approved for treatment of PNH. It has similar efficacy as eculizumab but has four times longer half-life, which reduces the frequency of dosing and the annual cost.
- Pegcetacoplan is a C3 inhibitor that is effective at treating persistent anemia due to C3-mediated extravascular hemolysis. It should be considered in patients with remaining symptomatic or transfusion-dependent anemia due to extravascular hemolysis despite optimal treatment with C5 inhibitors. It is important to note that there is risk of brisk intravascular hemolysis with this agent.
- Allogenic HSC transplantation is the only cure for PNH, but due to serious complications it should not be offered as initial treatment and is generally reserved for patients who are refractory to complement inhibition.

3. What are the reasons for failure of eculizumab therapy and is it managed?
- As the maintenance dosing of eculizumab is not weight-based, breakthrough hemolysis can occur, and increasing the dose or administering more frequently can restore the response.
- As eculizumab does not affect the increased formation and stability of the C3 convertase, activation and degradation products of C3 deposited on the red cells can initiate extravascular hemolysis. Rituximab and splenectomy are not useful as the opsonization is C3-mediated, resulting in extravascular hemolysis that occurs predominantly in the liver.
- Increased complement activation from a viral infection can cause breakthrough hemolysis. If the trigger is transient, there is no indication to change treatment.
- A polymorphism in C5 found in some Asian patients (particularly Japanese patients) prevents binding of eculizumab to C5.

4. What is the role of anticoagulation in PNH?

- There is no indication for prophylactic anticoagulation in PNH patients on eculizumab if they have never had a thromboembolic event prior to starting treatment with eculizumab.
- All patients who have a thrombotic episode while on eculizumab should be anticoagulated indefinitely.
- Patients who were started on eculizumab in the setting of an acute thrombotic episode but with poor control of intravascular hemolysis should be anticoagulated indefinitely.
- If a patient has a PNH clone >50% but no indication for eculizumab, they should be prophylactically anticoagulated with warfarin. Studies using other anticoagulants, including direct oral anticoagulants, have not been reported for patients with PNH.

Paroxysmal Cold Hemoglobinuria

EPIDEMIOLOGY

1. What is the epidemiology of paroxysmal cold hemoglobinuria (PCH)?

- PCH is a rare form of autoimmune hemolytic anemia that is most commonly seen in children after viral infections.
- PCH was previously strongly associated with congenital and tertiary syphilis but now is rarely seen due to lower rates of syphilis.
- PCH in adults has been associated with viral infections and with lymphoproliferative disorders.

2. What is the pathophysiology of PCH?

- PCH is mediated by the Donath–Landsteiner antibody, an IgG antibody with biphasic properties. Polyclonal IgG antibodies are directed against the P antigen on the RBC surface, leading to activation of the classical pathway of complement, resulting in intravascular hemolysis.
- The IgG antibody attaches to RBCs and binds complement at temperatures <37°C in the cooler peripheral circulation. As the IgG-coated RBCs flow to the core areas of the body where the temperature is >37°C, complement is activated via the classical pathway and the RBCs undergo brisk complement-mediated intravascular hemolysis.

3. What are the clinical manifestations of PCH?

- Sudden onset of symptoms including hemoglobinuria, chills, rigors, myalgia, back and pelvic pain, nausea, fatigue, and jaundice. In severe cases, acute renal failure can occur as a result of massive hemoglobinuria.
- In chronic PCH, episodes of hemolysis are precipitated by exposure to cold temperatures.
- Physical exam reveals jaundice without splenomegaly or lymphadenopathy.

4. What are the laboratory features of PCH?

- Antibody appears 7 to 10 days after onset of febrile illness and may persist for 6 to 12 weeks after.
- Signs of intravascular hemolysis as evidenced by high serum LDH; low haptoglobin; high levels of free plasma hemoglobin, hemoglobinuria, and hemosiderinuria; and indirect hyperbilirubinemia.

- Serum complement levels decreased.
- Unlike CAD, there is no red cell agglutination seen in the peripheral blood smear as the antibody in PCH is an IgG (IgM in CAD).
- *Neutrophil erythrophagocytosis* on peripheral smear is a specific finding.
- The DAT test is positive for C3 and negative for IgG during hemolytic episodes.
- The Donath–Landsteiner test is specific for PCH. Patient serum is cooled to 4°C and incubated with P antigen-positive RBCs. At 4°C, the Donath–Landsteiner IgG antibody binds to the RBCs, and when the sample is warmed to 37°C the classical pathway of complement is activated and the cells undergo complement-mediated hemolysis, resulting in positive test.

TREATMENT

1. What is the treatment for PCH?
- Hemolysis is usually self-limited.
- Supportive measures include keeping the patient warm and avoiding cold exposure.
- If blood transfusions are indicated, use a blood warmer. Most donors are P anti-gen-positive, so P-negative donor blood may not be available. Therefore, trans-fusion with P-positive blood may be the only option.
- As PCH is usually transient, immunosuppression is not usually required, but steroids and rituximab can be used in refractory cases. Data to support complement-mediated drugs such as eculizumab have been limited but can be considered.
- Plasmapheresis can be used in severe cases, but the response is short-lived because the IgG antibody in the extravascular space reequilibrates with the plasma.

Microangiopathic Hemolytic Anemia

Microangiopathic hemolytic anemia is discussed in Chapter 8.

Metabolic Enzyme Deficiency Hemolytic Anemia

1. How is enzyme deficiency hemolytic anemia classified?
- The enzyme deficiencies that can lead to hemolytic anemia can be divided into three groups:
  - Disorders of the enzymes involved in the antioxidant pathway necessary to protect RBC proteins and hemoglobin from oxidation
  - Disorders of anaerobic glycolysis that is the source of ATP
  - Disorders of nucleotide purine and pyrimidine metabolism
- Most of the enzyme disorders are autosomal recessive except for glucose-6-phosphate dehydrogenase (G6PD) deficiency, which is X-linked.

GLUCOSE-6-PHOSPHATE DEHYDROGENASE DEFICIENCY

- Glucose-6-phosphate dehydrogenase B (G6PD B) is the normal wild-type enzyme and is not associated with hemolysis.

- It has a half-life of 62 days, providing sufficient enzyme activity to protect RBCs from oxidative damage throughout their life span.

1. **What are the different variants of G6PD deficiency?**
   - World Health Organization (WHO) classification of G6PD deficiency variants:
     - Class I: severe enzyme deficiency with <10% activity characterized clinically by chronic hemolysis.
     - Class II: severe enzyme deficiency with <10% activity and intermittent hemolysis precipitated by drugs, infection, or chemicals. G6PD Mediterranean (B [−] genotype), the mutant form that causes favism, has a half-life that is measured in hours. Therefore, the enzyme activity is markedly reduced in all red cells irrespective of their age and leads to severe disease. Favism (caused by eating fava beans) occurs most frequently in children under 5 years of age and can be fatal.
     - Class III: moderate deficiency with 10% to 60% activity and intermittent hemolysis only with precipitating factors and is usually limited to older RBCs. G6PD A− is found in 10% to 15% of African Americans and is primarily responsible for primaquine sensitivity and typically causes only mild hemolysis. Its half-life is ~13 days and so the older red cells are particularly susceptible to oxidative damage.
     - Class IV: no enzyme activity deficiency. G6PD A+ has normal enzyme function and therefore does not cause hemolysis.
     - Class V: mutants with increased enzyme activity.

2. **What is the inheritance of G6PD deficiency?**
   - The gene that encodes G6PD is located on the X chromosome. Therefore, males who inherit the mutant X chromosome from their mothers are affected. Females may be homozygous, compound heterozygous, or heterozygous with unfavorable inactivation of the wild-type G6PD chromosome depending on the degree of skewing of X inactivation.
   - Most of the mutations are missense mutations that impact enzymatic activity variably, explaining the heterogeneity of the disease.

3. **What is the pathophysiology of G6PD deficiency?**
   - G6PD catalyzes the first step in the hexose monophosphate pathway that converts glucose-6-phosphate to 6-phosphogluconate and, in the process, reduces NADP to NADPH. In G6PD-deficient RBCs, hemolysis occurs due to failure to generate adequate NADPH.
   - NADPH is important for maintaining glutathione in the reduced state.
   - Glutathione is the major antioxidant in the RBC. Therefore, when G6PD activity is deficient, hemoglobin and other RBC proteins are oxidized, leading to precipitation of the damaged proteins. Binding of the precipitated proteins to the cytoskeleton distorts the red cell, reducing its life span.
   - The oxidized, denatured hemoglobin forms insoluble complexes that attach to the membrane, creating Heinz bodies that are seen as membrane blebs on Wright stain and visualized specifically with methyl violet staining.
   - The oxidized hemoglobin also undergoes cross-linking that leads to puddling of hemoglobin in the cytoplasm, forming the bite cells that are characteristic of G6PD deficiency seen in the Wright-stained peripheral blood smear.
   - Oxidation also causes disulfide bond formation between membrane and cytoskeletal proteins that makes the RBCs rigid and leads to destruction within the spleen.

4. What are the clinical features of G6PD deficiency?

- Most are asymptomatic and without biochemical evidence of hemolysis or anemia at baseline.
- Only individuals with the Class I variant have ongoing, chronic hemolytic anemia.
- Episodes of acute hemolysis are precipitated by drugs, infections, or certain foods including fava beans (favism is an imprecise alternative name for G6PD deficiency). Commonly offending medications include antimalarials, aspirin, dapsone, nitrofurantoin, NSAIDs, quinine, quinidine, rasburicase, and sulfa-containing medications.
- Both intravascular and extravascular hemolysis lead to a fall in hemoglobin concentration and onset of jaundice 2 to 4 days after a precipitating event.
- In cases due to G6PD A- with onset of reticulocytosis, the symptoms abate as the reticulocytes have near-normal G6PD activity, but in G6PD Mediterranean and other Class II variants the anemia is usually more severe and longer lasting, persisting even after the precipitating event has passed.

5. Who should be tested for G6PD deficiency?

- Patients with chronic DAT-negative hemolysis or infants with neonatal jaundice
- Prior to giving medications, such as dapsone or rasburicase, which can cause severe hemolysis in patients with G6PD deficiency
- Can be omitted in patients starting on sulfonylurea or antibiotics such as nitrofurantoin that cause only mild hemolysis

6. When and how should you test for G6PD deficiency?

- During an episode of acute hemolysis, the G6PD-deficient red cells are lysed; therefore, the results of testing for enzyme deficiency can be falsely negative, especially in patients with Class III variants. Testing 3 months after the inciting event is recommended in order to reduce false negative results.
- The basic principle of all screening and confirmatory testing in G6PD deficiency is assessment of reduction of NADP to NADPH by the enzyme.
- The fluorescent spot test is the most sensitive and reliable initial assay, and for confirmation NADPH production is assessed quantitatively by spectrophotometry.
- Confirmation of the diagnosis by molecular studies is available but not routinely done as the information does not affect management decisions.

7. How do we manage G6PD deficiency?

- Avoid fava beans and oxidant medications that can precipitate a hemolytic crisis.
- RBC transfusions are safe and indicated in acute, severe hemolysis.
- Adequate hydration and good urine output should be maintained to prevent renal insufficiency as a consequence of hemoglobinuria.
- As acute, severe hemolysis is mostly intravascular, splenectomy is typically not effective.

PYRUVATE KINASE DEFICIENCY

- Although the disease is rare, pyruvate kinase (PK) deficiency is the most common cause of congenital nonspherocytic, chronic hemolytic anemia.
- Inheritance is autosomal recessive.

- PK deficiency leading to hemolytic anemia is due to mutation in the *PKLR* (liver, red cell) gene located in chromosome 1q21, leading to marked reduction of enzyme activity in RBCs.

1. **What is the mechanism of hemolysis in PK deficiency?**
   - The mechanism of hemolysis in PK deficiency is incompletely understood. Decrease in ATP production alone has not been clearly shown to be causative.
   - As the deficiency leads to a block in the glycolytic pathway, 2,3 DPG levels are increased, consequently shifting the oxygen dissociation curve to the right. This increase in 2,3 DPG improves oxygen delivery, and anemia from PK deficiency is better tolerated than anemias from other causes.

2. **What are the clinical features of PK deficiency?**
   - The severity of hemolysis is variable, from mild compensated anemia to transfusion-dependent anemia, to hydrops fetalis.
   - Typical signs of extravascular hemolysis, including pallor, icterus, splenomegaly, reticulocytosis, and symptoms related to anemia.
   - Peripheral smear may show contracted echinocytes, but there are no specific diagnostic morphologic findings.
   - The diagnosis is made by assaying the PK enzyme activity in RBCs and detecting gene mutations in the *PKLR* gene.

3. **What is the treatment for hemolytic anemia due to PK deficiency?**
   - Folic acid
   - Splenectomy is beneficial in patients with severe symptomatic anemia by ameliorating hemolysis and decreasing transfusion requirements.
   - A recently FDA-approved drug, mitapivat, is a PK activator that reduces the hemolysis in patients with PK deficiency of certain genotypes.
   - HSC transplantation is an option in patients with very severe disease.

PYRIMIDINE 5′ NUCLEOTIDASE DEFICIENCY

- Pyrimidine 5′ nucleotidase (P5′N-1) deficiency is an autosomal recessive disorder characterized by accumulation of pyrimidine nucleotides in the RBCs.
- The characteristic morphologic feature on review of the peripheral blood film is *coarse basophilic stippling* due to precipitation of nondegraded RNA.
- Similar findings are observed in lead poisoning as lead is an inhibitor of the enzyme.

Red Cell Membrane Defects

HEREDITARY SPHEROCYTOSIS

1. **What is the inheritance pattern and prevalence of HS?**
   - The most common mode of inheritance is autosomal dominant, accounting for 75% of HS.
   - De novo mutations or autosomal recessive mutations account for the remaining 25% of cases.

- The severe forms of HS due to mutations in alpha-spectrin are autosomal recessive.
- HS is the most common among people of Northern European descent, with a prevalence of 1 in 2,000.

2. What is the pathophysiology of HS?

- Defect in proteins that are important in the vertical linkage of the lipid membrane to the underlying membrane skeleton is the cause of spherocytosis.
- Defects in ankyrin, spectrin, band 3, and protein 4.2 can lead to the formation and release of microvesicles from the lipid bilayer, causing destabilization of the lipid bilayer, which leads to the generation of microspherocytes.
- These spherocytes are not able to deform and negotiate the interendothelial fenestrations separating the red pulp and the sinuses of the spleen.
- In addition, HS red cells are trapped in an environment with low nutrients and low pH that lead to their eventual phagocytosis by splenic macrophages.
- Some of these conditioned red cells remain viable, escape the spleen, and contribute to the tail seen in the osmotic fragility test.

3. What are the different protein defects that lead to HS?

- The clinical manifestations of HS are widely variable.
- Beta-spectrin defects account for 15% to 30% of HS patients. They typically have mild to moderate disease and are transfusion independent.
- Alpha-spectrin defects account for 5% of patients with HS. Alpha-spectrin is normally produced in amounts that are three to four times greater than the amount of beta-spectrin. Therefore, HS due to defects in alpha-spectrin is usually autosomal recessive. Patients can be compound heterozygotes or homozygotes, and in these cases the clinical manifestations are usually severe.
- The most common cause of HS is a combined spectrin and ankyrin deficiency, accounting for 40% to 65% of HS patients of Northern European descent.
- Ankyrin primarily mediates binding of the cytoskeleton to the lipid moiety of the red cell membrane by linking band 3 to spectrin. Ankyrin deficiency leads to a proportional decrease in spectrin assembly in spite of normal production of the latter.
- Band 3 deficiency accounts for 33% of HS and presents with mild to moderate disease that follows an autosomal dominant inheritance pattern. Mushroom-shaped red cells are characteristically seen on review of the peripheral blood film.
- Protein 4.2 defects are usually autosomal recessively inherited and are a common cause of HS in Japan, but rare in other populations.
- Rh proteins along with the Rh-associated glycoproteins interact with ankyrin and link the membrane cytoskeleton to the lipid bilayer of the red cell. Absence or deficiency of these proteins can produce the HS phenotype.

DIAGNOSTIC CRITERIA

1. What are the clinical features of HS?

- Clinical manifestations can be divided into asymptomatic trait, and mild, moderate, and severe disease.
- Patients in the same family usually have similar disease manifestations unless complicated by additional mutations.

- Patients with HS trait have normal hemoglobin concentration, normal peripheral blood morphology, and no biochemical evidence of hemolysis. On testing, a slight increase in osmotic fragility may be observed if the red cells are incubated for 18 to 24 hours in nutrient-poor medium prior to osmotic fragility testing. The eosin 5'-maleimide (EMA) binding test is usually negative.
- Mild HS is seen in 20% to 30% of patients. These patients have evidence of compensated hemolysis with normal hemoglobin, mild splenomegaly, mild reticulocytosis (usually less than 6%), and infrequent spherocytes observed in the peripheral blood film.
- Moderate HS is seen in 60% to 70% of patients. Symptoms usually present during childhood but can manifest at any age. They present with mild to moderate anemia, splenomegaly, intermittent indirect hyperbilirubinemia, and reticulocytosis. Patients may have fatigue and mild pallor secondary to the anemia or they may be asymptomatic.
- Patients with severe HS have evidence of florid hemolysis and require intermittent or regular blood transfusion to treat the anemia.

SIGNS AND SYMPTOMS

1. What are the complications of HS?
- Gallbladder disease due to bilirubinate stones
- Leg ulcers and chronic dermatitis
- Aplastic crisis due to viral infections, most commonly parvovirus B19 infection
- Megaloblastic crisis due to folate deficiency as a consequence of increased folate demand, as in pregnancy or recovery from an aplastic crisis
- Thrombosis, especially after splenectomy

2. What are the laboratory features of HS?
- The degree of anemia depends on the severity of the HS defect. MCHC can be increased due to cellular dehydration.
- Depending on the severity of the disease, spherocytes with varying degree of anisopoikilocytosis with bizarre-shaped red cells are observed in the most severe forms. Pincer- or mushroom-shaped cells are typically seen in band 3 defects and spherocytic acanthocytes can be seen in beta-spectrin defects.
- Markers of hemolysis including elevated LDH, indirect hyperbilirubinemia, reticulocytosis, and decreased haptoglobin may be present depending on the severity of the disease.
- EMA: EMA is a fluorescent dye that binds to red cell membrane proteins including band 3, Rh protein, Rh glycoprotein, and CD47. Irrespective of the underlying defect, most patients with HS exhibit decreased binding of EMA. However, decreased binding of EMA is also seen in patients with hereditary elliptocytosis, hereditary pyropoikilocytosis, some red cell enzymopathies, and congenital dyserythropoietic anemia type II.
- The most commonly used diagnostic assay for HS is the osmotic fragility test, wherein RBCs are incubated in test tubes containing solutions of incrementally decreasing saline concentration. Because of the decreased relative surface area of spherocytes, they undergo osmotic lysis at a higher saline concentration than normal red cells. The osmotic fragility test is not specific for HS as spherocytes in patients with warm antibody autoimmune hemolytic anemia also produce an abnormal result. The osmotic fragility test can be negative in HS patients with

few spherocytes, recent blood transfusion, iron deficiency, or in the recovery phase from an aplastic crisis.
- As noted earlier, the incubated osmotic fragility test may be more sensitive and specific for detection of HS compared with the standard osmotic fragility test.
- The reduced red cell surface area can be measured by ektacytometry, but this test is available only in a few research labs.
- Other tests that may have more sensitivity and specificity include the acidified glycerol lysis test and the cryohemolysis test.
- To characterize the molecular defect in HS is challenging due to the multiple gene mutations that can produce the same phenotype.
- As a first step, erythrocyte proteins can be subjected to analysis by sodium dodecyl sulfate polyacrylamide gel electrophoresis (SDS-PAGE). Using this method, quantitative abnormalities in red cell cytoskeletal proteins can be identified in 75% to 93% cases.
- The gene encoding the abnormal protein can then be sequenced to identify the molecular abnormality.

TREATMENT

1. How is HS diagnosed clinically?
- Family history (however, 15%–25% of cases arise de novo)
- Hemolytic anemia with spherocytes and negative DAT
- Positive screening test: EMA-binding assay or the incubated osmotic fragility test

2. What is the treatment for HS?
- The indications for splenectomy include patients who have transfusion-dependent anemia and patients who have symptomatic anemia, including growth failure, leg ulcers, and extramedullary hematopoietic tumors.
- As the red cells are sequestered and destroyed in the spleen, splenectomy will improve the anemia in most patients with HS, rendering the RBC life span to near-normal duration. Splenectomy does not change the morphology of the peripheral RBC.
- Splenectomy also decreases the incidence of gallstones. If patients have symptomatic gallstones causing acute cholecystitis or biliary obstruction, a combined cholecystectomy and splenectomy can be performed.
- As the risk of postsplenectomy sepsis is high in patients with immature immune systems, the procedure should be delayed until the patient reaches the age of 5 to 9 years.
- Delaying splenectomy beyond 10 years of age increases the risk of cholelithiasis significantly.
- Immunization against encapsulated organisms including pneumococcus, *Haemophilus influenzae*, and meningococcus should be administered at least 2 weeks before splenectomy. Penicillin prophylaxis is controversial; some physicians give penicillin V for at least 5 years after splenectomy, while others treat for the lifetime of the patient.
- Splenectomy failure is uncommon, but an accessory spleen can develop in 15% to 40% of patients and would be accompanied by the absence of Howell–Jolly bodies in the peripheral blood film.

OTHER RED CELL MEMBRANE DEFECTS

1. What is hereditary elliptocytosis (HE)?
- The incidence is 1 in 2,000 to 4,000 and is more common in individuals of West African descent as it may confer resistance to malaria.
- Pathophysiology is due to defective interaction between the horizontal components of the membrane cytoskeleton.
- Mutations in spectrin (most common), protein 4.1, and glycophorin lead to HE.
- Red cells exhibit elliptical shapes.

2. What is hereditary pyropoikilocytosis (HPP)?
- HPP is a subtype of HE in which the spectrin mutation is present in the homozygous or compound heterozygous state. And the mutations lead both to abnormalities of the horizontal interaction due to defects in spectrin self-association and to abnormalities of the vertical interaction due to spectrin deficiency.
- This combination leads to severe poikilocytosis with bizarre shapes and fragmentation, microspherocytes, and clinically significant hemolysis.
- Splenectomy is indicated to reduce transfusion requirements.

3. What is spur cell anemia?
- Spur cell anemia is seen in severe liver disease, where abnormal lipoproteins and excess cholesterol are produced in the liver. The abnormal and excess lipids are acquired by red cells and lead to an increase in the cellular surface area. After passage through the spleen, the red cells acquire projections seen as exaggerated forms of acanthocytes called spur cells because of the resemblance of the projections to spurs.
- Patients present with hemolytic anemia with spur cell acanthocytes in the peripheral blood and signs of florid liver failure.
- Treatment should focus on liver failure, which is usually end-stage when the spur cell anemia develops.

QUESTIONS

1. A 47-year-old female with a recently diagnosed warm antibody hemolytic anemia (WAHA) currently on steroid taper presents with chest pain. She is taking 30 mg prednisone and 1 mg folic acid daily and her hemoglobin (Hgb) last week was 10. Labs today show Hgb of 5.9, haptoglobin <8, LDH 790, reticulocyte count 0.8%, and positive IgG DAT. What is the best first step in management?
A. IVIG 0.4g/kg daily × 5 days
B. Increasing prednisone to 1 mg/kg/day
C. ABO-matched blood transfusion
D. Asking the patient about prior transfusions and pregnancy before proceeding with blood transfusion

2. Which of the following is false regarding cold agglutinin disease?
A. Rituximab with fludarabine leads to higher response rates than rituximab alone.
B. Splenectomy is rarely effective in cold agglutinin disease treatment.
C. Neutrophil erythrophagocytosis is a specific finding on smear.
D. IgM autoantibodies are directed against carbohydrate I/i on RBCs.

3. **Which of the following statements is false regarding paroxysmal nocturnal hemoglobinuria (PNH)?**
   A. PNH is caused by a germline mutation in the *PIGA* gene.
   B. PNH clones are seen in about 50% of patients with aplastic anemia and 15% of patients with low-risk myelodysplastic syndrome.
   C. Evaluation of PNH clone size should be done on WBCs.
   D. The direct antiglobulin test is typically negative in PNH.

4. **Which of the following is true regarding the treatment of PNH?**
   A. Eculizumab reduces extravascular hemolysis but does not affect intravascular hemolysis.
   B. After 6 months of eculizumab therapy, if no evidence of hemolysis, a trial off eculizumab should be attempted.
   C. All patients who have a thrombotic episode while receiving eculizumab should be anticoagulated indefinitely.
   D. Normalization of reticulocyte count is the first indication of effective eculizumab therapy.

5. **Which of the following would you not expect to see in cold agglutinin disease?**
   A. Elevated MCHC
   B. DAT positive for C3 and IgM
   C. Erythroid hyperplasia on bone marrow
   D. Red cell agglutination on the peripheral blood smear

6. **Which of the following statements is false?**
   A. PNH clones >50% have an increased risk of thrombosis.
   B. High doses of penicillin are associated with the hapten mechanism of hemolytic anemia.
   C. Allogenic hematopoietic stem cell transplant is the only cure for PNH.
   D. Hemoglobinuria is classically seen in warm antibody hemolytic anemia.

7. **Which of the following statements is false regarding enzyme deficiency hemolytic anemia?**
   A. Class III glucose-6-phosphate dehydrogenase (G6PD) patients have normal enzyme activity and no hemolysis.
   B. Inheritance of pyruvate kinase deficiency is X-linked.
   C. Testing for G6PD deficiency during episode of hemolysis can result in false negative result.
   D. It is appropriate to test for G6PD deficiency prior to giving dapsone.

8. **Which of the following statements is false regarding paroxysmal cold hemoglobinuria (PCH)?**
   A. PCH is mediated by the immunoglobulin M Donath–Landsteiner antibody.
   B. PCH is strongly associated with congenital and tertiary syphilis.
   C. During hemolytic episodes, the direct antiglobulin test is usually positive for C3 and negative for immunoglobulin G.
   D. PCH is a complement-mediated intravascular hemolysis.

9. **Which of the following is false regarding the treatment of hereditary spherocytosis (HS)?**
   A. Splenectomy is indicated in HS patients with transfusion-dependent anemia.
   B. Splenectomy decreases the incidence of gallstones.
   C. Immunization against encapsulated organisms should be done 2 weeks prior to splenectomy.
   D. Morphology of red blood cells will normalize 2 weeks after splenectomy.

10. **Which of the following statements is false?**
    A. Decreased binding of eosin 5'-maleimide is seen in both hereditary spherocytosis and hereditary elliptocytosis.
    B. *Mycoplasma pneumoniae* is a secondary cause of cold agglutinin disease.
    C. Steroids are first-line treatment in warm antibody hemolytic anemia and should be continued until direct antiglobulin test is negative.
    D. Erectile dysfunction and esophageal spasm in paroxysmal nocturnal hemoglobinuria are due to smooth muscle dystonia.

11. **Which of the following is true regarding pyruvate kinase (PK) deficiency?**
    A. The anemia in PK deficiency is better tolerated than the anemia in other conditions because 2,3 disphosphoglycerate (DPG) levels are reduced, consequently shifting the oxygen dissociation curve to the left.
    B. PK deficiency is an autosomal dominant disease.
    C. PK deficiency is a genetic disease characterized by basophilic stippling on peripheral smear.
    D. Mitapivat is a PK activator that reduces the hemolysis in patients with PK deficiency of certain genotypes.

ANSWERS

1. **C. ABO-matched red blood cell transfusion.** A dropping Hgb in the setting of reticulocytopenia is life threatening and transfusion should not be delayed or withheld.

2. **C. Neutrophil erythrophagocytosis is a specific finding on smear.** Neutrophil erythrophagocytosis is a specific finding seen on the peripheral smear in paroxysmal cold hemoglobinuria (PCH) not CAD.

3. **A. PNH is caused by a germline mutation in the *PIGA* gene.** PNH is caused by a somatic mutation in the PIGA gene located on the X chromosome not a germline mutation.

4. **C. All patients who have a thrombotic episode while receiving eculizumab should be anticoagulated indefinitely.** Eculizumab reduces intravascular hemolysis but does not affect extravascular hemolysis therefore patients will have a persistently elevated reticulocyte count. Treatment with ecluziumab does not address the underlying cause of PNH and therefore should be administered indefinitely. Patients with a history of thrombosis while recieving eculizumab should be on anticoagulation indefinitely.

5. **B. DAT positive for C3 and IgM.** In cold agglutinin disease the DAT is positive for C3 only. IgM antibody is not detected because the DAT reagent does not contain anti-IgM.

6. **D. Hemoglobinuria is classically seen in warm antibody hemolytic anemia.** Hemolysis in WAHA is predominantly extravascular. Signs of intravascular hemolysis, including hemaglobinuria is rare.

7. **B. Inheritance of pyruvate kinase deficiency is X-linked.** Inheritance of pyruvate kinase deficiency is autosomal recessive, not X-linked.

8. **A. PCH is mediated by IgM Donath–Landsteiner antibody.** The Donalth-Landsteiner antibody is of the IgG subtype, not IgM.

9. **D. Morphology of red blood cells will normalize 2 weeks after splenectomy.** Splenectomy is indicated for transfusion dependent anemia in patients with HS. While splenectomy leads to improvement in anemia it does not affect the morphology of the peripheral RBC.

10. **C. Steroids are first-line treatment in warm antibody hemolytic anemia and should be continued until direct antiglobulin test is negative.** Steroids are first-line treatment in WAHA. The goal for treatment is transfusion independence and symptom improvement which can be achieved regardless of DAT. A negative DAT is not essential for sucsessful treatment.

11. **D. Mitapivat is a PK activator that reduces the hemolysis in patients with PK deficiency of certain genotypes.** The remainder of answers are incorrect as anemia in PK deficency is actually better tolerated when compared to anemia of other causes, it is inherited in autosomal recessive pattern (not autosomal dominant) and is not characterized by basophilic stipppling (which is often seen in pyrimidine 5' nucleotidase deficiency).

Hemoglobinopathies

4

Victoria Wytiaz and Sharon Singh

Thalassemia

DEFINITION

1. **What is thalassemia?**
   - Thalassemia is a group of disorders associated with defective synthesis of either alpha- or beta-globin subunits of hemoglobin, inherited as pathologic alleles of the globin genes on chromosomes 11 (beta-globin) and 16 (alpha-globin).
   - Syndromes are classified based on which globin chains are affected; this includes both absent and reduced globin chain synthesis.
     - Absent is denoted by $\alpha°$ or $\beta°$ and reduced is denoted by $\alpha+$ or $\beta+$.
   - Clinical manifestations (discussed subsequently) are diverse.
   - Thalassemias as a whole are one the most common monogenetic disorders worldwide.
     - Thalassemia trait does confer protection against severe malaria, leading to a high incidence in areas where malaria is prevalent.

PATHOPHYSIOLOGY

1. **What is the pathophysiology of ineffective erythropoiesis in thalassemia?**
   - Overall, decreased hemoglobin production and red blood cell (RBC) survival is due to excess of unaffected globin chains, which form unstable homotetramers that precipitate as cytotoxic inclusion bodies.
   - In beta-thalassemia, alpha-homotetramers cause severe impairment of erythroid maturation, resulting in ineffective erythropoiesis, premature hemolysis of mature red cells, and extramedullary hematopoiesis.
     - As such, severe beta-thalassemia can manifest as expanded marrow cavities and proliferation in extramedullary hematopoietic sites (spleen, liver).
     - In beta-thalassemia, coinheritance of alpha-thalassemia or hereditary persistence of fetal hemoglobin (HPFH) can result in a milder disease phenotype, whereas coinheritance of alpha-globin gene triplication/quadruplication can increase the alpha-globin chain imbalance and result in a more severe disease phenotype.

ALPHA-THALASSEMIA

1. How is alpha-thalassemia diagnosed and treated?

- It is more common in patients of the following ethnic background: Middle East, North Africa, and Southeast Asia.
- Patients present with microcytic hypochromic anemia with normal hemoglobin A2 (HbA2) levels on hemoglobin electrophoresis.
- It requires DNA analysis to accurately diagnose.
- Patients with one to two alpha-globin gene deletions are generally asymptomatic/have mild microcytic anemia and do not require treatment, but prenatal genetic counseling is recommended.
- Deletion of three alpha-globin genes results in hemoglobin H disease, while deletion of four genes results in fetal hydrops and leads to maternal pregnancy complications.
- Nondeletional mutations are less common than deletional variants, but lead to a more severe phenotype.
- Treatment is only indicated in the setting of severe and/or symptomatic anemia.

BETA-THALASSEMIA

1. What is beta-thalassemia minor?

- β^0/β, $\beta+/\beta$
- Electrophoresis with variable increased HbA2 and hemoglobin F (HbF; $\delta\beta$ variant [i.e., deletion of delta- and beta-globin genes] can have normal HbA2; iron deficiency can falsely lower HbA2)
- Microcytosis and hypochromia present
- Minor manifestations with few indications for treatment
  - Pregnant patients may require supportive transfusions as hemoglobin can fall below 7 g/dL.

2. What is beta-thalassemia intermedia?

- $\beta^0/\beta+$, $\beta+/\beta+$
- Hemoglobin E (HbE)/beta-thalassemia can lead to either thalassemia intermedia or a major phenotype.
- Patients have moderate hemolytic anemia but can have later complications of chronic anemia and will have transfusion needs at some point in life.
- Ferritin monitoring should occur given the increased gastrointestinal tract absorption that can occur due to ineffective erythropoiesis.
  - Levels >500 indicate need for further monitoring with liver MRI and possible iron chelation.

3. What is beta-thalassemia major?

- β^0/β^0
- Severe anemia and ineffective erythropoiesis
- Manifestations seen in infancy (failure to thrive, poor feeding, hepatosplenomegaly)
- Transfusions with leukocyte-depleted, extended antigen-matched (at least to Rh [Cc, Ee] and Kell) RBCs recommended with a pretransfusion goal hemoglobin (Hb) of 9 to 10.5 g/dL, to be achieved with scheduled program
- Close attention to bone health given ineffective erythropoiesis
- Increased iron burden inevitable and three classes of iron chelators are used

- Hexadentate (deferoxamine), bidentate (deferiprone), and tridentate (defer-asirox)
■ Other complications: cardiac failure due to iron overload, infections, ongoing poor growth, and endocrinopathies

TREATMENT

1. **What treatments, aside from transfusion and iron chelation, exist?**
   ■ Hematopoietic stem cell transplant
   - Curative allogeneic stem cell transplant (SCT) with a human leukocyte anti-gen (HLA)-matched sibling donor, first completed in 1982; indicated for severe form of thalassemia
   - Best outcomes seen with matched sibling donor in patients <17 years old and without significant iron overload

2. **Are there newer therapies to consider?**
   ■ Gene therapy
   - Betibeglogene autotemcel is approved for transfusion-dependent beta-thalas-semia patients. It is prepared from autologous CD34+ cells transduced with a self-inactivating lentiviral vector encoding a modified beta-globin (β^{A-T87Q}-globin) gene and is transplanted (autologous hematopoietic stem cell trans-plant) in recipients following myeloablative conditioning.
   - Other gene therapy strategies are currently being investigated, including genome editing to inhibit BCL11A (involved in HbF repression in adults).
   ■ Luspatercept
   - Luspatercept is an erythroid maturation agent approved for adults with trans-fusion-dependent anemia in the setting of myelodysplastic syndrome (MDS) as well as beta-thalassemia.
   - Mechanism of action is inhibition of growth factor-beta superfamily ligands and ultimately the Smad2/3 signaling pathway to promote bone marrow erythroid maturation.
   - The phase 3 BELIEVE trial showed that patients receiving luspatercept had overall reduction in RBC transfusion burden.
   ■ Other agents
   - Fetal hemoglobin inducers: hydroxyurea is used frequently in sickle cell ane-mia but has more limited efficacy in thalassemia; decitabine and other novel fetal globin inducers are currently being studied.
   - Other agents are currently being investigated to ameliorate ineffective eryth-ropoiesis and target iron dysregulation.

The Sickle Cell Syndromes

DEFINITIONS AND NOMENCLATURE

1. **What is the genetic basis and the spectrum of clinical syndromes associ-ated with the sickle cell gene?**
   ■ Hemoglobin S (HbS) arises from a DNA point mutation, resulting in a single amino acid substitution, glutamic acid to valine, at the sixth amino acid of beta-globin.

- HbS is codominant with hemoglobin A1 and other hemoglobin variants.
- Heterozygosity for HbS alone is known as sickle cell trait.
- Sickle cell disease (SCD) is defined as homozygosity for HbS or HbS in the compound heterozygote state with another pathologic beta-globin variant (C, D, E, O^{Arab}, Lepore) or when associated with beta-thalassemia.

DEMOGRAPHICS

1. **Describe the frequency of SCD in the United States and worldwide.**
   - HbS is the most common, clinically significant structural hemoglobin variant worldwide.
   - In endemic regions, heterozygosity for HbS confers protection from severe falciparum malaria infection, resulting in a survival advantage among carriers.
   - There is no reliable global SCD estimate, but there are an estimated 300,000 babies with SCD born every year (75.5% born in sub-Saharan Africa, 16.9% Arab-India, 4.6% Americas, 3% Eurasia).
   - SCD occurs in approximately 1 in every 360 African American newborns in the United States. There are an estimated 100,000 Americans living with SCD.

2. **What is the median overall survival of a patient with SCD?**
   - The estimated median survival of patients with SCD in the United States is not clearly defined and depends on several factors, with one report showing a median overall survival of 58 years and another report showing a median age of death of 43 years.
   - The infant and childhood mortality decreased substantially with the introduction of newborn screening, prophylactic penicillin, and pneumococcal vaccination.
   - Although death related to organ failure does occur in SCD, most deaths occur during a vaso-occlusive crisis related to acute chest syndrome, stroke, or venous thromboembolism (VTE).
   - Elevated HbF levels are associated with improved outcomes.
     - Coinheritance of alpha-thalassemia reduces the risk of stroke in SCD.

PATHOPHYSIOLOGY

1. **What effect does the sickle cell mutation have on RBCs?**
   - When deoxygenated, the HbS molecule undergoes a conformational change that results in decreased solubility and polymerization. This is worsened by reduced oxygen tension and acidosis.

2. **What is the mechanism of anemia in SCD?**
   - Sickled cells undergo hemolysis leading to a chronic hemolytic anemia.
   - The average life span of a sickle cell is 17 days (~1/7 that of a normal RBC).

3. **What causes the acute vaso-occlusive pain crisis typical of SCD?**
   - Entrapment of erythrocytes and leukocytes in the microcirculation leads to vascular obstruction and tissue ischemia.

4. **What factors contribute to the pathophysiology of vaso-occlusion?**
   - Impaired RBC deformability (hemoglobin polymerization and sickling)
   - Red cell adhesion to endothelial cells
   - Endothelial cell damage

- Prothrombotic state (thrombin activation)
- Leukocytosis and other inflammatory mediators

THE SICKLE CELL SYNDROMES

1. **What factors determine the clinical manifestations and disease severity in SCD?**
   - Clinical manifestations and severity depend on the beta-globin genotype (AS, S-beta-thalassemia, SC, and SS; see Table 4.1).
   - Higher concentration of HbF reduces severity (HPFH or hydroxyurea).
   - Coexisting alpha-thalassemia reduces the severity of some hemolytic disease manifestations but may increase the risk of vaso-occlusive complications like pain crisis and osteonecrosis.
   - Based on anthropologic and molecular data, there are five separate founder mutations resulting in distinct beta-globin haplotypes. The African haplotypes have a more severe disease phenotype.

2. **What is the role of coinherited hemoglobin C in SCD?**
   - Hemoglobin C is caused by the substitution of lysine for glutamic acid at the sixth amino acid of the beta-globin gene
   - Hemoglobin C carrier state (AC) is asymptomatic.
   - Homozygosity for hemoglobin C (CC) results in mild anemia and splenomegaly with minimal associated symptoms.
   - Compound heterozygosity for hemoglobin C and HbS results in a symptomatic sickle cell syndrome.

3. **What is the role of coinherited beta-thalassemia in SCD?**
   - Beta-thalassemia represents a variety of genetic mutations that result in decreased beta-globin production. The severity ranges from a mild/moderate decrease in beta-globin production (beta [+] thalassemia) to complete absence of beta-globin production (beta [0] thalassemia).
   - Impaired production of beta-globin chains leads to a relative excess of alpha-globin chains that may be unstable and precipitate.
   - Compound heterozygosity for HbS and beta-thalassemia results in symptomatic SCD.

DIAGNOSIS

1. **List the various sickle cell syndromes.**
   - Sickle cell trait (heterozygous HbS; AS)
   - Sickle cell disease (homozygous HbS; SS)
   - Hemoglobin SC disease (SC)
   - Sickle beta (+) thalassemia
   - Sickle beta (0) thalassemia

2. **How is SCD diagnosed?**
   - Hemoglobin electrophoresis, isoelectric focusing, or high-performance liquid chromatography allows the identification and quantification of the various beta hemoglobin variants. These methods are not diagnostic of alpha-thalassemia trait (loss of two of the four alpha chains) or alpha-thalassemia silent carrier state (loss of one of the four alpha chains).

TABLE 4.1 ■ Sickle Cell Genotypes

Syndrome Name	Genotype	Beta-Globin Variant	Severity of Disease
Sickle cell trait	AS	60% A, 40% S	Largely asymptomatic
Sickle cell anemia	SS	>90% S	Most severe disease
Hemoglobin SC disease	SC	50% S, 50% C	Severe
Sickle beta (+) thalassemia	S-Beta +	>50% S, <50% A	Intermediate
Sickle beta (0) thalassemia	S-Beta 0	>90% S	Most severe disease
Sickle cell anemia with HPFH	SS-HPFH	65%–85% S, 15%–45% F	Intermediate/less severe

HPFH, hereditary persistence of fetal hemoglobin.

3. **What can be seen on the peripheral smear?**
   - Polychromasia due to reticulocytosis
   - Howell–Jolly bodies due to hyposplenia
   - Drepanocytes (sickle-shaped cells) in syndromes with >50% HbS
   - Codocytes (target cells) in thalassemia
   - Codocytes and hemoglobin crystals in hemoglobin C disease

4. **What is HbA2?**
   - HbA2 is a normal and minor hemoglobin variant.
   - HbA2 is increased in beta-thalassemia and sickle beta-thalassemia.
   - HbA2 is composed of two alpha and two delta chains ($\alpha2\delta2$) as compared with hemoglobin A1, which is composed of two alpha and two beta chains ($\alpha2\beta2$).
   - Sickle beta (0) thalassemia will have higher levels of HbA2 on hemoglobin electrophoresis and can thereby be distinguished from homozygous SCD.

CAVEATS IN THE CLINICAL PRESENTATION OF THE VARIOUS SICKLE CELL SYNDROMES

1. **Describe the clinical presentation of the sickle cell trait.**
   - Sickle cell trait is typically asymptomatic, but RBCs can become deformed/sickled with extreme physical exertion, severe dehydration, and at high altitude.
   - Sickle cell trait can be associated with gross hematuria due to papillary necrosis, which may be precipitated by dehydration and/or physical exertion.
   - Sickle cell trait is associated with increased risk of renal medullary carcinoma.

2. **Which sickle cell syndromes have the most severe clinical symptoms?**
   - Homozygous SS disease and sickle beta (0) thalassemia are the most severe.

3. **List two symptoms that are more common in hemoglobin SC disease.**
   - Retinopathy and avascular necrosis are more common in SC disease.

4. **What are the most common manifestations of a vaso-occlusive crisis?**
   - Bone pain

- Dactylitis, primarily in children
- Acute chest syndrome
- Osteonecrosis

5. **Patients with SCD are at higher risk for what types of infections?**
   - Bacteremia with encapsulated organisms (*Streptococcus pneumoniae, Haemophilus influenzae, Neisseria meningitidis*), *Escherichia coli*, staphylococcal species, and *Salmonella*
   - Pneumonia with *Mycoplasma, Chlamydia,* and *Legionella*
   - Osteomyelitis with *Staphylococcus aureus* and *Salmonella*

6. **Why is infection a major cause of morbidity/mortality for patients with SCD?**
   - Functional hyposplenism/asplenia
     - Of note, severe SCD commonly results in functional asplenia from autoinfarction. Milder genotypes may lead to chronic splenomegaly and risk for splenic sequestration in adult patients.
   - Decreased tissue perfusion
   - Indwelling catheters (for chronic transfusions)
   - Skin ulceration/bone infarction

7. **List several of the chronic complications that occur in patients with SCD.**
   - Avascular necrosis
   - Cognitive and developmental delay related to cerebral infarctions
   - Pulmonary hypertension
   - Chronic restrictive lung disease
   - Chronic renal failure
   - Osteoporosis
   - Heart failure
   - Proliferative retinopathy
   - Chronic pain

MANAGEMENT OF ACUTE EPISODES

MANAGEMENT OF ACUTE CHEST SYNDROME

1. **Define acute chest syndrome.**
   - Requires a new pulmonary infiltrate on chest x-ray (CXR) and at least one of the following: fever >38.5°C, hypoxemia, respiratory symptoms, or chest pain

2. **What percentage of patients with SCD will have an episode of acute chest syndrome in their lifetime?**
   - 50%

3. **List common presenting symptoms in acute chest syndrome.**
   - Fever, cough, chest pain, and shortness of breath
   - Hypoxemia: can be seen in more severe presentations and is more common in adults

4. **List potential triggers for acute chest syndrome.**
   - Acute vaso-occlusive pain episode, which is the most common trigger in adults
   - Infection, pulmonary embolism, bone marrow or fat embolism, fluid overload, and opioid narcosis with hypoventilation

5. **List tests in the diagnostic evaluation of acute chest syndrome.**
   - CXR, complete blood count (CBC), comprehensive metabolic panel, type and screen, blood cultures, and respiratory viral panel; consider CT angiogram if clinically appropriate (e.g., concern for pulmonary embolism)

6. **List general treatment measures for acute chest syndrome.**
   - Antibiotics, incentive spirometry, supplemental oxygen, intravenous fluids, pain control, and simple or automated exchange transfusion

7. **What treatment has been shown to decrease the frequency of acute chest syndrome?**
   - Hydroxyurea

MANAGEMENT OF VASO-OCCLUSIVE PAIN CRISIS

1. **Describe the management of vaso-occlusive pain crises.**
   - Prompt assessment, administration of analgesia, and frequent evaluation to optimize pain management

2. **What preventive treatments have been shown to decrease the frequency of acute pain crises?**
   - Hydroxyurea
     - The 1995 Multicenter Study of Hydroxyurea in Sickle Cell Anemia (MSH) randomly assigned 299 adults with sickle cell anemia and at least three painful episodes in 1 year to receive placebo or hydroxyurea. Compared with controls, the hydroxyurea-treated individuals had a decrease in painful events.
   - L-glutamine
     - L-glutamine was approved by the Food and Drug Administration in 2017 based on a phase 3 clinical trial of 230 patients. Patients were randomized to daily treatment with L-glutamine or placebo. Those who received L-glutamine had fewer acute pain events, fewer hospitalizations, fewer days in the hospital, and fewer episodes of acute chest syndrome.
   - Crizanlizumab
     - Crizanlizumab is a humanized monoclonal antibody against P-selectin which is involved in pathogenic adhesion of sickled red cells and leukocytes to the endothelium during vaso-occlusion.
     - The SUSTAIN trial (Safety and Efficacy of Crizanlizumab [SelG1] With or Without Hydroxyurea Therapy in Sickle Cell Disease Patients With Sickle Cell-Related Pain Crises) was a placebo-controlled, double-blind, phase 2 trial that randomized patients to high-dose or low-dose crizanlizumab or placebo.
     - Patients treated with high-dose crizanlizumab had 45.3% lower median rate of pain crisis and longer median time to first and second crisis compared with placebo.

PREVENTIVE CARE IN SICKLE CELL DISEASE

1. **What are the recommendations for infectious prophylaxis in children with SCD?**
   - Administer oral penicillin prophylaxis twice daily until 5 years of age in all children with sickle cell anemia to reduce the risk of pneumococcal infections.
   - Vaccinate against *S. pneumoniae.*

2. **Describe the data and recommendations for stroke screening in children with sickle cell anemia.**
   - Children should be screened annually with transcranial Doppler (TCD) beginning at 2 years of age and continuing until 16 years of age.
   - Data are from the STOP trial (Stroke Prevention Trial in Sickle Cell Anemia. Children with elevated TCD velocities were randomly assigned to either receive transfusions to maintain HbS concentrations of less than 30% or remain on standard supportive care with transfusion only when clinically indicated. This study demonstrated that chronic transfusions reduced the risk of primary stroke by 90%, which led to the early termination of the trial.

3. **What is the treatment for secondary prevention of recurrent stroke?**
   - Monthly simple or exchange transfusion to keep hemoglobin >9 g/dL and HbS <30%

4. **In addition to standard screening for hypertension, what should SCD patients who are >10 years of age be annually evaluated for?**
   - Proteinuria
   - Dilated eye exam to evaluate for retinopathy

5. **List the benefits of hydroxyurea.**
   - Improved overall survival
   - Decrease in the frequency and severity of vaso-occlusive crises
   - Decrease in the incidence of acute chest syndrome
   - Decrease in the need for transfusions

6. **What is the effect of hydroxyurea?**
   - Increases levels of HbF
   - Lowers the number of circulating leukocytes and reticulocytes and alters the expression of adhesion molecules, all of which contribute to vaso-occlusion

7. **List the side effects of hydroxyurea.**
   - Myelosuppression, nausea, diarrhea, skin ulcers, mouth sores, and hair thinning

8. **How long does it take for hydroxyurea to lead to a clinical response?**
   - It may take up to 3 to 6 months.
   - A 6-month trial is recommended prior to declaring a treatment failure.
   - Monitor mean corpuscular volume, reticulocyte count, and white blood cells/absolute neutrophil count for index of adherence, response, and dosing.

TRANSFUSIONS IN SICKLE CELL DISEASE

1. **What are the benefits of exchange transfusion for patients with SCD?**
   - Increases the percent of normal (donor) hemoglobin A-containing RBCs
   - Permits transfusion of increased volumes of donor blood without increasing blood viscosity
   - Reduces rate of iron accumulation

2. **What are the risks of exchange transfusion?**
   - Increased alloimmunization risk (extended antigen matching is recommended at least to Rh [Cc, Ee] and Kell to reduce risk)

- High cost
- Need for permanent venous access

3. **What are the indications for chronic exchange/prophylactic transfusions in SCD?**
   - Primary or secondary prevention of stroke, recurrent acute chest syndrome despite hydroxyurea, severe vaso-occlusive crisis not responsive to hydroxyurea, recurrent priapism, and pulmonary hypertension not responsive to hydroxyurea

4. **What is the HbS goal in patients undergoing chronic exchange/prophylactic transfusions in SCD?**
   - Reduce the HbS to <30%

5. **What are the indications and data for preoperative transfusions in patients with SCD?**
   - Transfuse RBCs to bring the hemoglobin level to 10 g/dL prior to undergoing a surgical procedure involving general anesthesia.
   - The TAPS trial (Transfusion Alternatives Preoperatively in Sickle Cell Disease) randomized 70 patients with SCD to no preoperative transfusion or preoperative transfusion with a target hemoglobin of 10 g/dL. The study was terminated early due to an increased incidence of serious adverse events in the no-transfusion arm.

6. **When should transfusion NOT be used in patients with SCD?**
   - Uncomplicated vaso-occlusive pain episodes without symptomatic anemia due to lack of evidence of benefit

IRON OVERLOAD IN SICKLE CELL DISEASE

1. **Why are patients with SCD at risk for iron overload?**
   - For every 3 to 4 units of RBCs that a patient receives, 1 g of iron enters the body (adults normally have only 4–5 g of iron in the body).
   - There is no physiologic means to remove excess iron as regulation of iron homeostasis normally occurs at the level of absorption through the hormone hepcidin, which inhibits the transport of gastrointestinal iron into the body. As transfused blood represents iron that circumvents the normal pathways of iron regulation, this excess iron accumulates in tissues and can result in organ dysfunction.

2. **How is iron overload diagnosed?**
   - Serum ferritin
     - Ferritin levels are nonlinear and do not correlate precisely with liver iron burden.
     - In general, ferritin level <1,500 ng/mL indicates lower liver iron concentration (LIC <7 mg/g dw) and ferritin >2,500 to 3,000 ng/mL is associated with higher LIC (>10–15 mg/g dw) and risk of liver fibrosis.
   - LIC by MRI (R2 or R2*)
     - MRI every 1 to 2 years in patients with SCD receiving chronic transfusion therapy

3. **List treatments for iron overload.**
   - Deferiprone, deferoxamine, and deferasirox

ADDITIONAL THERAPIES IN SICKLE CELL DISEASE

1. **What additional medications are available to patients with SCD?**
   - Voxelotor is a HbS polymerization inhibitor recently approved for patients ≥4 years. The HOPE trial (Hemoglobin Oxygen Affinity Modulation to Inhibit HbS Polymerization) was a double-blind, placebo-controlled, phase 3 trial that randomized patients to high-dose or low-dose voxelotor or placebo. Voxelotor significantly increased hemoglobin levels and decreased hemolytic markers.

2. **In whom would you consider a stem cell transplant for SCD?**
   - Patients with severe symptoms of SCD including frequent pain episodes, neurologic injury (including stroke history and elevated TCD), and recurrent acute chest syndrome unresponsive to treatment with transfusions and hydroxyurea and for whom there is an HLA-matched sibling donor
   - Better outcomes with stem cell transplant performed with patients <13 years old

3. **Are there other advanced therapies for SCD?**
   - Gene therapy (gene addition, editing): currently in clinical trial stages with long-term follow-up needed
   - Alternate donor allogeneic stem cell transplant (e.g., haploidentical-related donor) in clinical trial setting

QUESTIONS

1. **Which statement regarding thalassemia is false?**
   A. Deletional variants in alpha-thalassemia lead to a more severe phenotype than nondeletional mutations.
   B. It is inherited as pathologic alleles of globin genes on chromosomes 11 and 16.
   C. Thalassemia trait is considered protective against malaria.
   D. Iron overload leads to significant morbidity in severe thalassemia.

2. **What is the most likely phenotype of a child with β°/β+ genotype?**
   A. Silent carrier with no symptoms
   B. Not compatible with life
   C. Moderate hemolytic anemia with likely need for transfusions long term
   D. Severe anemia with early need for transfusions

3. **Which of the following represents a potential cure for severe beta-thalassemia?**
   A. Fetal hemoglobin inducers (hydroxyurea)
   B. Allogeneic stem cell transplant
   C. Luspatercept
   D. Gene therapy
   E. B and D

4. You suspect sickle cell disease in a patient and order a hemoglobin electrophoresis. The following is consistent with which diagnosis?

HbA	0%
HbS	87%–92%
HbC	0%
HbF	2%–15%
HbA2	>3.5%

HbA, hemoglobin A; HbA2, hemoglobin A2; HbC, hemoglobin C;
HbF, hemoglobin F; HbS, hemoglobin S.

A. Sickle cell disease (HbSS)
B. Sickle cell trait
C. Sickle beta (+) thalassemia
D. Sickle beta (0) thalassemia

5. Which lane on the following electrophoresis corresponds to a diagnosis
   of sickle cell trait?

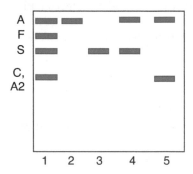

A. 1
B. 2
C. 3
D. 4
E. 5

6. A patient states they have a history of sickle cell disease. The periph-
   eral smear shows an abundance of target cells. What type of sickle cell
   disease may you suspect?
   A. SS
   B. Sickle beta-thalassemia
   C. SC
   D. Sickle cell trait

7. Which of the following is not recommended in children with sickle cell
   disease (SCD)?
   A. Annual transcranial Doppler
   B. Empiric iron chelation therapy at 10 years of age

C. Annual eye exam

D. Daily penicillin prophylaxis

8. **Which patient should not receive transfusion?**

    A. Preoperatively for a cholecystectomy with presenting hemoglobin of 8 g/dL

    B. Patient with a history of recurrent acute chest syndrome

    C. Patient with uncomplicated vaso-occlusive pain episode

    D. Patient with a history of stroke as secondary stroke prevention

9. **What level of ferritin would make you concerned your patient may be developing iron overload?**

    A. 250 ng/mL

    B. 500 ng/mL

    C. 750 ng/mL

    D. 2,500 ng/mL

10. **Which of the following is necessary for the diagnosis of acute chest syndrome?**

    A. Fever

    B. Chest pain

    C. Respiratory symptoms

    D. New infiltrate on chest x-ray (CXR)

11. **What mutation causes sickle cell disease?**

    A. Point mutation in the beta-globin gene

    B. Frameshift mutation in the beta-globin gene

    C. Deletion in the beta-globin gene

    D. Insertion in the beta-globin gene

12. **For a patient with sickle cell disease (SCD) at high risk for stroke, which is the appropriate initial treatment for primary prevention?**

    A. Hydroxyurea

    B. Chronic transfusion to maintain hemoglobin S <30%

    C. L-glutamine

    D. Aspirin

13. **Which of the following does not play a role in the clinical manifestations and disease severity of sickle cell disease (SCD)?**

    A. Beta-globin genotype

    B. Age at diagnosis

    C. Concentration of hemoglobin F

    D. Coexistence of alpha-thalassemia

14. **Which of the following is recommended for infectious prophylaxis in children with sickle cell disease (SCD)?**

    A. Oral penicillin prophylaxis BID until 3 years of age

    B. Oral penicillin prophylaxis BID until after 5 years of age

    C. Vaccinate with pneumococcal polysaccharide vaccine before 2 years of age

    D. Vaccinate with pneumococcal conjugate vaccine at birth

ANSWERS

1. **A. Deletional variants in alpha-thalassemia lead to a more severe phenotype than nondeletional mutations.** Nondeletional mutations in alpha-thalassemia usually lead to a more severe phenotype than deletional variants. In addition, since the alpha-2-globin gene produces two to three times more globin than alpha-1, nondeletional/deletional variants in the alpha-2-globin gene are more severe than alpha-1.

2. **C. Moderate hemolytic anemia with likely need for transfusions long term.** Beta-thalassemia intermedia is characterized by moderate hemolytic anemia, but affected individuals can have later complications of chronic anemia and will have transfusion needs at some point in life.

3. **E. B and D.** Allogenic stem cell transplant can be curative and best outcomes are seen with patients under age 17 and with an HLA-matched sibling donor. Gene therapy is also potentially curative for severe beta-thalassemia.

4. **D. Sickle beta (0) thalassemia.** The patient has ~90% hemoglobin S (HbS) and no hemoglobin A (HbA) or hemoglobin C (HbC); therefore, the patient either has HbSS or sickle cell beta (0) thalassemia. The elevated hemoglobin A2 (HbA2) is consistent with the latter.

5. **D. 4.** Patients with sickle cell trait have hemoglobin A and hemoglobin S (± hemoglobin F but with no hemoglobin C) on hemoglobin electrophoresis.

6. **C. SC.** Abundance of target cells is a characteristic feature of hemoglobin SC disease.

7. **B. Empiric iron chelation therapy at 10 years of age.** Empiric iron chelation is not routinely recommended in patients with SCD. Iron chelation should be done when there is evidence of iron overload.

8. **C. Patient with uncomplicated vaso-occlusive pain episode.** Preoperative transfusion to goal Hb of 10 g/dL as well as chronic transfusions for patients with a history of either stroke or acute chest syndrome are appropriate.

9. **D. 2,500 ng/mL.** A ferritin of 2,500 ng/mL or more is associated with higher liver iron concentrations (LIC >10–15mg/g dw); however, this should be confirmed by T2 or T2* MRI as ferritin levels do not correlate precisely with iron burden.

10. **D. New infiltrate on chest x-ray (CXR).** All other answers are part of the diagnosis and presentation but a new infiltrate is required.

11. **A. Point mutation in the beta-globin gene.** Sickle cell disease is caused by a mutation resulting in glutamic acid to valine substitution at the sixth amino acid of beta-globin.

12. **B. Chronic transfusion to maintain hemoglobin S <30%.** According to the STOP trial (Stroke Prevention Trial in Sickle Cell Anemia), patients at high risk of stroke based on transcranial Doppler are treated with transfusions to maintain hemoglobin S <30%. As per the TWiTCH trial (TCD With Transfusions Changing to Hydroxyurea), after at least 1 year of chronic transfusions, hydroxyurea treatment can be considered for low-risk children without severe vasculopathy on (magnetic resonance angiography [MRA]).

13. **B. Age at diagnosis.** Age at diagnosis does not play a role in the clinical manifestations of disease severity of SCD. Higher concentration of hemoglobin F is associated with reduced severity of clinical manifestations. Coexisting alpha-thalassemia reduces the severity of some disease manifestations for select sickle cell haplotypes, and the beta-globin genotype (AS, S-beta-thalassemia, SC, and SS) plays a significant role in clinical manifestations and disease severity.

14. **B. Oral penicillin prophylaxis BID until after 5 years of age.** Oral penicillin prophylaxis is recommended for children with SCD until age 5. Vaccination with pneumococcal conjugate vaccine per normal pediatric vaccination schedule (starting at 2 months of age) and with pneumococcal polysaccharide vaccine ≥ 2 years of age.

Erythrocytosis, Hemochromatosis, and Porphyrias

Richard King

5

Erythrocytosis

DEFINITION

1. **What is the World Health Organization (WHO) cutoff level for polycythemia vera?**
   - Males: hemoglobin >16.5 g/dL or hematocrit >49%
   - Females: hemoglobin >16.0 g/dL or hematocrit >48%

DIAGNOSTIC WORKUP

1. **What symptoms are important in the history?**
   - Symptoms are nonspecific, but might include headaches, fatigue, shortness of breath, fever, sweats, weight loss, pruritus, erythromelalgia, early satiety, or gout.
   - Explore any history of venous or arterial thromboembolism.
   - Ask about any use of testosterone, anabolic steroids, or erythropoietin (EPO).
   - Ask about family history of erythrocytosis.

2. **What physical exam findings are important to look for?**
   - Measure pulse oximetry.
   - Pay close attention to cardiopulmonary findings, abdominal masses, Cushingoid features, and telangiectasias.

3. **What diagnostic tests are important for erythrocytosis?**
   - First-line testing to investigate for polycythemia vera (see Chapter 12)
     - EPO level
     - *JAK2* V617F mutation
     - If *JAK2* V617F testing is negative, test for *JAK2* exon 12 mutation
   - Second-line testing if history is suggestive of an acquired erythrocytosis
     - Directed toward potential underlying etiologies (see causes in the next section)
   - Second-line testing if history is suggestive of a hereditary erythrocytosis
     - Venous P50 (oxygen tension at which hemoglobin is 50% saturated)
     - Consider germline mutation testing for causes of hereditary erythrocytosis (see next section)

CAUSES

1. **What are the causes of acquired erythrocytosis?**
   - Polycythemia vera (see Chapter 12)

- Secondary causes
  - EPO level normal or increased
    - High altitude
    - Carbon monoxide poisoning
    - Smoking
    - Drugs (anabolic steroids)
    - Cardiac disease
    - Pulmonary disease
    - Sleep apnea
    - Volume contraction
  - EPO level increased
    - EPO-secreting tumors
      - Cerebellar hemangioblastoma
      - Hepatocellular carcinoma
      - Meningioma
      - Parathyroid carcinoma or adenoma
      - Pheochromocytoma
      - Renal cell carcinoma
      - Uterine leiomyoma
    - Posttransplant erythrocytosis
    - Renal cysts
    - Renal artery stenosis
    - TEMPI (telangiectasias, erythrocytosis with increased EPO, monoclonal gammopathy, perinephric fluid collections, intrapulmonary shunting)
    - EPO administration

2. **What are the causes of hereditary erythrocytosis?**
   - Germline mutations in the Epo receptor (*EPOR*): low EPO level
   - Germline mutations in the oxygen-sensing pathway: normal or elevated EPO level
     - Von Hippel–Lindau (*VHL*)
     - Prolyl hydroxylase domain-2 (*PHD2*; also known as the *EGLN1* gene)
     - Hypoxia-inducible factor-2 alpha (*HIF2A*)
     - Erythropoietin (*EPO*)
   - Left shift in oxygen dissociation curve (decrease in venous P50)
     - High-oxygen affinity hemoglobin variants
     - Methemoglobinemia
     - 2,3-bisphosphoglycerate deficiency

MANAGEMENT

1. **See Chapter 12 for management of polycythemia vera.**

2. **How do you manage secondary erythrocytosis?**
   - General
     - Optimize cardiovascular risk factors and smoking cessation.
     - In the absence of symptoms, there are no good studies demonstrating benefits with phlebotomy.
     - If no history of thrombosis, consider low-dose aspirin for thrombosis prophylaxis in patients with cardiovascular risk factors.
     - If there is history of thrombosis, consider aspirin for arterial thrombosis history and anticoagulation for venous thrombosis history.

- Consider phlebotomy if it helps the symptoms.
- For other disease-specific considerations, see the following text.
■ Chronic obstructive pulmonary disease (COPD)
- There is no proven impact on phlebotomy and thrombosis rates.
- Restrict phlebotomy only to those whose symptoms are likely due to the erythrocytosis based on relief with phlebotomy.
- Defer other management to a pulmonary specialist.
■ Sleep apnea
- Optimization of sleep apnea with continuous positive airway pressure (CPAP) overnight
■ Cyanotic congenital heart disease
- There is no routine phlebotomy.
- Consider for symptom relief if hematocrit is very high (e.g., >65%).
■ Testosterone therapy
- Withhold or reduce dose for goal hematocrit in normal range.
- If stopping or reducing dose is undesired, therapeutic phlebotomy is used by some.
■ Post-renal transplant erythrocytosis
- Angiotensin converting enzyme (ACE) inhibitor or angiotensin receptor blocker (ARB) medication can result in reduced hematocrit.
- Theophylline is an alternative.

3. **How do you manage hereditary erythrocytosis?**
■ Follow general management strategies for secondary erythrocytosis.
■ Chuvash polycythemia (homozygous autosomal recessive VHL mutations)
- High risk of arterial or venous thrombotic events
- Thrombotic risk not reduced with phlebotomy
- Antiplatelet therapy and optimization of cardiovascular risk factors

Hemochromatosis

CAUSES OF ELEVATED FERRITIN

1. **What are the causes of elevated ferritin in the setting of iron overload?**
■ *HFE* hemochromatosis
■ Non-*HFE* hereditary hemochromatosis
■ Ferroportin disease
■ Iron-loading anemias (congenital or acquired)
■ Iatrogenic iron overload (red blood cell transfusion, parenteral iron administration)
■ Dysmetabolic iron overloading syndrome
■ African iron overload
■ Aceruloplasminemia/hypoceruloplasminemia
■ Atransferrinemia/hypotransferrinemia

2. **What are the causes of elevated ferritin in the absence of iron overload?**
■ Cellular damage
■ Inflammatory and infectious conditions
■ Metabolic syndrome and obesity
■ Insulin resistance/diabetes mellitus

- Excessive alcohol consumption
- Malignancy
- Hemophagocytic lymphohistiocytosis (HLH) and adult-onset Still disease
- Hereditary hyperferritinemia cataract syndrome
- Gaucher disease

3. **What conditions can be associated with elevated ferritin with or without iron overload?**
   - Chronic liver disease

HEMOCHROMATOSIS

1. **What are the characteristics of hemochromatosis?**
   - Patients have elevated transferrin saturation (>45%) with or without evidence of iron overload in the absence of a primary red blood cell disorder.
   - Iron deposition can lead to organ damage in the liver, pancreas, heart, endocrine glands, and joints.
   - Symptoms can include fatigue, weakness, weight loss, joint pain, symptoms of heart failure, symptoms of diabetes, abdominal pain, and decreased libido.

2. **What tests aid in the diagnosis of hemochromatosis?**
   - Ferritin and transferrin saturation
     - If ferritin and transferrin saturation are normal or low:
       - Hemochromatosis is unlikely.
       - There is no further evaluation for hemochromatosis.
     - If ferritin is normal or elevated and transferrin saturation is elevated:
       - Check genetic test for *HFE* p.Cys282Tyr (C282Y) variant.
       - With C282Y homozygosity, hemochromatosis is likely.
       - If C282Y homozygosity is not present:
         - Evaluate for other potential causes of iron overload (see the preceding section "Causes of Elevated Ferritin").
         - If ferritin is not elevated, then monitor ferritin annually.
         - If ferritin is elevated.
           - Determine the liver iron content by MRI.
           - Consider liver biopsy or FibroScan if the ferritin >1,000 or liver function tests are abnormal to stage fibrosis. Consult with a hepatologist.
           - Consider additional genetic testing for non–*HFE*-related hemochromatosis.
     - If ferritin is elevated and transferrin saturation is normal or decreased:
       - Evaluate for other causes of elevated ferritin (see preceding section "Causes of Elevated Ferritin").
       - Perform iron MRI of the liver and spleen.
         - If there is relatively weaker signal in the liver and strong signal in the spleen, then consider ferroportin disease.
   - Family testing
     - First-degree relatives of patients with *HFE*-related hemochromatosis should be screened with ferritin, transferrin saturation, and *HFE* genetic testing.

3. **Describe the genetics of hemochromatosis.**
   - *HFE*-related
     - *HFE* C282Y homozygosity
     - Other *HFE* variants

- *HFE* compound heterozygosity for C282Y/H63D may not be diagnostic of hemochromatosis and other causes of iron overload should be ruled out and managed first (e.g., management of diabetes or alcohol cessation).
- Patients with H63D or S65C variants in the absence of C282Y variant are not at increased risk of tissue iron overload, although they may have elevated ferritin or transferrin saturation.
- Non–*HFE*-related
  - Transferrin receptor 2 (*TFR2*): autosomal recessive
  - Hepcidin (*HAMP*): autosomal recessive
  - Hemojuvelin (*HJV*): autosomal recessive
  - Ferroportin (*SLC40A1*): autosomal dominant

4. How is hemochromatosis managed?
- Therapeutic phlebotomy
  - Start weekly or biweekly for ferritin >300 (transferrin saturation >50%) in males or >200 (transferrin saturation >45%) in females.
  - Target ferritin varies per guidelines (20–30 or 50–100).
- Screening for hepatocellular carcinoma
  - Follow cirrhosis screening guidelines for those who have cirrhosis or advanced fibrosis.

Porphyria

CLINICAL PRESENTATION

1. What porphyrias are associated with acute neurovisceral symptoms?
- Occur only in acute hepatic porphyria (AHP)
  - Acute intermittent porphyria (AIP): most common
  - Variegate porphyria (VP)
  - Hereditary coproporphyria (HCP)
  - ALA dehydratase porphyria (ADP): extremely rare

2. What are the neurovisceral symptoms associated with AHP?
- Nonspecific symptoms are thought to be due to the toxic effects of elevated aminolevulinic acid (ALA).
  - Visceral symptoms
    - Generalized severe abdominal pain
    - Nausea, vomiting, constipation, and anorexia
  - Neurologic symptoms
    - Muscle weakness (can be profound)
    - Peripheral neuropathy and extremity pain
    - Seizures
    - Autonomic dysfunction (hypertension and tachycardia)
  - Psychiatric symptoms
    - Anxiety, insomnia, and restlessness
    - Hallucinations and paranoia

3. What porphyrias are associated with chronic blistering photosensitivity?
- Porphyria cutanea tarda (PCT)
- Hepatoerythropoietic porphyria (HEP): more severe, hereditary form of PCT

- VP
- HCP
- Congenital erythropoietic porphyria (CEP): severe, nonpainful blistering photo-sensitivity and skin mutilation from birth or very early childhood

4. **What porphyrias are associated with nonblistering photosensitivity and how do they present?**
   - Acute, painful, nonblistering photosensitivity presenting in early childhood
     - Acute burning skin pain, swelling, and erythema
     - Occurs within 15 to 30 minutes of sun exposure
     - Usually presents early in childhood
     - Causes:
       - Erythropoietic protoporphyria (EPP)
       - X-linked dominant protoporphyria (XLP)

DIAGNOSTIC TESTING

Testing depends on the clinical presentation.

1. **What tests are done for acute neurovisceral symptoms?**
   - First-line tests to obtain when symptoms are present.
     - Random urine for:
       - Urine porphobilinogen (PBG)
       - Fractionated porphyrins
       - ALA
   - Second-line tests for determining the type of AHP:
     - Erythrocyte PBG deaminase
     - Plasma or serum porphyrins
     - Fecal porphyrins
   - Genetic testing aids in confirmation and family member counseling.

2. **What tests are performed for chronic blistering photosensitivity?**
   - First-line testing

TABLE 5.1 ■ Summary of Diagnostic Findings in the Acute Hepatic Porphyrias

	Urine Testing	Plasma Porphyrins	Fecal Porphyrins	Other Testing	Genetics
AIP	↑↑↑ ALA ↑↑↑ PBG	Normal or mild ↑ (nonspecific pattern)	Normal in most cases	Erythrocyte PBG deaminase decreased ~50% in most but not all	*HMBS* (AD)
VP	↑ ALA ↑ PBG	↑ (if skin lesions)	↑ coproporphyrin III (III to I ratio <10) ↑ protoporphyrin		*PPOX* (AD)

(continued)

TABLE 5.1 ■ Summary of Diagnostic Findings in the Acute Hepatic Porphyrias (*continued*)

	Urine Testing	Plasma Porphyrins	Fecal Porphyrins	Other Testing	Genetics
HCP	↑ ALA ↑ PBG	↑ (if skin lesions)	↑ coproporphyrin III (III to I ratio >10)		*CPOX* (AD)
ADP	↑ ALA Normal PBG	Normal	Normal	Erythrocyte zinc protoporphyrin increased	*ALAD* (AR)

ADP, ALA dehydratase porphyria; AIP, acute intermittent porphyria; ALA, aminolevulinic acid; HCP, hereditary coproporphyria; PBG, porphobilinogen; VP, variegate porphyria.

- ● Plasma porphyrins or random urine fractionated porphyrins
- ■ Second-line testing
  - ● Urine PBG
  - ● Fecal porphyrins if VP or HCP is suspected
  - ● If PCT is diagnosed, consider evaluation for hereditary form by testing erythrocyte uroporphyrinogen decarboxylase (UROD) activity, which will be decreased in the hereditary form, or *UROD* gene sequencing.

TABLE 5.2 ■ Summary of Diagnostic Findings in the Cutaneous Blistering Porphyrias

	Urine Testing	Plasma Porphyrins	Fecal Porphyrins	Other	Genetics
PCT	Normal ALA Normal PBG ↑ in predominantly uroporphyrins and heptacarboxyporphyrins	↑ in predominantly uroporphyrins and heptacarboxyporphyrins	Complex pattern	Erythrocyte UROD activity decreased in hereditary form	20% are hereditary *UROD* (AR/AD)
HEP	Similar to PCT but more pronounced elevations	Similar to PCT but more pronounced elevations	Complex pattern	Erythrocyte UROD activity decreased	*UROD* (AR)
VP	↑ ALA ↑ PBG	↑ coproporphyrin III ↑ protoporphyrin	↑ coproporphyrin III (III to I ratio <10) ↑ protoporphyrin		*PPOX* (AD)
HCP	↑ ALA ↑ PBG	↑ coproporphyrin III (if skin lesions)	↑ coproporphyrin III (III to I ratio >10)		*CPOX* (AD)
CEP	↑ uroporphyrin I and coproporphyrin I	↑ uroporphyrin I and coproporphyrin I	↑ coproporphyrin I	Increase in erythrocyte porphyrins May have hemolysis	*UROS* (AR)

ALA, aminolevulinic acid; CEP, congenital erythropoietic porphyria; HCP, hereditary coproporphyria; HEP, hepatoerythropoietic porphyria; PBG, porphobilinogen; PCT, porphyria cutanea tarda; UROD, uroporphyrinogen decarboxylase; VP, variegate porphyria.

3. **What tests are performed for acute nonblistering photosensitivity (which most often presents in early childhood)?**
   - Erythrocyte protoporphyrin (metal-free and zinc protoporphyrin)
     - Increased erythrocyte total protoporphyrin with metal-free protoporphyrin >85% of total protoporphyrin
       - Diagnostic of EPP
         - Protoporphyrins are released from erythrocytes into the plasma, taken up by skin, and upon sun exposure results in skin damage.
         - Protoporphyrins are taken up by hepatocytes and excreted in bile (5% develop liver failure).
         - Autosomal recessive *FECH* mutations
     - Increased erythrocyte metal-free (50%–85%) and zinc protoporphyrin (15%–50%)
       - Suggests XLP
         - XLP with the same phenotype as EPP
         - Gain-of-function mutation in *ALAS2*
     - Total erythrocyte protoporphyrins also elevated (<50% metal-free) in iron deficiency, lead poisoning, hemolysis, and anemia of chronic disease

MANAGEMENT

1. **How is acute AHP managed?**
   - Urgent treatment required in acute attacks
     - Hemin: 3 to 4 mg/kg intravenously once daily for 4 days
       - Hemin replenishes the regulatory heme pool, leading to negative feedback inhibition of ALAS1 synthesis in hepatocytes and significant decrease in porphyrin precursors.
       - Reconstitution in albumin may decrease risk of phlebitis.
     - Glucose loading: can be used until hemin is available
     - Supportive measures
       - Correction of hyponatremia and hypomagnesemia
       - Opioid analgesics for severe pain
       - Antiemetics for nausea
       - Beta-blockers for tachycardia and hypertension
     - Addressing the triggers that induce hepatic ALAS1 synthesis
       - Medications
       - Alcohol
       - Tobacco smoking
       - Fasting/carbohydrate restriction
       - Hormones (progesterone, luteal phase of menstrual cycle)
       - Infections or other physiologic stresses (e.g., surgery)
   - Prevention in AHP patients with recurrent attacks
     - Givosiran
       - Mechanism: small interfering RNA targeted to hepatocytes leading to cleavage of ALAS1 mRNA and reduced porphyrin synthesis
       - Dosing: 2.5 mg subcutaneous injection once monthly
       - Outcomes:
         - Reduces urinary ALA and PBG
         - Reduces attack rate
       - Adverse effects:

- Anaphylaxis
- Injection site reaction and rash
- Fatigue
- Nausea
- Increases in serum creatinine or liver function tests
- Elevations in homocysteine
- Hemin prophylaxis
  - Variable frequency from twice weekly to once monthly
  - Monitoring of iron stores
- Long-term care
  - Hepatocellular carcinoma screening starts at age 50 (alpha fetoprotein [AFP] and ultrasound).
  - Monitor for renal insufficiency.
- Skin manifestations in VP and HCP
  - Hemin, phlebotomy, or hydroxychloroquine are not beneficial treatments.
  - Management is avoidance of triggers and protection from sunlight.

2. How is PCT treated?
- Identification and management of predisposing factors
  - Iron overload, hemochromatosis
  - Alcohol, smoking
  - Hepatitis C, HIV
  - Estrogen
- Treatment
  - Therapeutic phlebotomy with goal ferritin <20
  - Alternative to phlebotomy is hydroxychloroquine 100 mg two times per week

3. How are EPP and XLP treated?
- Avoidance of sunlight (protective clothing, topical zinc oxide)
- Beta carotene
  - Might quench activated free radicals
  - Usually turns the skin yellow/orange
  - Variable results
  - 30 to 300 mg orally daily (titrate to serum levels of 600–800 mcg/dL)
- Afamelanotide
  - Alpha-melanocyte-stimulating hormone analog
  - Increases skin melanin and improves sun tolerance
  - 16 mg implant subcutaneous every 2 months

CAUSES OF SECONDARY PORPHYRINURIA

1. What are the causes of secondary porphyrinuria?
- Isolated elevated (1.5–2x upper limit normal) urine coproporphyrin not specific for a primary porphyria
- Causes of secondary coproporphyrinuria:
  - Alcohol intoxication
  - Heavy metal toxicity
  - Occupational toxins/chemicals (benzene, polyhalogenated aromatic hydro-carbons, vinyl chloride, dioxin)
  - Cirrhosis or other hepatobiliary disease
  - Hereditary hyperbilirubinemia

- Anemia (iron deficiency, hemolysis, pernicious) or myelodysplastic syndrome (MDS)
- Fasting, diabetes, and pregnancy

PSEUDOPORPHYRIA

1. What is pseudoporphyria?

- Chronic blistering skin lesions are histologically similar in appearance to porphyria, but with negative biochemical porphyrin testing.
- Skin biopsy cannot differentiate cutaneous porphyria from pseudoporphyria or other bullous disorders and is not helpful in differentiating the types of blistering cutaneous porphyrias.
- Causes of pseudoporphyria:
  - UV exposure (such as tanning beds)
  - Medications
  - Dialysis

QUESTIONS

1. A 30-year-old female is referred to the clinic for a hemoglobin of 17.8 and hematocrit of 53%. The white blood cell and platelet counts are normal. Labs over the prior 12 years showed persistent hemoglobin of around 17 to 18 without any symptoms. Family history is notable for similar elevations in the hemoglobin and hematocrit in her older brother and father. Erythropoietin (EPO) level is below the reference range. Peripheral blood testing did not reveal a *JAK2* V617F mutation or *JAK2* exon 12 mutation. Which of the following genes would be most likely to have a pathogenic variant identified if tested in this individual?
   A. *BPGM*
   B. *EPOR*
   C. *HIF2A*
   D. *PHD2*
   E. *VHL*

2. A 40-year-old male who had a renal transplant 2 years earlier is referred to the clinic for a hemoglobin of 18.4 and hematocrit of 56%. There are no other abnormalities in the blood counts and no history of prior erythrocytosis in the patient or family members. Erythropoietin level is on the high end of the normal reference range. Imaging studies do not show any evidence of renal or hepatic tumors. What is the best next step in management?
   A. Observe.
   B. Start therapeutic phlebotomy.
   C. Start an angiotensin converting enzyme (ACE) inhibitor.
   D. Perform genetic testing to evaluate for hereditary erythrocytosis.

3. A 26-year-old asymptomatic male underwent genetic testing and was found to have heterozygous *HFE* variant S65C. Ferritin and transferrin saturation are normal and the patient has no family history of hemochromatosis. What is the most accurate statement regarding counseling this patient?

A. The genetic testing shows the patient has hemochromatosis and should start therapeutic phlebotomy.
B. The genetic testing shows the patient has hemochromatosis and should be monitored closely for symptoms or elevations in the ferritin and transferrin saturation.
C. The patient does not have hemochromatosis now but is at an increased risk for iron overload in the future.
D. The patient does not have hemochromatosis and has no increased risk for iron overload compared with the general population.

4. A 47-year-old male is found to have a transferrin saturation of 64% and ferritin of 932 when evaluated by his primary care physician for fatigue. The patient's father passed away from liver failure. The patient's younger sister is also found to have an elevated transferrin saturation and ferritin. Which of the following results of *HFE* gene analysis would be diagnostic of hemochromatosis?
   A. *HFE* C282Y homozygosity
   B. *HFE* S65C heterozygosity
   C. *HFE* H63D heterozygosity
   D. *HFE* C282Y/S65C compound heterozygosity

5. A 34-year-old male is referred to the clinic for a family history of hemochromatosis. The patient is found to have a transferrin saturation of 53%, ferritin of 410, and *HFE* C282Y homozygosity. The patient is asymptomatic and has normal liver function tests. In addition to counseling, what is the next best step in management?
   A. Observation with annual monitoring of lab tests
   B. Liver biopsy
   C. Iron chelation therapy
   D. Therapeutic phlebotomy

6. A 61-year-old female is referred from her dermatologist after biopsy of blistering hand skin lesions suggested possible porphyria. Urine porphyrin testing shows elevations in uroporphyrin and heptacarboxyporphyrins and normal porphobilinogen levels. Hemoglobin is normal and ferritin is elevated at 800. The patient has no family history of porphyria. You suspect porphyria cutanea tarda and order tests for underlying potential risk factors. What is the best initial management for porphyria cutanea tarda for this patient?
   A. Intravenous (IV) hemin therapy
   B. Glucose loading
   C. Givosiran
   D. Therapeutic phlebotomy

7. An 18-year-old female presents to the ED for severe abdominal pain, nausea, constipation, and anxiety. She is unable to eat or drink anything due to her symptoms. She has mild hypertension and tachycardia. Lab testing shows a sodium of 128 and mild elevations in aspartate aminotransferase (AST) and alanine aminotransferase (ALT). CT of the abdomen and pelvis is only notable for ileus. You suspect an acute hepatic porphyria. Which of the following tests would be most helpful to obtain first?

A. Erythrocyte porphobilinogen (PBG) deaminase
B. Urine porphobilinogen and aminolevulinic acid (ALA)
C. Fecal porphyrins
D. Plasma porphyrins

8. **A 20-year-old male was diagnosed with acute intermittent porphyria at the age of 18 and has required hospitalizations and intravenous (IV) hemin treatment three times in the past 6 months despite twice-monthly prophylactic IV hemin. You recommend initiating treatment with givosiran. What is the most accurate statement about the mechanism of this treatment?**
   A. Givosiran reduces porphyrin levels by binding excessive porphyrins.
   B. Givosiran replenishes the regulatory heme pool, leading to negative feedback inhibition of ALAS1 synthesis in hepatocytes.
   C. Givosiran is a small interfering RNA targeted to hepatocytes leading to cleavage of ALAS1 mRNA and reduced porphyrin synthesis.
   D. Givosiran replaces deficient porphobilinogen deaminase.

9. **An 18-year-old female is referred for blistering hand lesions and scarring. Symptoms are worse after sun exposure. The patient has no other symptoms. Urine porphyrins show mild elevations in coproporphyrin III. Urine porphobilinogen is moderately elevated. Fecal porphyrins show very high levels of coproporphyrin III and protoporphyrin. Variegate porphyria is suspected and a pathogenic heterozygous variant in the *PPOX* gene is identified. What is the best recommendation about the patient's skin lesion?**
   A. Treatment with therapeutic phlebotomy should be started.
   B. Intravenous (IV) hemin therapy should be initiated.
   C. Hydroxychloroquine therapy should be initiated.
   D. Protect the skin from sun exposure and avoid potential triggers such as alcohol, progestins, and other medications.

10. **A 26-year-old female was diagnosed in early childhood with erythropoietic protoporphyria and has avoided outdoor activities in the summer to prevent skin symptoms. She previously tried beta carotene but did not like how it turned her skin orange. She wants to be able to enjoy summer outdoor activities and asks what treatments are available. Which of the following might best improve sun tolerance?**
    A. Starting a diet low in carbohydrates
    B. Receiving an afamelanotide implant
    C. Starting givosiran
    D. Starting hydroxychloroquine

11. **You suspect hereditary erythrocytosis in a patient. You obtain P50 level and it is low. Which of the following is the most likely diagnosis?**
    A. High-oxygen affinity hemoglobin variant
    B. *VHL* mutation
    C. *PHD2* mutation
    D. *HIF2a* mutation

12. **Mutations in which genes can result in autosomal dominant hereditary hemochromatosis?**
    A. Transferrin receptor 2
    B. Hepcidin
    C. Hemojuvelin
    D. Ferroportin
    E. *HFE*

ANSWERS

1. **B. *EPOR*.** The history and testing suggest a hereditary erythrocytosis, and a subnormal EPO level is suggestive of an *EPOR* mutation. The other genes listed can cause a hereditary erythrocytosis, but would be expected to have a normal or elevated EPO level.

2. **C. Start an angiotensin converting enzyme (ACE) inhibitor.** The patient has posttransplant erythrocytosis, and the first-line therapy to reduce the hematocrit is an ACE inhibitor or angiotensin receptor blocker (ARB). Therapeutic phlebotomy could be considered if the patient does not respond to first-line treatment. Since the patient previously had normal hematocrit levels, a hereditary erythrocytosis is less likely.

3. **D. The patient does not have hemochromatosis and has no increased risk for iron overload compared with the general population.** When no *HFE* C282Y mutation is present, nor any elevations in transferrin saturation or ferritin or family history of iron overload, this person is not considered at any elevated risk of iron overload regardless of the presence of any combination of heterozygosity, homozygosity, or compound heterozygosity for *HFE* H63D and S65C variants.

4. **A. *HFE* C282Y homozygosity.** This patient's history and lab testing are highly suspicious for hemochromatosis, and in such cases homozygosity for *HFE* C282Y is diagnostic of hemochromatosis. The other genetic testing results are not diagnostic alone, and other testing to confirm iron overload, such as iron MRI testing, should be sought to confirm iron overload.

5. **D. Therapeutic phlebotomy.** In this patient with hemochromatosis, ferritin >300 but <1,000, and no signs of liver abnormalities on blood testing, therapeutic phlebotomy can be started without any additional testing. Observation alone would be inappropriate because this would leave the patient at risk of developing complications from iron overload. Liver biopsy is not required prior to initiating therapy and is reserved for staging fibrosis if the ferritin is >1,000 or liver function tests are abnormal. Therapeutic phlebotomy is preferred over iron chelation therapies.

6. **D. Therapeutic phlebotomy.** Therapeutic phlebotomy is first-line treatment in porphyria cutanea tarda. IV hemin, glucose loading, and givosiran are treatments in acute hepatic porphyria, not porphyria cutanea tarda. If therapeutic phlebotomy is not tolerated in porphyria cutanea tarda, low-dose hydroxychloroquine twice weekly can be helpful.

7. **B. Urine porphobilinogen and aminolevulinic acid (ALA).** In a patient presenting with acute neurovisceral symptoms, urine porphobilinogen and ALA are the most helpful initial tests. Urine porphobilinogen greater than four times the upper limit of the reference range is diagnostic of an acute hepatic porphyria, while negative urine porphobilinogen and ALA testing during acute symptoms rules out acute hepatic porphyria as a

cause of the symptoms. Erythrocyte PBG deaminase can be helpful as a second-line test to suggest acute intermittent porphyria if it is reduced along with elevated porphobilinogen levels, but it can be normal in a small percentage of patients with acute intermittent porphyria and is often normal in other types of acute hepatic porphyria, so it is not helpful as a first-line test. Fecal and plasma porphyrins can be helpful to distinguish between the types of acute hepatic porphyria, but could be non-specific in acute intermittent porphyria and thus not helpful as first-line tests in someone presenting with acute neurovisceral symptoms.

8. **C. Givosiran is a small interfering RNA targeted to hepatocytes leading to cleavage of ALAS1 mRNA and reduced porphyrin synthesis.** Hemin, not givosiran, works by replenishing the regulatory heme pool leading to negative feedback inhibition of ALAS1 synthesis in hepatocytes.

9. **D. Protect the skin from sun exposure and avoid potential triggers such as alcohol, progestins, and other medications.** In patients with variegate porphyria and only skin symptoms, the mainstay of management is avoidance of sunlight and triggers. IV hemin only temporarily lowers porphyrin production and is not helpful for long-term management of chronic skin symptoms. Therapies for porphyria cutanea tarda, such as phlebotomy and hydroxychloroquine, are not helpful for skin symptoms in variegate porphyria.

10. **B. Receiving an afamelanotide implant.** Afamelanotide is a subcutaneous implant that has been shown to improve sun tolerance in patients with erythropoietic protoporphyria. A diet higher, not lower, in carbohydrates is sometimes advised in patients with porphyria. Givosiran is used to prevent acute neurovisceral attacks in patients with an acute hepatic porphyria, but has not been studied in patients with erythropoietic protoporphyria. Hydroxychloroquine is used as an alternative to phlebotomy in patients with porphyria cutanea tarda.

11. **A. High-oxygen affinity hemoglobin variant.** Mutations in *VHL*, *PHD2*, or *HIF2a* result in hereditary erythrocytosis with normal P50 level. High-oxygen affinity hemoglobin variant, methemoglobinemia, and 2.3-BPG deficiency result in hereditary erythrocytosis with reduced P50 level.

12. **D. Ferroportin.** Mutation in ferroportin results in autosomal dominant hereditary hemochromatosis, while mutations in the other genes listed result in autosomal recessive hereditary hemochromatosis.

White Blood Cell Disorders

6

Thomas Michniacki and Kelly Walkovich

Granulocyte Disorders

NEUTROPHIL OVERVIEW

1. **How are neutropenia and neutrophilia defined?**
   - Neutropenia is typically defined as absolute neutrophil count (ANC) below 1,500 cells/microL (1.5×10^9/L).
     - Mild neutropenia: ANC greater than 1,000 but less than 1,500 cells/microL
     - Moderate neutropenia: ANC greater than 500 but less than 1,000 cells/microL
     - Severe neutropenia: ANC less than 500 cells/microL
     - Very severe neutropenia: ANC less than 200 cells/microL
   - ANC = white blood cells/microL × (percent [polymorphonuclear cells + bands] / 100)
   - Be aware of Duffy-associated neutrophil count (DANC; formerly known as benign ethnic neutropenia), with individuals of certain ethnic descent (especially African, West Indian, Sephardic Jews, and Yemenites) having lower baseline ANCs with values typically greater than 1,200 cells/microL (although they might be less than 1,000 cells/microL). Low ANC is correlated with a Duffy antigen/receptor null (FyA-/FyB-) phenotype in these individuals.
   - Neutrophilia leukocytosis is defined as a total white blood cell count greater than 11,000 cells/microL along with an ANC greater than 7,700 cells/microL in adults (more than 2 *SD* above the mean).

2. **What is the maturation process and life cycle of neutrophils?**
   - Steps of maturation: myeloblast → promyelocyte → myelocyte → metamyelocyte → band → neutrophil
   - Neutrophils spend approximately 14 days within the bone marrow, including retention of mature cells within a large, nonmitotic storage pool that can be released into circulation rapidly if needed (e.g., secondary to infection).
   - The chemokine receptor CXCR4 is an important regulator of neutrophil release from the marrow.
   - Once released, neutrophils typically last 24 to 48 hours within the circulation.
   - Neutrophils depart the circulation and move into inflamed/injured tissue via chemotaxis and ultimately diapedesis across or between endothelial cells. This process occurs via three main classes of proteins: selectins, integrins, and chemokines. Initial vessel adhesion and transient rolling across the endothelial wall by the neutrophils occur through the selectins. Further actions by the integrins and chemokines ultimately lead to movement arrest and migration across the vessel wall into the tissues.

- Once within the tissues, neutrophils are believed to not undergo phagocytosis by macrophages or apoptosis for another few days.

3. How do neutrophils function?

- Neutrophils assist in the recruitment and activation of additional cells of the immune system.
- Neutrophils have three direct antimicrobial functions: degranulation, phagocytosis, and creation of neutrophil extracellular traps (NETs).
- Degranulation results in the release of azurophilic, specific, and tertiary granules.
- Phagocytosis ultimately generates reactive oxygen species (the "respiratory burst").
- The respiratory burst involves the activation of the enzyme nicotinamide adenine dinucleotide phosphate (NADPH) oxidase, which helps create superoxide. Superoxide is converted to hydrogen peroxide by superoxide dismutase, with hydrogen peroxide next undergoing enzymatic reaction with myeloperoxidase (MPO) to create the bactericidal hypochlorous acid.
- NETs: These are weblike extracellular structures, extruded by dying neutrophils, consist of granule proteins and chromatin which can further facilitate microbe killing.

ACQUIRED NEUTROPHIL DISORDERS

1. What are the acquired causes of neutropenia?

- Medications:
  - Neutropenia usually begins within 3 months of starting the medication, with the pathogenesis felt to be secondary to either drug-dependent autoimmune destruction of neutrophils and/or their precursors, or as a result of direct bone marrow toxicity.
  - Numerous medications are implicated, but the most commonly reported include clozapine, thionamides (antithyroid medications), nonsteroidal anti-inflammatory drugs (NSAIDs), dapsone, antibiotics, sulfa-containing drugs, angiotensin-converting enzyme (ACE) inhibitors, histamine blockers, and ticlopidine.
  - Be aware of levamisole-tainted cocaine and heroin causing neutropenia in illicit drug users.
- Infections:
  - Bacterial infections commonly described include *Shigella* enteritis, typhoid fever, tuberculosis, brucellosis, and rickettsial pathogens.
  - Fungal infections include histoplasmosis.
  - Malaria is a known cause, as are numerous viral agents, most notably HIV, Epstein–Barr virus (EBV), COVID-19, cytomegalovirus (CMV), hepatitis viruses, human herpesvirus 6 (HHV-6), and varicella.
- Nutritional deficiencies:
  - Deficiencies in vitamin B_{12}, folate, and copper
  - Anorexia nervosa and/or severe malnutrition
- Autoimmune disorders:
  - Systemic lupus erythematosus and rheumatoid arthritis are the most commonly associated autoimmune disorders.

- Increasingly, genetic sequencing is being used to screen chronic "idiopathic" neutropenia patients for underlying inborn errors of immunity (e.g., GATA2 haploinsufficiency).
- Bone marrow disorders such as myelodysplastic syndromes (MDS)
- Large granular lymphocyte (LGL) leukemia:
  - May fall within the same disease spectrum as Felty syndrome with splenomegaly, neutropenia, and rheumatoid arthritis, but is clonal in nature

2. What are the acquired causes of neutrophilia?

- Can be secondary to increased production, reduced margination, enhanced release from the marrow storage pool, and decreased removal from the circulation
- Increased production due to infection, autoimmune conditions, malignancy, myeloproliferative disease, chronic idiopathic neutrophilia, post-neutropenia recovery, and medications (lithium and quinidine)
- Increased marrow storage pool release secondary to corticosteroids, stress, infection, endotoxin stimulation, and hypoxia
- Reduced margination from stress, exercise, epinephrine, and infection
- Decreased circulation clearance of neutrophils due to corticosteroids or splenectomy

3. What are the acquired qualitative disorders of neutrophils?

- Numerous acquired conditions can affect the functional abilities of neutrophils.
- These include diabetes mellitus, trauma, severe burns, renal failure, liver disease, alcoholism, infections (most commonly HIV and influenza), and autoimmune conditions.

INHERITED NEUTROPHIL DISORDERS

1. What are the inherited causes of neutropenia?

- DANC, as noted earlier
- Shwachman–Diamond syndrome:
  - Mutations in the *SBDS* gene (or less commonly *DNAJC21*, *EFL1*, or *SRP54*) that lead to bone marrow failure, exocrine pancreatic insufficiency, and skeletal abnormalities. Pancreatic and skeletal features may be mild and not clinically apparent. Neutropenia can progress to pancytopenia with bone marrow failure/leukemia.
- Cyclic neutropenia:
  - Recurrent neutropenia every 14 to 35 days, but most patients exhibit a 21-day cycle period with 7 to 10 days of profound neutropenia
  - Reciprocal monocytosis during times of neutropenia
  - Recurrent infections, fevers, and/or mouth ulcers during times of neutropenia, with signs of chronic inflammation of the gingiva and oral mucosa
  - Patients are also at risk of *Clostridium septicum* infections.
  - Diagnosis requires monitoring neutrophil counts two to three times per week for 6 to 8 weeks.
  - Ninety percent of patients have mutations in the elastase gene (*ELANE*) that lead to cyclic arrest in myelocyte maturation and selective apoptosis of neutrophil precursors.

- Treatment involves recombinant granulocyte colony stimulating factor (G-CSF) and supportive care.
- Severe congenital neutropenia:
  - Increased apoptosis of myeloid cells leading to severe neutropenia and risk of death from infection
  - Can be due to various mutations, including elastase/*ELANE* (autosomal dominant, 50%–60% of cases) and *HAX1* (formerly known as Kostmann syndrome; autosomal recessive)
  - At risk of malignant transformation into MDS and acute myeloid leukemia (AML); following 10 years of G-CSF therapy, the annual risk of MDS/AML is reported at 2.3% per year, with a cumulative MDS/AML incidence after 15 years on G-CSF of 22%; annual bone marrows are thus recommended for malignancy screening
  - Treatment with escalating doses of G-CSF until an ANC of 1,000 to 3,000 cells/microL is reached
  - Hematopoietic cell transplantation should be considered in those unable to tolerate G-CSF, with continued infections despite G-CSF usage, or requiring high doses of G-CSF (greater than 15 mcg/kg/d)
- Can also be associated with WHIM (warts, hypogammaglobulinemia, infections, and myelokathexis) syndrome and GATA2 haploinsufficiency

2. **What are the inherited functional disorders of neutrophils?**
- MPO deficiency:
  - MPO is the most common primary phagocyte disorder, but may also be acquired.
  - MPO catalyzes hydrogen peroxide into hypochlorous acid.
  - Greater than 95% of patients are asymptomatic, but may be unmasked in the setting of poorly controlled diabetes mellitus.
  - Symptomatic individuals have an increased risk of *Candida* species infections and vasculitis.
  - Diagnosis is obtained by histochemical staining for MPO.
  - Complete MPO deficiency may lead to abnormal dihydrorhodamine (DHR) testing, possibly resulting in an incorrect diagnosis of chronic granulomatous disease (CGD) for the patient.
  - Treatment is supportive.
- CGD:
  - CGD is caused by defects in NADPH oxidase, which leads to inability of phagocytes to kill certain microbes.
  - Most pathogenic variants are X-linked, although female carriers have increased autoimmune features and may have skewed lionization, leading to infection susceptibility.
  - Patients are particularly susceptible to catalase-positive organisms, with the most common pathogens being *Staphylococcus aureus*, *Aspergillus*, *Burkholderia* (*Pseudomonas*), *Serratia*, and *Nocardia*.
  - The lung, skin, lymph nodes, and liver are most frequently infected, with recurrent abscesses common.
  - Diagnosis is made via neutrophil function testing (nitroblue tetrazolium [NBT] or DHR 123 tests) and confirmed via genetic studies.

- Treatment involves antimicrobial prophylaxis with trimethoprim-sulfameth-oxazole and itraconazole, with consideration for use of interferon-gamma.
- Treat all acute infections aggressively.
- Corticosteroids may be used to control the inflammatory manifestations of CGD.
- Hematopoietic stem cell transplantation is curative.
- Leukocyte adhesion deficiencies affect the ability of neutrophils to emigrate to sites of inflammation due to mutations in key integrins and selectins.
  - May cause neutrophilia
- Neutrophil dysfunction is associated with numerous other syndromes, including Chediak–Higashi syndrome, Griscelli syndrome, and *STAT3* loss of function.

TREATMENT OF NEUTROPENIA

1. **How are neutropenic conditions associated with an increased risk of infection treated?**
   - See preceding text for disease-specific recommendations, but most involve the use of G-CSF and aggressive supportive therapy.
   - G-CSF:
     - Initial dosing of G-CSF is 5 mcg/kg/d, with escalation until appropriate ANC is reached (of note, patients with cyclic neutropenia typically respond to lower dosing of 2–3 mcg/kg/d).
     - It may be associated with bone pain, neutrophilia, splenomegaly, and rarely splenic rupture.
   - Those with severe chemotherapy or bone marrow transplantation-associated neutropenia and life-threatening infections may occasionally benefit from granulocyte transfusions.
   - Infection prophylaxis:
     - Prophylaxis includes trimethoprim-sulfamethoxazole, itraconazole, and interferon-gamma in CGD patients.
     - Prophylactic antibiotics have not been found to be of value in most cases of nonchemotherapy-related neutropenia (this should be individualized).
     - Emphasize excellent hand and dental hygiene to reduce the risk of serious infections, including bacteremia.

MONOCYTE OVERVIEW

1. **What is the life cycle and function of monocytes?**
   - Following the development from monoblasts within the marrow, monocytes move to the circulation for 1 to 3 days prior to moving to the tissue, where they differentiate into macrophages or dendritic cells.
   - Monocytes and their progeny serve three main functions within the immune system: phagocytosis, cytokine production, and antigen presentation.

2. **What is the definition of monocytosis and monocytopenia?**
   - Monocytosis is defined as a total monocyte count of more than 500 cells/microL.
   - Monocytopenia is a rare isolated finding and is usually associated with additional cytopenias.

CAUSES OF MONOCYTOSIS AND MONOCYTOPENIA

1. What are the major causes of monocytosis?
- Infectious causes: subacute bacterial endocarditis, tuberculosis, syphilis, and protozoal and rickettsial infections (Rocky Mountain spotted fever and kala-azar)
- Autoimmune conditions: systemic lupus erythematosus, sarcoidosis, inflammatory bowel disease, and rheumatoid arthritis
- Malignancy: chronic myelomonocytic leukemia, chronic myeloid leukemia (CML), AML, and lymphoma
- Miscellaneous conditions: post-neutropenia recovery, postsplenectomy, cyclic neutropenia (reciprocal monocytosis during times of neutropenia), corticosteroids, tetrachloroethane poisoning, and alcoholic liver disease

2. What are the causes of monocytopenia?
- Typically found with other immune cytopenias, but may be additionally observed with corticosteroid usage, infections with endotoxin production, stress, and GATA2 deficiency
- Hairy cell leukemia (a monocyte count of 0 should raise suspicion for this disorder in the right clinical setting)

EOSINOPHIL OVERVIEW

1. What is an eosinophil?
- Eosinophils are granulocytes that play a vital role in combating viral and parasitic infections, along with mediating the body's response to allergens (in addition to mast cells and basophils).
- Activated eosinophils may damage tissues through recruitment of other inflammatory cells, cytokine release, and toxic granule production.

2. What defines eosinophilia?
- Eosinophilia is defined as a total eosinophil count of greater than 500 cells/microL.
- Eosinophilia can be further classified as mild (500–1,500 cells/microL), moderate (1,500–5,000 cells/microL), or severe (>5,000 cells/microL).
- Hypereosinophilia (HE) is defined as moderate-to-severe eosinophilia (greater than or equal to 1,500 cells/microL).
- Keep in mind that the level of peripheral blood eosinophilia does not always predict the risk of organ damage.

CAUSES OF EOSINOPHILIA AND EOSINOPENIA

1. What are the major causes of eosinophilia?
- Allergic disorders: asthma, acute urticaria, atopic dermatitis, allergic bronchopulmonary aspergillosis, eosinophilic gastroenteritis, food allergy, and atopic rhinitis
- Parasites and infections: invasive helminths, EBV, malaria, toxoplasmosis, tuberculosis, amebiasis, cat scratch fever, coccidioidomycosis, fungal rhinosinusitis, and scabies

- Hereditary disorders: hyperimmunoglobulin E syndrome, familial eosinophilia, and hereditary angioedema
- Drug reactions, including drug reaction with eosinophilia and systemic symptoms (DRESS)
- Miscellaneous: adrenal insufficiency, graft-versus-host disease (GVHD), and peritoneal/hemodialysis
- Rheumatologic disorders: eosinophilic fasciitis, eosinophilic granulomatosis with polyangiitis, polyarteritis nodosa, sarcoidosis, and scleroderma
- Hypereosinophilic syndrome and clonal eosinophilia:
  - Eosinophilia associated with *PDGFRA*, *PDGFRB*, *FGFR1*, or *PCM1-JAK2* rearrangements. These rearrangements could be tested for by fluorescence in situ hybridization (FISH), polymerase chain reaction (PCR), or bone marrow cytogenetics.
  - If other cytogenetic abnormalities or excess blasts are present, the diagnosis could be chronic eosinophilic leukemia or other World Health Organization (WHO)-defined myeloid neoplasm.
  - The lymphocytic variant of hypereosinophilic syndrome is associated with abnormal or clonal lymphocytes.
  - In the absence of all the above clonal findings, the diagnosis could be idiopathic eosinophilia, including hypereosinophilic syndrome. The latter two disorders do not have clonal findings.
    - Hypereosinophilic syndrome is characterized by absolute eosinophil count of 1,500 cells/microL or greater for at least 6 months, with evidence of organ damage from infiltrating eosinophils. In the absence of end-organ damage, the diagnosis of hypereosinophilic syndrome cannot be made.
    - Patients with hypereosinophilic syndrome may present with fever, fatigue, weight loss, hepatosplenomegaly, pulmonary infiltrates, and skin manifestations.
    - Cardiac damage is the leading cause of morbidity and mortality, with Loeffler endocarditis a possible complication.
  - Treat the underlying condition if one can be found, with consideration for corticosteroids in symptomatic patients.
  - Imatinib therapy has been successfully used in those found to have *PDGFRA* rearrangements. If cardiac involvement is present, concomitant steroid therapy should be considered.
  - In those severely affected with clonal eosinophilic disorder, consider hematopoietic stem cell transplantation.
- Mastocytosis:
  - Mastocytosis is a clonal expansion of mast cells causing cutaneous (urticaria pigmentosa) or systemic multiorgan (bone marrow, spleen, liver, and lymph node) infiltration.
  - Infiltrating mast cells typically express CD2 and/or CD25, in addition to normal mast cell markers.
  - Patients are often found to have a somatic mutation involving *KIT*.
  - Patients may present with episodic signs/symptoms of mast cell activation, including hypotension, syncope, urticaria, flushing, fatigue, Darier sign, diarrhea, and musculoskeletal pain.
  - Adults presenting with skin manifestations should be evaluated for presence of systemic disease.

- Patients are often found to have elevated serum tryptase levels (persistently exceeds 20 ng/mL).
- Cytopenias may occur due to marrow infiltration.
- Abnormal liver enzymes are found in case of liver infiltration.
- Patients should have ready access to epinephrine injections given the risk of anaphylaxis.
- Treatment is aimed at preventing mast cell mediator release through the use of antihistamines, cromolyn sodium, and antileukotriene agents.
- Imatinib can be used if the systemic mastocytosis is not *KIT*-mutated.
- Advanced systemic mastocytosis can be treated with midostaurin or avapritinib.
- Severe cases may require cytoreductive therapies. Hematopoietic stem cell transplantation can be considered as part of a clinical trial (experimental).
  - Many malignancies are associated with eosinophilia:
    - Eosinophilia is notably present in adenocarcinomas, primary (neoplastic) hypereosinophilic syndrome, Sezary syndrome, acute and chronic eosinophilic leukemia, CML, and myeloproliferative neoplasms.

2. **What are the causes of eosinopenia?**
   - May be secondary to conditions causing release of adrenal corticosteroids, prostaglandins, and epinephrine
   - Exposure to corticosteroids or epinephrine

BASOPHIL OVERVIEW

1. **What is a basophil?**
   - Basophils are the least common but the largest granulocytes.
   - They assist in the formation of inflammatory reactions during immune and allergic responses.
   - They are capable of phagocytosis and release of heparin, serotonin, and histamine.

CAUSES OF BASOPHILIA AND BASOPHILOPENIA

1. **What are the major causes of basophilia?**
   - Malignant disorders, most notably CML, AML, MDS, and myeloproliferative neoplasms
   - Hypersensitivity reactions to drugs and foods
   - Infections: smallpox, tuberculosis, varicella, helminths, and influenza
   - Allergic syndromes
   - Mastocytosis
   - Autoimmune conditions, most notably rheumatoid arthritis and ulcerative colitis
   - Severe hypothyroidism and administration of estrogen

2. **What are the major causes of basophilopenia?**
   - Glucocorticoids
   - Thyrotoxicosis

Lymphocyte Disorders

CAUSES OF LYMPHOPENIA AND LYMPHOCYTOSIS

1. **What are the major acquired causes of lymphopenia?**
   - Infections:
     - Bacterial: tuberculosis, severe bacterial sepsis, brucellosis, and typhoid fever
     - Viral: HIV, measles, severe acute respiratory syndrome (SARS), and hepatitis
     - Severe fungal sepsis and histoplasmosis
     - Malaria
   - Autoimmune disorders, including systemic lupus erythematosus, Sjögren syndrome, and rheumatoid arthritis
   - Iatrogenic: corticosteroid usage, immunosuppressive therapy, and radiation
   - Miscellaneous: thoracic leak, protein-losing enteropathy, Cushing syndrome, alcoholism, stress, trauma, zinc deficiency, malnutrition, and renal failure

2. **What are the major acquired causes of lymphocytosis?**
   - Numerous malignancies, including chronic lymphocytic leukemia and other lymphoproliferative neoplasms, and thymoma
   - Infections (notably viral), pertussis, hypersensitivity reactions (including drug reactions), and autoimmune conditions
   - Miscellaneous: postsplenectomy, trauma, stress, cigarette smoking (persistent polyclonal B-cell lymphocytosis), and hyperthyroidism

QUESTIONS

1. **You are referred a 45-year-old African American for evaluation of persistent neutropenia. Over the past 3 months, he has had absolute neutrophil count (ANC) values of 1,250 cells/microL, 1,300 cells/microL, and 1,205 cells/microL. There is no reciprocal monocytosis with his neutropenia and he states that he has been told throughout his life that his neutrophils have always been slightly low. He denies any history of recurrent serious infections. What should be your next step in his care?**
   A. Perform a bone marrow evaluation
   B. Place him on prophylactic antibiotics
   C. No need for continued monitoring
   D. Prescribe daily granulocyte colony stimulating (G-CSF) factor injections

2. **A woman is placed on a course of high-dose corticosteroids by her primary care physician for a case of severe atopic dermatitis. What complete blood count (CBC) abnormality would one likely find if a CBC was obtained on this patient while receiving her corticosteroids?**
   A. Neutrophilia
   B. Anemia
   C. Eosinophilia
   D. Thrombocytopenia

3. You are taking over the care of a 25-year-old man from your pediatric hematology colleague. He has a history of recurrent liver abscesses and *Aspergillus* pulmonary infection in the past but is now doing well. He is currently receiving prophylaxis with itraconazole, trimethoprim-sulfamethoxazole, and interferon-gamma. What is the underlying inherited cause of his condition?
   A. Lack of myeloperoxidase (MPO)
   B. Pathogenic variants affecting the nicotinamide adenine dinucleotide phosphate (NADPH) oxidase complex
   C. *SBDS* gene mutations
   D. Duffy antigen/receptor null phenotype

4. You are the consulting hematologist for a patient found to have an absolute eosinophil count of 4.5 × 10⁹/L, along with urticarial rash, persistent cough with hypoxia, and a mild transaminitis. CT of the chest/abdomen shows pulmonary and hepatic infiltrates. Genetic testing reveals the presence of a *FIP1L1-PDGFRA* fusion within clonal marrow cells. Based on the patient's genetic analysis results, what medication should be included in the patient's treatment regimen?
   A. Imatinib
   B. Ipilimumab
   C. Ivermectin
   D. Trametinib

5. A 27-year-old Caucasian woman is seen in your clinic for an evaluation of neutropenia. Her past medical history is notable for a diagnosis of rheumatoid factor-positive rheumatoid arthritis for which she was recently evaluated by a rheumatologist. She states she was prescribed a course of scheduled prednisone and naproxen as needed by her rheumatologist but has yet to begin the medications. A complete blood count (CBC) reveals an absolute neutrophil count (ANC) of 950 cells/microL, platelet count of 135,000 cells/microL, and a microcytic anemia with a hemoglobin value of 10.5 g/dL. Eosinophil count is normal. Physical exam is notable for numerous swollen and painful joints and splenomegaly. What is the most likely diagnosis for this patient?
   A. Systemic mastocytosis
   B. Duffy-associated neutrophil count (DANC)
   C. Severe congenital neutropenia
   D. Felty syndrome

6. A 24-year-old woman is receiving propylthiouracil (PTU) treatment for her Graves disease. What hematologic lab abnormality is the patient at the highest risk of suffering from due to her medication history?
   A. Thrombocytosis
   B. Neutropenia
   C. Eosinophilia
   D. Anemia

7. You are evaluating a 22-year-old man who was referred to your clinic for workup of monomorphic urticaria pigmentosa and intermittent episodes of flushing, pruritus, abdominal pain, and diarrhea. His history is additionally notable for apparent episodes of anaphylaxis in association with alcohol ingestion or emotional stress. His workup thus far at other providers has not yielded a causative allergy. What laboratory study may be helpful in making a correct diagnosis for this patient?
    A. Dihydrorhodamine (DHR) 123 test
    B. Screening for mutations in the elastase gene
    C. Serum tryptase
    D. Serum lipase

8. A 32-year-old woman smokes two packs of cigarettes a day. She is currently relatively healthy despite her high tobacco usage. What benign proliferative hematologic condition is this patient at risk for given her history of cigarette smoking?
    A. Persistent polyclonal B-cell lymphocytosis
    B. Hemophagocytic lymphohistiocytosis (HLH)
    C. Autoimmune lymphoproliferative syndrome (ALPS)
    D. Primary myelofibrosis

9. A man is seen by an endocrinologist for hypertension, insulin resistance, and central obesity with prominent striae. Following a thorough evaluation, he is ultimately diagnosed with Cushing syndrome. Given his new diagnosis, what value would one expect to find when a complete blood cell count is obtained on the patient?
    A. Absolute neutrophil value of 750 cells/microL
    B. Platelet count of 35,000 cells/microL
    C. Absolute lymphocyte value of 0.8×10^9/L
    D. Hemoglobin of 9.0 g/dL

10. A 42-year-old woman is receiving treatment with pegylated interferon-alfa and ribavirin for a history of hepatitis C infection. Her treating physician has decided to begin treatment with granulocyte colony stimulating factor (G-CSF) to help lessen neutropenia associated with her antiviral regimen. What adverse reaction can commonly be seen with G-CSF administration?
    A. Hyperactivity
    B. Thrombocytosis
    C. Hirsutism
    D. Ostealgia

11. You have recently taken over the care of a 34-year-old woman with a diagnosis of systemic mastocytosis. Which genetic alteration is most often found associated with this disorder?
    A. *BCR-ABL*
    B. *KIT*
    C. *JAK2*
    D. *TET2*

12. A 25-year-old male with a history of cocaine usage is found to have significant neutropenia with an absolute neutrophil count of 100 cells/microL. Which substance now known to be frequently found as a contaminant in cocaine has strongly been associated with neutropenia?
    A. Levofloxacin
    B. Methylamphetamine
    C. Levamisole
    D. Mannitol

ANSWERS

1. **C. No need for continued monitoring.** This patient most likely has Duffy-associated neutrophil count (DANC) and thus requires no further monitoring or treatment. There is no evidence of cyclic neutropenia with reciprocal monocytosis or episodes of severe infections. Chronic idiopathic neutropenia is a consideration, but patients typically have ANC values ranging from 500 to 1,000 cells/microL with an associated monocytosis. Given his lack of recurrent severe infections, he does not require prophylactic antibiotics or G-CSF.

2. **A. Neutrophilia.** Patients placed on corticosteroids often manifest neutrophilia. Anemia and thrombocytopenia should not be seen. Additionally, corticosteroids often cause eosinopenia rather than eosinophilia.

3. **B. Pathogenic variants affecting the nicotinamide adenine dinucleotide phosphate (NADPH) oxidase complex.** This patient is suffering from chronic granulomatous disease (CGD), which is caused by various mutations leading to alterations in the NADPH oxidase protein complex. A lack of MPO is seen in myeloperoxidase deficiency, with these patients typically being asymptomatic. *SBDS* mutations most commonly cause Shwachman–Diamond syndrome, and the Duffy antigen/receptor null phenotype is observed in those with DANC.

4. **A. Imatinib.** *PDGFRA* rearrangement is the diagnosis given the patient's eosinophilia and presence of *FIP1L1-PDGFRA* fusion. Such patients can be treated with imatinib. Ipilimumab and trametinib are cytotoxic T-lymphocyte-associated antigen 4 (CTLA-4) and MEK inhibitors, respectively, and do not seem to play a role in this disease. Ivermectin is used to treat parasitic infections which may lead to eosinophilia.

5. **D. Felty syndrome.** The triad of neutropenia, splenomegaly, and rheumatoid arthritis is classic for a diagnosis of Felty syndrome. The patient additionally has anemia and mild thrombocytopenia, which can also be found with the syndrome. The patient's cytopenias may be partially explained by splenic sequestration, but with microcytic anemia a concurrent diagnosis of anemia of chronic disease should be considered. With Felty syndrome, neutropenia cannot be explained by concurrent illnesses or medications and is often persistent. Benign ethnic neutropenia is characterized by lifelong mild neutropenia with normal hemoglobin and platelet counts. Severe congenital neutropenia typically presents in early childhood, with ANC values of less than 200 cells/microL, and requires granulocyte colony stimulating factor injections to help prevent serious infections.

6. **B. Neutropenia.** Thionamides, such as methimazole, carbimazole, and PTU, are used in the treatment of Graves hyperthyroidism, but may cause agranulocytosis. PTU appears to more likely cause the condition compared with methimazole. Neutropenia often occurs within the first 1 to 3 months of treatment and is dose-dependent with methimazole usage. Thionamides may be associated with aplastic anemia, but this complication is less common than agranulocytosis.

7. **C. Serum tryptase.** The patient's history is concerning for systemic mastocytosis, which can be associated with an elevation of serum tryptase (>20 ng/mL). Serum tryptase should be measured when the patient is at baseline state and not during or immediately following an apparent mast cell mediator release episode. Values obtained following a symptomatic incident indicate mast cell activation but cannot distinguish between mastocytosis and anaphylaxis secondary to another cause. DHR 123 testing is used for diagnostic evaluation of chronic granulomatous disease. Elastase gene mutations may be found in cyclic neutropenia and severe congenital neutropenia but have no apparent association with mastocytosis. Patients with systemic mastocytosis can present with pancreatitis and thus serum lipase may be elevated, but serum tryptase is more specific for mastocytosis.

8. **A. Persistent polyclonal B-cell lymphocytosis.** Persistent polyclonal B-cell lymphocytosis is significantly associated with cigarette smoking and is characterized by a persistent elevation in peripheral blood polyclonal binucleated atypical-appearing lymphocytes. Serum Immunoglobulin M (IgM) is often elevated and there appears to be an association with the Human Leukocyte Antigen (HLA)-DR7 allele. Women are more at risk of the condition than men. ALPS is more commonly seen in pediatric patients and does not appear to be associated with cigarette smoking. HLH and primary myelofibrosis additionally do not have a clear association with tobacco exposure.

9. **C. Absolute lymphocyte value of 0.8 × 10⁹/L.** Lymphocytopenia often accompanies Cushing syndrome. Polycythemia has been associated with Cushing syndrome rather than anemia. There is additionally no association of thrombocytopenia with the condition.

10. **D. Ostealgia.** Musculoskeletal discomfort is a frequent finding following G-CSF administration. Alopecia, thrombocytopenia (possibly due to splenomegaly, a rare side effect of G-CSF), and fatigue have been reported rather than hirsutism, thrombocytosis, and hyperactivity.

11. **B. *KIT*.** The majority of systemic mastocytosis patients possess a gain-of-function mutation in the tyrosine kinase receptor *KIT*. *JAK2* and *TET2* mutations may be found in those with systemic mastocytosis, but are much less common than *KIT* alterations. *BCR-ABL* gene fusions are most often associated with chronic myelogenous and acute lymphoblastic leukemias.

12. **C. Levamisole.** Numerous reports have now noted cocaine laced with levamisole, an agent historically used to treat malignancies and parasitic infections, as a cause of neutropenia in illicit drug users. Mannitol and methylamphetamine are additional substances that may be found in altered cocaine but are not associated with reports of significant agranulocytosis. Levofloxacin has not reportedly been associated with cocaine manufacturing or with neutropenia.

Bone Marrow Failure/ Aplastic Anemia

James Yoon and Kristen Pettit

7

Bone Marrow Failure/Aplastic Anemia

DEFINITION

- Cytopenias and failure of hematopoiesis resulting from stem cell injury

EPIDEMIOLOGY

- Varied but usually biphasic age distribution: teens to 20s (inherited/constitutional) and age > 60 yrs (acquired); men and women equally affected
- Incidence: ~2 persons per million, higher in East Asia (~4 persons per million)

BONE MARROW FAILURE SYNDROMES

1. **What are the two main categories of bone marrow failure (BMF)?**
   - Acquired
   - Inherited

2. **What are the major clinical manifestations?**
   - Typically cytopenia-related
     - Anemia: fatigue and dyspnea
     - Leukopenia: infection
     - Thrombocytopenia: mucosal bleeding (menorrhagia, epistaxis, easy bruising)

3. **What are the major peripheral blood morphologic findings?**
   - Pancytopenia with normocytic to macrocytic red blood cells (RBCs)
   - Reticulocytopenia

4. **What are the typical bone marrow biopsy findings?**
   - Paucity of hematopoietic cells (hypocellular)
     - <25% bone marrow cellularity in severe aplastic anemia (SAA) *or*
     - 25% to 50% bone marrow cellularity if less than 30% of the cells are hematopoietic
       - Preponderance of adipocytes
     - Usually normal karyotype—as opposed to hypoplastic myelodysplastic syndrome (MDS)
     - Low frequency of somatic mutations in *BCOR/BCORL1, DNMT3A,* and *ASXL1*

5. **What historical findings are indicative of an inherited BMF process?**
   - Inherited/constitutional
     - Young age at onset, abrupt onset of manifestations

- Lack of symptoms unrelated to cytopenias (no symptoms suggestive of rheumatologic disease such as arthritis/serositis/rash *or* malignancy/infection/granulomatous disease, i.e., constitutional symptoms)
- Lack of known exposures to insults such as chemotherapy/radiation, drugs (nonsteroidal anti-inflammatory drugs [NSAIDs], sulfonamides, antihistamines, anticonvulsants), and alcohol

6. What clinical features may be indicative of an inherited BMF process?

TABLE 7.1 ■ Inherited Bone Marrow Failure Syndromes

Syndrome	Clinical and Hematologic Features
Fanconi anemia	■ Short stature, radius/thumb anomaly, café au lait spots, microcephaly, malformed/absent kidneys, GI and heart defects, infertility ■ Pancytopenia
Dyskeratosis congenita and other telomeropathies	■ Oral leukoplakia, nail dystrophy, abnormal skin hyperpigmentation, pulmonary fibrosis ■ Pancytopenia
Shwachman–Diamond	■ Exocrine pancreatic insufficiency, steatorrhea ■ Neutropenia, anemia, thrombocytopenia

7. What are some of the genetic aberrations present in inherited BMF?

TABLE 7.2 ■ Genetic Mutations in Inherited Bone Marrow Failure Syndromes

Syndrome	Mutations
Fanconi anemia	■ ≥22 genes: *FANCA, FANCB, FANCG* (95% of cases; mostly autosomal recessive)
Dyskeratosis congenita	■ *DKC1* (X-linked) ■ *TERC* and *TERT* (autosomal dominant) ■ *TINF2* (autosomal dominant)
Shwachman–Diamond	■ *SBDS* (autosomal recessive)

8. How is Fanconi anemia diagnosed?

- Chromosome breakage testing: diepoxybutane or mitomycin C testing (on peripheral blood lymphocytes or skin fibroblasts) to assess chromosome fragility

9. How is dyskeratosis congenita confirmed?

- Telomere length testing on peripheral blood cells and confirmatory genetic testing

APLASTIC ANEMIA

1. What are the etiologies of aplastic anemia (AA)?

- Acquired or idiopathic
- Inherited BMF syndrome

2. What are some acquired causes of AA?

TABLE 7.3 ■ Acquired Causes of Aplastic Anemia

Etiology	Description
Drugs	■ Antibiotics: chloramphenicol, sulfonamides ■ NSAIDs (e.g., phenylbutazone, indomethacin) ■ Antiepileptic drugs: carbamazepine, phenytoin ■ Chemotherapy (expected) ■ Antithyroid medications: methimazole, propylthiouracil
Toxins	■ Benzene ■ Solvents ■ Pesticides, insecticides
Viral infections	■ EBV ■ HIV ■ Hepatitis
Acquired hematologic disorders	■ PNH (acquired mutation in *PIG-A*, deficient expression of CD55 and CD59 on RBCs) ■ Myelodysplastic syndrome
Other	■ Radiation injury ■ Pregnancy ■ SLE, rheumatoid arthritis ■ Anorexia

EBV, Epstein–Barr virus; NSAIDs, nonsteroidal anti-inflammatory drugs; PNH, paroxysmal nocturnal hemoglobinuria; SLE, systemic lupus erythematosus; RBCs, red blood cells.

3. How is severity of AA determined?
- ■ **SAA**
  - ● Bone marrow cellularity <25% (or 25%–50% if <30% of the cells are hematopoietic) *and* at least two of the following:
    - ■ Absolute reticulocyte count <60,000/microL
    - ■ Absolute neutrophil count <500/microL
    - ■ Platelets <20,000/microL
- ■ **Very severe SAA (vSAA)**
  - ● Blood counts meeting the SAA criteria *and*
  - ● Neutrophil count <200/microL
- ■ **Non-SAA**
  - ● Bone marrow cellularity <30%
  - ● Not meeting the cytopenia criteria for SAA or vSAA

TREATMENT

1. What conditions should be ruled out before starting treatment for idiopathic AA?
- ■ Inherited BMF syndrome
- ■ Hypoplastic MDS

- Removal of offending drug or toxin if identified
- Viral infection

2. **When is treatment indicated in idiopathic AA?**
   - Treatment indicated in SAA and vSAA
   - Treatment indicated in non-SAA with transfusion dependence

3. **What first-line systemic therapies are used to treat acquired AA?**
   - Patients <40 years old with a matched related donor: allogeneic hematopoietic cell transplant (alloHCT)
   - Patients <40 years old without a matched related donor or those >40 years old and fit: immunosuppressive therapy (IST)
     - IST consists of the following:
       - Horse antithymocyte globulin (hATG)
       - Cyclosporine (CSA), goal trough 200 to 400 ng/mL
       - Eltrombopag
   - Patients who are frail: supportive care alone
   - Supportive care measures crucial to the treatment of all patients with AA

4. **What management options are available for relapsed or refractory acquired AA?**
   - AlloHCT recommended in patients eligible for transplantation with suitable and available donor
   - If not eligible for alloHCT:
     - Rabbit antithymocyte globulin (rATG) with CSA; repeat hATG not recommended in patients previously treated with hATG due to high incidence of serum sickness
     - Eltrombopag if not incorporated in previous treatment
     - Romiplostim, a thrombopoietin agonist
     - Alemtuzumab, an anti-CD52 monoclonal antibody

5. **What toxicities are anticipated from IST?**
   - Antithymocyte globulin (ATG): serum sickness, a type III hypersensitivity reaction characterized by rash, arthralgias, and fevers
   - CSA: acute kidney injury, infection, hepatotoxicity, hypertension, posterior reversible encephalopathy syndrome, and osteopenia
   - Eltrombopag: hepatotoxicity and thromboembolism

6. **How is hematologic response assessed?**
   - Achievement of transfusion independence
   - Peripheral blood counts no longer meet the SAA criteria
   - Taper CSA if response achieved at 3 to 6 months

7. **When is alloHCT indicated in acquired AA?**
   - Patients <40 years of age meeting the SAA criteria with a readily available matched related donor should proceed directly to alloHCT.
   - The role of alloHCT is not defined in patients older than 40 years.
   - Bone marrow (as opposed to peripheral blood) is the preferred source of hematopoietic stem cells in AA.

8. **What supportive care measures are given in AA?**
   - Blood product transfusion support
   - Management of iron overload: chelation therapy for those with longer life expectancy or therapeutic phlebotomy after recovery from HCT or IST
   - Eltrombopag for thrombocytopenia
   - Infection prevention and treatment: varies depending on treatment plan
   - Usually no role for granulocyte colony-stimulating factor (G-CSF) or erythropoiesis-stimulating agents (ESAs) in patients with AA

9. **What are some special considerations for transfusions in AA?**
   - Transfuse blood products judiciously to prevent alloimmunization.
   - Transfuse cytomegalovirus (CMV)-negative, leukoreduced, irradiated blood products whenever possible.
   - Avoid blood products from related donor to minimize risk of graft failure caused by immune reaction to donor antigens.

10. **How is AA secondary to BMF treated?**
   - Allogeneic stem cell transplantation is the treatment of choice for AA secondary to BMF.

QUESTIONS

1. **The patient is a 9-month-old boy who is seen by his pediatrician for failure to thrive and diarrhea. The patient's parents have changed his formula from milk-based to a soy-based formula without improvement. He is currently on an elemental formula without improvement in greasy foul-smelling stools and with little appreciable weight gain. The child is in less than the fifth percentile for height and weight. Physical examination is remarkable for short stature and abdominal distension without peritoneal signs.**

   Laboratory testing is as follows:

Laboratory Test	Patient's Result	Reference Range
Hematocrit	30.9%	33.0%–39.0%
Hemoglobin	10 g/dL	11.0–13.0 g/dL
Mean corpuscular volume	100.5 fL	76–90 fL
White blood cell count	4.17×10^9/L	4–10×10^9/L
Segmented neutrophils	9%	20%–45%
Lymphocytes	80.3%	40%–65%
Monocytes	10.2%	1%–3%
Platelet count	402×10^9/L	150–400×10^9/L

Fecal elastase is undetectable.

Which of the following diagnostic tests should be ordered next?
A. Chromosome breakage analysis
B. High-resolution karyotyping
C. *SBDS* gene sequencing
D. Bone marrow biopsy/aspirate
E. Telomere length analysis

2. The patient is a 17-year-old man who presents to the ED with 1 week of fever at home of >39°C. Examination demonstrates short stature, conjunctival pallor, and polydactyly of the thumb on the right hand. No other abnormalities on physical examination were noted.

Laboratory Test	Patient's Result	Reference Range
Hemoglobin	6.4 g/dL	13.5–17.0 g/dL
Mean corpuscular volume	100 fL	79–99 fL
White blood cell count	1.9×10^9/L	$4.0–10.0 \times 10^9$/L
Absolute neutrophil count	0.3×10^9/L	$1.5–7.2 \times 10^9$/L
Absolute reticulocyte count	10×10^9/L	$20–80 \times 10^9$/L
Platelet count	8×10^9/L	$150–400 \times 10^9$/L

The patient is started on broad-spectrum antibiotics and transfused appropriately with packed red blood cells (PRBCs) and platelets. Bone marrow evaluation was hypocellular at <10%. Bone marrow cytogenetics revealed 46,XY. What would be the best test to confirm the diagnosis of the underlying condition?
A. Chromosome breakage analysis
B. High-resolution karyotyping
C. *SBDS* gene sequencing
D. Erythrocyte adenosine deaminase level
E. Telomere length analysis

What is the most appropriate likely next step in the management of this patient?
A. Horse antithymocyte globulin (ATG) plus cyclosporine plus eltrombopag
B. Rabbit ATG plus cyclosporine
C. Alemtuzumab
D. Human leukocyte antigen (HLA) typing of older sibling for possible matched related hematopoietic stem cell transplantation
E. Matched unrelated hematopoietic stem cell transplantation
F. Single agent eltrombopag

3. The patient is a 50-year-old man with severe acquired aplastic anemia who achieved a hematologic response 4 months after initiating immunosuppressive therapy with horse antithymocyte globulin (ATG), cyclosporine, and eltrombopag. Cyclosporine and eltrombopag are able to be gradually tapered off, with sustained response. One year later at a routine return visit, he has the following laboratory studies:

Laboratory Test	Patient's Result	Reference Range
Hemoglobin	6.8 g/dL	13.5–17.0 g/dL
Mean corpuscular volume	76.8 fL	79–94 fL
White blood cell count	3.25×10^9/L	$4.3–11.3 \times 10^9$/L
Absolute neutrophil count	0.4×10^9/L	$1.5–7.5 \times 10^9$/L
Platelet count	63×10^9/L	$150–400 \times 10^9$/L
Absolute reticulocyte count	30×10^9/L	$20–80 \times 10^9$/L

Bone marrow biopsy confirms relapse of aplastic anemia with ~5% marrow cellularity and no evidence of dysplasia or other marrow process. The patient has no siblings and no human leukocyte antigen (HLA)-matched donors are available at this time. What is the most appropriate likely next step in the management of this patient?
A. Horse ATG, cyclosporine, and eltrombopag
B. Rabbit ATG and cyclosporine
C. Single agent eltrombopag
D. HLA-mismatched unrelated donor transplant

4. A 22-year-old man presented to urgent care with a 5-day history of sore throat and malaise. He reports no medical history other than "nail fungus," which he has never been evaluated for. He has no allergies and takes no medications. On physical examination, whitish plaques were noted on his tongue, which could not be scraped off with a tongue blade. The nails on the hands demonstrate atrophy and splitting. His skin seems spotted with pigmentation on the anterior chest and neck. The patient reported family history of leukemia and "lung problems." His rapid strep test was negative; however, his complete blood count demonstrated anemia and thrombocytopenia. Which of the following diagnostic tests should be ordered next/would confirm diagnosis?
A. Chromosome breakage analysis
B. High-resolution karyotyping
C. *SBDS* gene sequencing
D. Telomere length analysis
E. Soluble interleukin-2 receptor level

5. The patient is an 89-year-old female with multiple medical comorbidities and a long-standing history of severe aplastic anemia who relapsed after antithymocyte globulin (ATG) and cyclosporine in the past. She remains transfusion-dependent, requiring packed red blood cell transfusion every 1 to 2 months for symptomatic anemia. Her last transfusion was 2 weeks ago. She presents for further management. Physical exam reveals a frail, chronically ill-appearing female in no acute distress with conjunctival pallor. No hepatosplenomegaly was appreciated. Laboratory studies are as follows:

Laboratory Test	Patient's Result	Reference Range
Hemoglobin	10.8 g/dL	12.0–16.0 g/dL
Mean corpuscular volume	101.8 fL	79.0–99.0 fL
White blood cell count	5.25 × 10⁹/L	4.0–10.0 × 10⁹/L
Absolute neutrophil count	1.25 × 10⁹/L	1.5–7.5 × 10⁹/L
Platelet count	23 × 10⁹/L	150–400 × 10⁹/L

Serum creatinine is 2.25 mg/dL. Ferritin is 1,300 ng/mL. Liver iron quantification is calculated at 10 mg/g. What is the most appropriate likely next step in the management of this patient?
A. Rabbit ATG and cyclosporine
B. Alemtuzumab
C. Evaluation for matched related hematopoietic stem cell transplantation
D. High-dose cyclophosphamide
E. Single agent eltrombopag

6. The patient is a 68-year-old Caucasian male who was referred to hematology for pancytopenia with a white blood cell count of 2.2 × 10⁹/L, hemoglobin of 11.3 g/dL, and platelets of 105 × 10⁹/L. Reticulocyte percentage was 5.4%, absolute neutrophil count (ANC) 0.9 × 10⁹/L, and absolute lymphocyte count 0.8 × 10⁹/L . Coombs test was negative. Nutritional studies were performed: B$_{12}$ level and folate were within reference range, ferritin was 295 ng/mL, and transferrin saturation was 55%. His indirect bilirubin was 1.2 mg/dL (upper limit of normal 1.1 mg/dL). Lactate dehydrogenase was 932 U/L and haptoglobin was low at 2.0 mg/dL (lower limit of normal 30 mg/dL). He was started on folic acid, and Paroxsymal nocturnal hemoglobunuria (PNH) flow cytometry was sent, which demonstrated 17.63% glycophosphatidylinositol (GPI)-deficient granulocytes, 66.79% deficient monocytes, 1.56% type II red blood cells (RBCs), and 17.25% type III RBCs. He was started on eculizumab. He has two siblings: a sister and a brother. He is referred for a second opinion. Labs after four doses of eculizumab are provided in the following:

Laboratory Test	Patient's Result	Reference Range
Hemoglobin	8.5 g/dL	14.8–17.8 g/dL
Mean corpuscular volume	110.1 fL	81.9–101 fL
White blood cell count	2.32 × 10⁹/L	4.3–11.3 × 10⁹/L
Absolute neutrophil count	1.08 × 10⁹/L	2.0–7.4 × 10⁹/L
Platelet count	82 × 10⁹/L	159–439 × 10⁹/L
Absolute reticulocyte count	98.5 × 10⁹/L	47–152 × 10⁹/L
Lactate dehydrogenase	367 U/L	100–253 U/L

Peripheral blood smear: RBCs with 1+ anisocytosis, 2+ poikilocyto-sis with a few tear drops and paucity of polychromatophilic cells. Neutropenia is present with a few of the neutrophils with segmentation abnormalities (hyposegmented). No large granular lymphocytes are appreciated. No left shift, basophilia, eosinophilia, or blasts are seen. Platelet count is decreased and morphologically normal. What is the next best step in therapy/evaluation?

A. Discontinuation of eculizumab and rechecking PNH flow cytometry
B. Addition of horse antithymocyte globulin and cyclosporine to eculizumab
C. Bone marrow biopsy and aspirate
D. Human leukocyte antigen typing of siblings for possible matched related hematopoietic stem cell transplantation
E. Telomere length analysis

7. The patient is a 38-year-old male who presents to the ED with a rash on bilateral lower extremities. The ED physician identified the rash as petechiae and a complete blood count was obtained and is noted as follows:

Laboratory Test	Patient's Result	Reference Range
Hemoglobin	11.6 g/dL	13.5–17.0 g/dL
Mean corpuscular volume	88.2 fL	79.0–99.0 fL
White blood cell count	3.22×10^9/L	$4.0–10.0 \times 10^9$/L
Absolute neutrophil count	0.44×10^9/L	$1.5–7.5 \times 10^9$/L
Platelet count	6×10^9/L	$150–400 \times 10^9$/L
Absolute reticulocyte count	27.4×10^9/L	$20–80 \times 10^9$/L
Lactate dehydrogenase	173 U/L	120–246 U/L

Paroxysmal nocturnal hemoglobinuria flow cytometry was sent, which demonstrated 2.7% glycophosphatidylinositol (GPI)-deficient mono-cytes, 2.6% deficient neutrophils, and 0.041% deficient red blood cells. A bone marrow biopsy was performed, which demonstrated variably cellular marrow (overall hypocellular) with decreased trilineage hemato-poiesis. No dysplasia was identified. Karyotype was normal male, XY. The patient has one sibling who is not a human leukocyte antigen (HLA) match, and has no HLA matched unrelated donors identified in the national registry.

What is the most appropriate likely next step in the management of this patient?

A. Matched unrelated hematopoietic stem cell transplantation
B. Rabbit antithymocyte globulin (ATG) and cyclosporine
C. Horse ATG, cyclosporine, and eltrombopag
D. High-dose cyclophosphamide

Which of the following clinical/laboratory features would be predictive of a better response to immune suppressive therapy in this patient?
A. Age of the patient
B. Pretreatment hemoglobin level
C. Pretreatment reticulocyte count
D. Presence of a PNH clone

ANSWERS

1. **C. *SBDS* gene sequencing.** The patient has pancreatic insufficiency and severe aplastic anemia, which go along with Shwachman–Diamond syndrome. Shwachman–Diamond syndrome is the second leading cause of exocrine pancreatic insufficiency. Patients typically present early in life with failure to thrive and signs and symptoms of exocrine pancreatic insufficiency. The test of choice is sequencing the *SBDS* gene, which is abnormal in roughly 90% of cases. Karyotyping would not identify this genetic anomaly. Bone marrow aspirate and biopsy would likely demonstrate a hypoplastic bone marrow but this would be a nonspecific finding. Telomere length analysis would be helpful if there was concern for dyskeratosis congenita; however, this patient does not have stigmata that would raise suspicion for the disease (oral leukoplakia, skin hyperpigmentation, and dystrophic nails).

2. **A. Chromosome breakage analysis; D. Human leukocyte antigen (HLA) typing of older sibling for possible matched related hematopoietic stem cell transplantation.** Thumb abnormalities, short stature, and severe aplastic anemia are suggestive of Fanconi anemia. The diagnostic test of choice is chromosome breakage analysis. *SBDS* gene sequencing would be useful in Shwachman–Diamond syndrome, which is characterized by pancreatic insufficiency, short stature, and skeletal dysostosis. Erythrocyte adenosine deaminase levels can be elevated in Diamond–Blackfan anemia but not Fanconi anemia. Telomere length analysis would be helpful in dyskeratosis congenita, which is characterized by oral leukoplakia, hyperpigmented skin, nail dystrophy, and aplastic anemia.

   Current standard of care for younger patients (<40 years) is to proceed directly to allogeneic stem cell transplantation with a matched sibling donor, as long as the sibling does not have Fanconi syndrome (*Blood* 2006 Oct 15; 108(8):2509–2519). Horse ATG, cyclosporine, and eltrombopag would be reasonable should the patient have comorbidities or geographic and donor constraints that would make transplantation not feasible. Horse and rabbit ATG were compared head-to-head with superior response rates and overall survival in the horse ATG arm (*N Engl J Med* 2011; 365:430–438). Alemtuzumab would be considered in the relapsed/refractory setting and is not recommended for upfront treatment outside of a clinical trial (*Blood* 2012; 119:345–354). Single agent eltrombopag is not curative therapy and should not be used in otherwise healthy individuals fit for transplant or intensive immune suppression.

3. **B. Rabbit ATG and cyclosporine.** In patients who have previously been treated with horse ATG, second induction with rabbit ATG in combination with cyclosporine yielded overall response rates of 30% in the primary refractory setting and 65% in the relapsed setting (*Br J Haematol.* 2006; 133:622–7). Repeat doses of horse ATG may increase the risk of serum sickness and is therefore not recommended. Single agent eltrombopag can be considered in patients with no prior eltrombopag treatment history in the relapsed/refractory setting (*N Engl J Med* 2012; 367:11–19).

Alternative donor transplantation (haploidentical, unmatched, core blood) is considered investigational. Matched sibling donor transplant is the most preferred, followed by matched unrelated donor transplant (*Blood* 2017; 129:1428–1436).

4. **D. Telomere length analysis.** Oral leukoplakia, dystrophic nails, hyperpigmented skin, and cytopenias are suggestive of dyskeratosis congenita in this case. The family history of leukemia and pulmonary disease underscores the spectrum of disease manifestations of telomeropathies, with dyskeratosis congenita (DC) being one of the more severe manifestations. Telomere length analysis, usually of peripheral blood leukocytes, will confirm the diagnosis. High-resolution karyotyping will not give information on telomere length. *SBDS* gene sequencing would be appropriate if there was suspicion for Shwachman–Diamond syndrome. The patient does not have stigmata of Schwachman–Diamond syndrome— short stature and pancreatic insufficiency. Soluble IL-2 receptor is usually elevated in hemophagocytic lymphohistiocytosis (HLH). Although he has bicytopenia, he does not have other clinical findings typical of HLH, such as fever or splenomegaly. In addition, there are other lab findings with short turnaround times, such as hypertriglyceridemia, hypofibrinogenemia, or ferritinemia, that would typically support the diagnosis of HLH prior to testing for soluble interleukin-2 receptor.

5. **E. Single agent eltrombopag.** The patient is an elderly infirm female with symptomatic anemia related to severe aplastic anemia and secondary hemochromatosis with significant liver iron deposition by liver MRI. Given her general state of health, single agent eltrombopag would likely be the best choice of the options provided. Hematologic response rate was 44% with single agent eltrombopag, with 3 of 25 patients becoming red blood cell transfusion independent (*N Engl J Med* 2012; 367:11–19). In patients who relapse after horse ATG and cyclosporine, 65% respond to rabbit ATG and cyclosporine (*Br J Haematol* 2006 Jun;133(6):622–627). However, given her age and comorbidities, in particular renal insufficiency, she would unlikely tolerate intensive immunosuppression. The same argument can be made for high-dose cyclophosphamide, stem cell transplant, and single agent alemtuzumab.

6. **C. Bone marrow biopsy and aspirate.** PNH can be thought of as a spectrum disorder with the classic PNH on one end of the spectrum, with high PNH clone burdens and brisk intravascular hemolysis, and bone marrow failure on the other end, with relatively smaller PNH clones and limited to absent intravascular hemolysis. This case clearly demonstrates a case of an overlap between classic PNH and bone marrow failure (*Blood* 2006; 108(8):2509–2519). While the patient has evidence of classic PNH with evidence of intravascular hemolysis (elevated lactate dehydrogenase [LDH], indirect bilirubin, reticulocyte count, and decreased haptoglobin), he also has evidence of concomitant bone marrow failure with significant cytopenias not confined to the red cell lineage. His inappropriately normal reticulocyte response and dysplasia on peripheral blood smear are most concerning for myelodysplastic syndrome (MDS) underlying his bone

marrow failure. While these aforementioned features are suggestive, they are not diagnostic of MDS and a bone marrow biopsy and aspirate should be performed next. Stopping eculizumab would not be advised for the purposes of repeating PNH studies, if the therapy is mitigating hemolysis. Telomere length would be helpful in a younger patient with aplastic anemia for which there was a concern for a telomeropathy.

7. **C. Horse ATG, cyclosporine, and eltrombopag; D. Presence of a PNH clone.** The current standard of care for younger patients (<40 years of age) is to proceed directly to allogeneic stem cell transplantation with a matched related donor. A matched sibling donor is only available, however, in 20% to 30% of cases (*Blood* 2006; 108(8):2509–2519). If the patient does not have a matched related donor, as in this scenario, the next best answer would be horse ATG, cyclosporine, and eltrombopag. Horse and rabbit ATG were compared head-to-head with superior response rates and overall survival in the horse ATG arm (*N Engl J Med* 2011; 365:430–438). Cyclophosphamide was compared with ATG in a phase 3 trial, which was terminated prematurely due to excess mortality. It is not considered a first-line therapy option (*Lancet* 2000; 356(9241):1554–1559). Matched unrelated donor transplant has roughly twice the mortality rates as a matched sibling donor, with 5-year survival estimated to be around 39%, and is also not preferred front-line therapy (*Blood* 2006; 108(8):2509–2519).

In an analysis performed in 97 patients with severe aplastic anemia treated with immune suppressive therapy, the presence of an absolute neutrophil count (ANC) >0.2 × 10^9/L and a PNH clone at diagnosis predicted a better response to immune suppression (*Ann Hematol* 2015; 94(7):1105–1110). While age is important in regard to transplantation-related complications, it has not been associated with responses to immune suppressive therapy. In the aforementioned trial, pretreatment hemoglobin level and reticulocyte count were not associated with improved responses with immunosuppressive therapy.

Platelet and Megakaryocyte Disorders

8

Samuel B. Reynolds and Asra Ahmed

Platelet and Megakaryocyte Overview

1. **What are the features of megakaryocytes?**
   - Megakaryocytes are large polypoid cells derived from megakaryocyte colony-forming cells (Meg-CFCs) and are responsible for the formation of platelets.
   - The average diameter of a megakaryocyte is 50 to 100 microns.
   - Megakaryocytes make up approximately 0.05% to 1% of all nucleated cells in the human bone marrow.
   - One of the key features of megakaryocytes is the presence of granules, including alpha granules, which contain proteins such as platelet factor 4 (PF4) or von Willebrand factor (vWF).
   - Surface markers and granules associated with megakaryocytes, including CXCR4 and GPIIb/IIIa, are identical to those present on mature platelets.

2. **Describe the process of megakaryocyte maturation.**
   - Megakaryocytes undergo endomitosis, a process by which DNA replicates without division of the nucleus, followed by progressive expansion and maturation of the cytoplasm. Once mature, anucleate cytoplasmic fragments bud off the megakaryocyte pseudopods, resulting in the formation of anucleate platelets. This entire process occurs over 5 to 7 days within the bone marrow.
   - A single megakaryocyte is responsible for the formation of 1,000 to 3,000 individual platelets.

3. **How is megakaryocytopoiesis regulated under physiologic circumstances? What other factors affect platelet production?**
   - Thrombopoietin (TPO) is a glycoprotein hormone consisting of 332 amino acids and is responsible for megakaryocytic differentiation, maturation, and proliferation. The N-terminal end has 144 amino acid homology with erythropoietin. The TPO gene is located on the long arm of chromosome 3 (q 26.3–27).
   - TPO is primarily produced in hepatocytes. The TPO levels in the blood are inversely correlated to megakaryocyte and platelet mass. A decline in circulating platelets results in increased plasma TPO level, resulting in enhanced platelet production and thus maintenance of platelet mass.
   - The entire process of megakaryocytopoiesis is regulated by signaling through the c-mpl receptor, which is present on both megakaryocytes and circulating platelets. Specifically, TPO secreted by the liver is quickly taken up by circulating platelets (via the c-mpl receptors). Residual circulating TPO provides basal stimulation for megakaryocytes, resulting in the stimulation of megakaryocytic growth and endomitosis (ploidy).

- Interleukin-3 (IL-3) and IL-11 promote Meg-CFC growth but have little impact on megakaryocyte endomitosis.
- Endomitosis, briefly, begins with enlargement of the megakaryocyte cytoplasm with diffuse filling of platelet-specific granules (alpha, dense), which are packaged into elongated "pro-platelets." Upon extension through bone marrow sinusoidal vessels, shear force leads to fragmentation of these pro-platelets, which are then released into the peripheral blood as circulating platelets.
- Cytokines IL-6 and IL-11 stimulate platelet production independently of TPO. This typically occurs in inflammatory conditions.

4. **What are the features of platelets?**
   - Platelets are anucleate cells made up of cytoplasmic fragments, which as noted above are generated following megakaryocytic endomitosis. Platelets are configured as flattened discs in the "inactive state."
   - The diameter of a platelet is 2 to 4 microns.
   - When activated, platelets transform from a flattened disc to a sphere with multiple projecting pseudopods that facilitate movement to areas of injury, adhesion to the vessel wall, and aggregation with other platelets.
   - Transmembrane receptors play a crucial role in platelet function.
     - Receptors include GPIb/IX/V, GPIa/IIa, integrin $\alpha_{IIb}\beta_3$ (formally known as GPIIb/IIIa).
   - The storage granules within platelets contain vital mediators of hemostasis.
     - Alpha granules contain vWF, PF4, thrombospondin, fibrinogen, beta-thromboglobulin, platelet-derived growth factor (PDGF), and various metalloproteinases (including MMP2 and MMP9).
     - Dense granules contain adenosine diphosphate (ADP), calcium, and serotonin.

5. **What are the key functions of platelets and how are they activated?**
   - Platelets are an integral component of the hemostatic system and are responsible for primary hemostasis at the site of endothelial injury.
   - Platelets are also active in modulating systemic inflammatory responses. Many systemic infections lead to peripheral circulating platelet activation, which then go on to facilitate a variety of processes, examples of which are summarized as follows:
     - Platelet aggregation: disseminated intravascular coagulation (DIC), thrombosis
     - Leukocyte aggregation: cytokine release/storm, neutrophil extracellular trapping
   - Under physiologic circumstances, platelets circulate in an inactive disc-shaped form as outlined earlier. When subjected to shear stress, collagen from the subendothelial tissue gets exposed and binds platelet GPIb/IX/V receptors via vWF. The GPVI and GPIa/IIa receptors are also bound by collagen. Collectively, this process results in the activation of platelets and release of granules. Platelets also undergo a series of conformational and biochemical changes, which culminate with the formation of a platelet plug (i.e., primary hemostasis).

6. **What is the life cycle of a platelet and how do anatomic/physiologic factors affect this cycle?**
   - Under normal physiologic conditions, the life span of a platelet is approximately 7 to 10 days.

- Once released into systemic circulation, approximately two-thirds of the platelets will enter the general circulation pool and one-third will remain in the spleen as a reserve population.
  - Platelets sequestered in the spleen contribute to the total platelet mass and can be demarginated via splenic contraction when the need for additional platelets arises.
- Senescent and damaged platelets are phagocytosed by the splenic macrophages, liver Kupffer cells, and other components of the reticuloendothelial system.

LABORATORY EVALUATION OF PLATELETS

1. How are platelets evaluated quantitatively?

- Complete blood count (CBC): quantified via an automated analyzer
  - Normal platelet count: 150,000 to 450,000/microL
- Thrombocytopenia: defined as platelet value <150,000/microL; further subdivided by severity as follows:
  - Mild: 100 to 150,000/microL
  - Moderate: 50 to 99,000/microL
  - Severe: <50,000/microL
  - Very severe <20,000/microL
- Thrombocytosis: defined as platelet >450,000/microL

2. How are platelets evaluated morphologically?

- Peripheral blood smear: provides morphologic information about platelets and, given clinical context, information about systemic processes and clues as to platelet-specific disorders
  - Large platelets: may reflect accelerated platelet turnover or a congenital disorder
  - Small platelets: found in some congenital platelet disorders
  - Gray platelets: hypogranular platelets due to deficiency of alpha granules (discussed later)
  - Schistocytes on peripheral smear: generally suggests underlying microangiopathic hemolytic anemia (MAHA)

3. How are platelets evaluated qualitatively?

- Platelet aggregation assays: These assays evaluate defects of platelet function, that is, platelet adhesion, activation, or aggregation. Platelet function defect is based on platelet response to exposure to various agonists, including ADP, arachidonic acid, thrombin, ristocetin, epinephrine, and collagen.
- Bleeding time (BT): BT provides a general assessment of general platelet function, although less commonly used in clinical practice given testing inconsistencies.
- Rotational thromboelastometry (ROTEM): ROTEM provides information on clotting time, clot formation, clot stability, and clot lysis for a comprehensive picture of whole blood hemostasis.

4. How is megakaryopoiesis evaluated?

- Bone marrow biopsy: This biopsy provides information on megakaryocytopoiesis and any disorders that affect early platelet production, including primary bone marrow disorder (e.g., myeloproliferative neoplasm [MPNs] or leukemias).

Quantitative Platelet Disorders

THROMBOCYTOPENIA

1. **What are the symptoms of thrombocytopenia?**
   - Clinical presentation is variable and ranges from mild symptoms, such as bruising, petechiae, and bleeding from mucosal surfaces (e.g., epistaxis, menorrhagia), to threatening central nervous system (CNS) and gastrointestinal (GI) hemorrhage.
   - The risk and severity of bleeding vary and depend on the degree of thrombocytopenia and the presence of concomitant coagulopathy or qualitative platelet disorder. Oral or parenteral administration of antiplatelet agents will also enhance the bleeding risk.

2. **What are the mechanisms of thrombocytopenia and the corresponding disease manifestations?**
   - Pseudothrombocytopenia (or "factitious" thrombocytopenia)
     - Idiosyncratic ex vivo agglutination of platelets is due to the presence of nonpathologic agglutinating immunoglobulins in the presence of ethylenediaminetetraacetic acid (EDTA) tubing reagent.
     - Platelet clumps are often identified on peripheral blood smear, example shown in Figure 8.1.

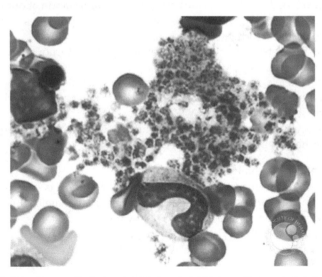

FIGURE 8.1 ■ Peripheral smear displaying platelet clumping, which manifests as pseudothrombocytopenia.
Source: Maslak, Peter. "Platelet Clump-1." *American Society of Hematology Image Bank*, 28 Sept 2011. Available at https://imagebank.hematology.org/image/3141/platelet-clump--1.

   - Incidence is estimated at 0.03% to 0.27% of the general population.
   - Patients are asymptomatic and do NOT have an increased bleeding risk.
   - When encountered, blood should be recollected with tubes using sodium citrate as the reagent for an accurate assessment of platelet counts.
     - Thrombocytopenia due to synthetic defects
       - Nutritional deficiencies

- Nutritional deficiencies may affect bone marrow proliferation across one or more cell lineage, including myeloid, erythroid, and megakaryocytic precursors.
  - Vitamin B_{12} and folic acid result in diminished megakaryocyte ploidy and thus reduced platelet production.
  - Copper deficiency is also associated with thrombocytopenia.
- Infection
  - Viral particles may directly suppress megakaryocytic development. The most common viruses implicated are Epstein–Barr virus (EBV), hepatitis C virus (HCV), cytomegalovirus (CMV), and hantavirus.
  - HIV can directly infect megakaryocytes through CXCR4 receptor signaling.
  - Viruses, including HIV and HCV, can also induce immune-mediated thrombocytopenia (see section on immune-mediated consumptive thrombocytopenia).
  - *Helicobacter pylori* infection can induce thrombocytopenia via molecular mimicry in an immune-mediated process (again see the "Immune Thrombocytopenic Purpura" section later in this chapter).
- Marrow disease
  - Infiltration of the bone marrow results in multilineage hematopoietic defects.
  - Common causes of infiltration include malignancy (e.g., lymphoma, solid organ tumors), severe disseminated infection (e.g., histoplasmosis), sarcoidosis, and enzyme storage diseases (e.g., Gaucher disease).
  - Primary hematopoietic stem cell disorders, such as myelodysplastic syndrome (MDS) and aplastic anemia, will also present with varying degrees of either single or multi-lineage dysplasia and/or pancytopenia. The pathophysiology varies by condition but generally involves either dyshematopoiesis or bone marrow aplasia.
  - Leukemogenesis, including high-grade myeloid neoplasms, can also diminish platelet production and may even be a presenting feature of the condition.
- Drug- and toxin-induced thrombocytopenia
  - Drug-induced thrombocytopenia (DITP) results from direct bone marrow and/or megakaryocyte toxicity. Chemotherapeutic agents, alcohol, gold, quinine, and thiazides are common causes.
  - Toxic bone marrow suppression following prolonged exposure to antimicrobials is also observed in both outpatient and hospital settings.
- Liver disease
  - In a state of chronic liver disease and/or cirrhosis, the liver's ability to produce TPO is compromised and platelet production is diminished accordingly.
  - Decompensated cirrhosis is also often marked by portal hypertension resulting in congestive splenomegaly with platelet sequestration and further thrombocytopenia.
- Thrombocytopenia due to platelet sequestration
  - Conditions that lead to platelet sequestration
    - In patients with splenomegaly, up to 90% of total body platelet mass can be sequestered in the spleen, whereas the normal spleen sequesters approximately one-third of the circulating platelet mass.
    - The most common cause of splenomegaly is passive congestion from portal venous hypertension.
    - Other causes of splenomegaly include the following:

- Chronic extravascular hemolysis due to various congenital anomalies, including thalassemia, hereditary red blood cell (RBC) cytoskeletal defects and pyruvate kinase deficiency
  - Hematologic neoplasms, lymphomas, and myeloproliferative disorders
  - Infections such as mononucleosis
  - Lysosomal storage diseases
- Approach to splenomegaly
  - Even in the setting of massive splenomegaly, the platelet count is rarely less than 30,000/microL. A lower platelet count, accordingly, should prompt a search for other causes of thrombocytopenia.
  - If feasible, treat the underlying condition.
  - In patients with cirrhosis who undergo liver transplant, splenomegaly and consequently platelet count both improve.
- Thrombocytopenia due to accelerated platelet consumption, with causes including immune-mediated thrombocytopenia and non–immune-mediated consumptive thrombocytopenia
  - Immune-mediated consumptive thrombocytopenia
    - This is a heterogeneous group of diseases characterized by immune-mediated destruction of platelets.
    - CBC reveals isolated thrombocytopenia.
    - On peripheral smear, platelets tend to be large and well-granulated, reflecting their young age from compensatory accelerated platelet production.
    - On bone marrow examination, morphologically normal megakaryocytes are increased, with otherwise normal erythropoiesis and myelopoiesis.
    - Causes include immune thrombocytopenic purpura (ITP), drug-induced thrombocytopenia, posttransfusion purpura (PTP), and antiphospholipid antibody syndrome (APAS). Each cause will be discussed separately in the next sections.
  - Non–immune-mediated thrombocytopenia
    - Causes include MAHAs (thrombotic thrombocytopenic purpura [TTP], hemolytic uremic syndrome [HUS], DIC, HELLP [hemolysis, elevated liver enzymes, low platelets] syndrome, malignant hypertension, vasculitis, hematopoietic stem cell transplantation, solid organ transplantation, malignancy).
    - TTP, DIC, HUS, and HELLP syndrome will be discussed in this chapter.

IMMUNE THROMBOCYTOPENIC PURPURA

1. What is ITP?

- ITP is thrombocytopenia that is due to autoantibodies directed against the platelet membrane receptors, resulting in accelerated platelet–antibody clearance. Autoantibodies are most commonly directed against the GPIb/IX and GPIIb/IIIa receptors. This process can occur in any part of the reticuloendothelial system but is primarily executed through splenic macrophages.

2. At what age does ITP occur and does spontaneous remission occur?

- ITP is seen in all age groups.
- Spontaneous remission in adults is low (<20% of patients) but is greater than 80% in children.

3. What causes ITP?

- For the majority of cases, an inciting event not identified
- Infections

- Viral infections (HCV, CMV, EBV, HIV, and SARS-Covid-19) have been implicated. It is postulated that viral antigens stimulate production of antibodies which then cross-react with platelet surface receptors.
- *Helicobacter pylori* can provoke a molecular mimicry response, whereby similarity between the bacterial molecular makeup and host antigen induces autoimmune thrombocytopenia. This is particularly true of the strains found in East Asia.
- Autoimmune diseases (such as systemic lupus erythematosus, rheumatoid arthritis and APAS, common variable immune deficiency, Hashimoto thyroiditis) also associated with ITP
- Chronic lymphocytic leukemia (CLL) or other lymphoproliferative disease
  - 1% percent of patients with CLL will develop ITP at some point during their disease course.
  - ITP seen in CLL needs to be differentiated from bone marrow infiltration and splenomegaly causing the thrombocytopenia.
- Evan syndrome
  - This is a disorder characterized by concomitant Coombs positive autoimmune hemolytic anemia and autoimmune thrombocytopenia.
  - Immune neutropenia may also be present.
  - It is often associated with other autoimmune diseases.

4. What are the symptoms of ITP?

- Symptoms are variable and depend on the degree of thrombocytopenia. Most patients are asymptomatic and have a low risk of spontaneous bleeding due to the presence of well-granulated functionally intact platelets.
- The risk of spontaneous bleeding increases significantly when the platelets are <10,000 to 20,000/microL.

5. How is ITP diagnosed?

- There is no gold standard diagnostic test for ITP; a diagnosis is obtained by first excluding the other causes of thrombocytopenia, including the aforementioned viral and nutritional etiologies.
- Bone marrow biopsy should be considered, especially in patients >50 years, to exclude a primary bone marrow failure, infiltrative process, or myeloid neoplasm.

6. What are the indications to treat ITP?

- The following are indications to treat ITP:
  - Bleeding
  - Platelets <30,000/microL
  - Need to increase the platelet count because of the need for anticoagulation of procedure
- If platelets are >30,000/microL without bleeding manifestations and without the need to increase the platelet count for a procedure, then monitoring is recommended.
- Although it may vary on a case-to-case basis, if the platelet count is <20,000/microL, hospital admission is generally recommended.

7. What is the approach to first-line treatment of ITP?

- The cornerstone of therapy is immunosuppression.
- The choice of therapy depends on several factors, including how fast the platelet count needs to be increased, prior response to therapeutic agents, and comorbidities.

- Corticosteroids suppress immune function and specifically impair the clearance of opsonized platelets by the reticuloendothelial system. Corticosteroids also dampen the effect of B and T lymphocytes, both of which are mediators of auto-immune processes.
  - The overall response rate with corticosteroids is >75%, with the duration of therapy depending on response and medication tolerability. Only 20% to 30% of patients, however, will remain in a sustained remission following steroid discontinuation.
  - Pharmacologic treatment of ITP **with corticosteroid** is recommended as follows:
    - Either prednisone (0.5 – 2.0 mg/kg/day) or dexamethasone (40 mg/day x 4 days) is recommended.
- Intravenous immunoglobulin (IVIG): There are multiple working theories as to the mechanism of IVIG in ITP. It is generally believed that IVIG interacts with the FcRII receptors on macrophages, ultimately inducing platelet clearance through the reticuloendothelial system.
  - IVIG is recommended when there is an immediate need to raise the platelet count as it raises platelet count within 1 to 2 days.
  - The overall response rate is 70% to 90%, with peak platelet levels achieved within 1 week of treatment.
  - The response is often temporary and there are significant financial toxicities to treatment with routine intravenous therapy.
  - IVIG is recommended in conjunction with steroids when a rapid increase in platelet count is required.
  - If utilized, several dosing strategies exist. One strategy is to administer IVIG initially at 1 g/kg as a one-time dose.
- Anti-Rh(D) is an alternative to IVIG for patients with Rh(D)-positive RBCs and works by saturating Fc receptor, similar to IVIG. Mild to moderate hemolysis is expected, so it should be avoided in patients prone to hemolysis or with existing hemolytic disorders (such as glucose-6-phosphate dehydrogenase [G6PD] deficiency).
- IVIG *or* anti-D may be used as monotherapies in the first-line setting when corticosteroid is contraindicated.

8. What are subsequent therapies for ITP?
- Rituximab is a monoclonal antibody directed against the CD20 antigen on B lymphocytes. Its utility in ITP, accordingly, is likely related to a depletion of CD20-positive lymphocytes and mitigation of platelet autoantibody production.
  - The overall response rate of rituximab is approximately 57% in both adults and children.
  - Rituximab is not considered a first-line therapy for ITP.
- Splenectomy eliminates a major site of platelet destruction as well as the primary site of autoantibody production.
  - Response rate is 50% to 70%.
  - Patients who undergo splenectomy have a lifelong risk of infection, specifically from encapsulated organisms, and require immunization against *Streptococcus pneumoniae*, *Haemophilus influenzae*, and *Neisseria meningitidis* prior to surgery.
- Thrombomimetic agents (or thrombopoietin receptor agonists, TPO-RAs). Romiplostim and eltrombopag are TPO analogues that stimulate different portions of the TPO receptors present on megakaryocytes, thus stimulating and promoting megakaryopoiesis.

- The thrombomimetic agents do not impact platelet clearance.
- Eltrombopag *or* romiplostim is recommended in adults who have been diagnosed with ITP for ≥ 3 months who are either dependent on or unresponsive to corticosteroid.
- Risks of thrombomimetic agents include thrombocytosis, thrombosis, and increased liver enzymes. Reversible increased reticulin fibrosis in the marrow may also be seen.
- Choice of treatment in adult patients with persistent ITP for ≥ 3 months is summarized as follows:
  - If dependent on or unresponsive to corticosteroid, TPO-RA is recommended over rituximab.
  - If dependent on or unresponsive to corticosteroid and TPO-RA is not an option, rituximab is preferred over splenectomy.
- Other immunosuppressive agents (generally reserved for relapsed/refractory ITP following failure of first-/second-line therapy) include the following:
  - Vinca alkaloid (e.g., vincristine)
  - Cyclophosphamide
  - Cyclosporine
  - Danazol
  - Fostamatinib: an oral spleen tyrosine kinase (Syk) inhibitor approved in 2018 in adults with an insufficient response to prior therapy (including corticosteroid, IVIG, TPO-RA, splenectomy)
- Platelet transfusions are supportive and may be administered in the setting of bleeding but should not be utilized as monotherapy.

9. **What autosomal dominant disease may present with thrombocytopenia and large platelets, but that can most often be differentiated from ITP by review of peripheral smear?**
   - *MYH9*-related disorders are a group of diseases characterized by mutations of the *MYH9* gene on chromosome 22, encoding nonmuscular myosin heavy chain. These disorders include Epstein syndrome, Fechtner syndrome, May–Hegglin anomaly, and Sebastian platelet syndrome.
   - *MYH9*-related disorders include the following symptoms:
     - Macrothrombocytopenia and leukocyte inclusions from myosin aggregates (Döhle-like inclusions) with moderate bleeding diathesis
     - May also see nephritis, sensorineural hearing loss, and cataracts

DRUG-INDUCED THROMBOCYTOPENIA

1. **What is the pathophysiology and presentation of DITP?**
   - Pathophysiology involves drug-dependent antibodies that bind to the Fab regions of platelets.
   - Thrombocytopenia generally develops 1 to 2 weeks of drug exposure and will generally begin resolving within 1 to 2 days of cessation.
   - Common precipitants include beta-lactam antibiotics, vancomycin, quinine, and antiepileptic drugs.
   - Bone marrow suppression is a separate phenomenon observed following receipt of various medications, such as chemotherapeutic agents, antibiotics, and immunosuppressive therapies.

2. **What is heparin-induced thrombocytopenia (HIT)?**
   - Type 1: Also known as heparin-associated thrombocytopenia, this is a *non–immune*-mediated drop in platelets in response to the direct effect of heparin on platelet activation. Mild thrombocytopenia usually occurs within the first 2 days of heparin exposure.
     - It is not associated with thrombosis.
     - Platelet counts normalize even with continuation of heparin.
   - Type 2: *Immune*-mediated HIT is a clinicopathologic syndrome associated with exposure to heparin or heparin derivatives; it develops in <5% of patients exposed to these products.
     - Type 2 HIT is driven by PF4 binding to heparin, triggering formation of a specific immunoglobulin G (IgG) that attaches to the heparin–PF4 complex, which in turn paradoxically induces platelet activation. The subsequent release of prothrombotic PF4 and thrombin leads to thrombosis and accelerated clearance of IgG-coated platelets.
     - If there is associated thrombosis, the condition is referred to as heparin-induced thrombocytopenia thrombosis syndrome (HITTS).
     - Disease characteristics:
       - Generally, at least a 50% drop in platelet count within 7 to 10 days of the first heparin exposure and within 1 to 3 days of subsequent heparin exposure is observed.
       - Patients are at lifelong risk of developing venous and arterial thrombi.

3. **How is HIT/HITTS diagnosed?**
   - Clinical likelihood is quantified using the "4Ts" score, which assigns points based on the following parameters:
     - Degree of Thrombocytopenia: 50% drop from baseline but with nadir ≥20,000/microL (2 points); 30% to 50% drop in platelet count or nadir platelet count of 10,000 to 20,000/microL (1 point)
     - Timing of platelet drop: within 5 to 10 days of present heparin exposure or platelet count drop within a day with prior heparin exposure within 30 days (2 points); onset after 10 days or within a day with prior heparin exposure between 30 and 90 days prior (1 point)
     - Thrombotic events: new thrombosis or skin necrosis or acute systemic reaction (2 points), venous more common than arterial; progressive or recurrent thrombosis, nonnecrotizing skin lesion, or suspected but not proven thrombosis (1 point)
     - Alternative cause of Thrombocytopenia: if no other cause is present, 2 points
   - The 4Ts score is then subclassified as low (0–3 points), intermediate (4–5 points), or high (6–8 points) risk. If intermediate- or high-risk suspicion is present, initiate empiric therapy for HIT and pursue further testing as follows:
     - Screen with immunoassay for antiheparin–PF4 complex, which is an enzyme-linked immunosorbent assay (ELISA) test that detects circulating antibodies. The PF4 assay is highly sensitive and specific at 97% to 99% and ≥90%, respectively.
     - If the PF4 assay is positive, confirm with a functional serotonin release assay (SRA), which measures release of radiolabeled serotonin from donor platelets after exposure to heparin and the patient's serum if heparin-induced antibody is present. The sensitivity and specificity of the SRA are both >95%.

4. How is HIT/HITTS treated?

- Discontinue all heparin products immediately, including flushes through peripheral and central intravenous access lines. Fractionated heparin products should also be discontinued.
- Start an alternative anticoagulant, such as parenteral direct thrombin inhibitor (DTI), either argatroban or bivalirudin. The DTI should be continued until the platelet count is >150,000/microL.
- If a thrombosis is identified, then the patient should undergo anticoagulation with warfarin for 3 to 6 months; longer durations may be utilized as indicated by clinical severity/persistence of thrombus.
- If no thrombosis is identified, anticoagulation with warfarin should be administered for 1 to 3 months. Warfarin should only be initiated after resolution of acute HIT as indicated by normalization of the platelet count due to the risk of thrombosis from protein C depletion.
- The efficacy of direct oral anticoagulants (DOACs) in HIT is still under investigation through several smaller studies; their routine use as frontline therapy is not advised at this time.
- Immunoassays can remain positive for several months after discontinuation of heparin. Care should be taken to avoid all future exposures to heparin products.

POSTTRANSFUSION PURPURA

1. What is the pathophysiology of PTP?

- Pathophysiology is driven by an anamnestic response of platelet alloantibodies (usually to human platelet antigen-1a [HPA-1a] antigen) that develop after exposure during a previous pregnancy or previous transfusion.

2. How do patients present and how is the diagnosis confirmed?

- Patients develop severe thrombocytopenia 1 to 2 weeks following blood product administration when these antibodies cross-react with native platelets.
- Diagnosis is made by serum detection of the HPA-1a antigen.

3. How is PTP treated?

- Most patients respond to treatment with IVIG, with platelet recovery occurring within 4 to 5 days of therapy.
- Plasma exchange may be required in refractory cases.
- Future blood products should be screened for HPA-1a-positive antigen.

ANTIPHOSPHOLIPID ANTIBODY SYNDROME

1. What is APAS?

- APAS is a hypercoagulable state driven by antiphospholipid antibodies that activate the coagulation pathway, resulting in both arterial and venous thrombosis and recurrent miscarriages or obstetric complications.

2. How is APAS diagnosed? (See Chapter 10 for further details.)

- At least one thrombotic event or pregnancy morbidity and one lab criterion.
- Lab criteria need to be confirmed on two separate occasions at least 12 weeks apart.
- Clinical criteria:
  - One or more episodes of venous, arterial, or small vessel thrombosis
  - Pregnancy complications:

- Three or more unexplained consecutive spontaneous abortions at <10 weeks' gestation
- One or more unexplained death of a morphologically normal fetus at or after 10 weeks' gestation
- One or more premature birth (<34 weeks) due to eclampsia, severe preeclampsia, or placental insufficiency
- Lab criteria:
  - Anticardiolipin antibodies (ACAs) or anti-beta-2 glycoprotein 1 (B2GP1) antibodies of the IgG and/or immunoglobulin M (IgM) isotype at medium or high titer (>40 or >99%)
  - Presence of a lupus anticoagulant (LA; such as prolonged dilute Russell's viper venom time), which is the strongest predictor of recurrent venous thromboembolism (VTE)

3. How is APAS treated?

- Indefinite anticoagulation is required; warfarin is a preferred agent.
- Patients who develop catastrophic antiphospholipid antibody syndrome (CAPS), characterized by widespread thrombosis, should undergo plasmapheresis with systemic immunosuppressive therapy. Consultation with rheumatology is critical for management.

THROMBOTIC THROMBOCYTOPENIC PURPURA

1. What is TTP?

- TTP is a clinical condition that results from deficiency of the *ADAMTS13* protease, which is a metalloprotease responsible for cleavage of large vWF multimers. In its absence, vWF multimers accumulate and promote the formation of small-vessel platelet-rich thrombi. These microthrombi then lead to vasoocclusion and shearing of RBCs, resulting in pronounced MAHA.
- Potentially fatal multiorgan dysfunction ultimately develops as platelet aggregates are deposited in the microcirculation, which notably induces small-vessel ischemia in the brain and renal arterioles.
- Typically, ADAMTS13 deficiency results from an acquired ADAMTS13 inhibitor. Rarely, ADAMTS13 deficiency results from mutations in *ADAMTS13*, resulting in congenital/familial TTP.
- Certain drugs (such as ticlopidine, clopidogrel, mitomycin-c, tacrolimus) have also been implicated in TTP.

2. How do patients with TTP present?

- The disease is sometimes characterized by a pentad of clinical findings that include fever, MAHA, thrombocytopenia, renal dysfunction, and mental status changes, including confusion and/or visual impairment.
- While the cornerstone of TTP diagnosis involves the presence of MAHA and thrombocytopenia, the other components of the pentad occur with varying frequency.

3. How is TTP diagnosed?

- The diagnosis requires a strong clinical suspicion in anyone who presents with MAHA, supported by laboratory studies showing elevated lactate dehydrogenase (LDH), low haptoglobin, and thrombocytopenia.

- A peripheral smear should be obtained immediately. The diagnosis is supported by the presence of ≥3 schistocytes/hpf.
- ADAMSTS-13 level of <10%, specifically in the presence of appropriate clinical history, is essentially diagnostic. For acquired/autoimmune TTP, the ADAMSTS-13 inhibitor will be elevated.
- TTP is a hematologic emergency and can be rapidly fatal if not diagnosed and expeditiously managed

4. How is TTP treated?

- Plasma exchange should be instituted as soon as the condition is suspected on the basis of clinical symptoms and laboratory and microscopic findings without waiting for confirmatory *ADAMSTS-13* testing.
- If plasma exchange is not available, the patient should be transfused with fresh frozen plasma (FFP), which contains some *ADAMSTS-13*, and transferred to a pheresis-capable facility.
- Platelet transfusion is generally contraindicated in TTP as it may further potentiate microthrombi formation on uncleaved vWF multimers and augment thrombocytopenia.
- Additional immunosuppression may also be required with corticosteroids and/or rituximab.
- In drug-induced TTP, the offending agent should be stopped; this subtype does not typically respond well to plasma exchange.
- Eculizumab may also be utilized in refractory cases if plasmapheresis, corticosteroids, and rituximab are unsuccessful. This agent is more commonly employed in complement-mediated thrombotic microangiopathy (also known as atypical HUS).
- Caplacizumab is a monoclonal antibody fragment that binds vWF and blocks its interaction with GPIb-IX-V on platelets. It is Food and Drug Administration-approved for acquired TTP but its optimal use remains debated, controversial, and not well-determined.

HEMOLYTIC UREMIC SYNDROME

1. What is HUS?

- HUS is a MAHA in the setting of either an infection or complement-mediated damage to the microvascular endothelium. End-organ dysfunction, including renal failure, is classically observed.

2. What are the types of HUS?

- Typical HUS: This occurs most commonly following GI infection with Shiga toxin-producing *Escherichia coli*, but can also be associated with other enteropathogenic illnesses.
- Complement-mediated (or atypical) HUS: This is driven by complement overactivation. Complement-mediated HUS can result from mutations in genes that control complement pathway and less commonly from an immune-mediated process. It has been associated with postpartum thrombotic microangiopathy and renal failure.

3. How does HUS present and how is it diagnosed?

- HUS is clinically characterized by hemolytic anemia, thrombocytopenia, and end-organ dysfunction stemming from microthrombi formation in capillaries, resulting in varying degrees of renal insufficiency. Fever may also be observed.

- A diagnosis of HUS is made clinically in the presence of various presenting afore-mentioned symptoms/syndromes, including renal failure, fever, abdominal pain, and in the setting of typical HUS hemorrhagic diarrhea often in the setting of antecedent infection. Laboratory studies will notably reveal MAHA (anemia, thrombocytopenia, elevated LDH, low haptoglobin, elevated reticulocyte production index and indirect bilirubin, and presence of schistocyte on peripheral smear evaluation). Renal failure is also common. Importantly, ADAMTS13 levels are normal, differentiating it from TTP. Advanced laboratory tests, including an alternative pathway/complement panel, may also be obtained if atypical HUS is suspected.

4. How is HUS treated?

- Typical HUS: Supportive care with intravenous fluids, antihypertensives, and dialysis as indicated is generally the mainstay of therapy. In general, antibiotics should not be administered as they may worsen/accelerate the disease process.
- Complement-mediated HUS: Eculizumab is recommend. This monoclonal antibody targets C5, thereby preventing C5 convertase to cleave the complement into C5a and b, ultimately inhibiting the respective vessel permeabilization and ultimate formation of the membrane attack complex. Eculizumab increases the risk of certain infections, such as *N. meningitidis*; therefore, vaccination is recommended before administration and periodically afterwards. Additionally, antibiotic prophylaxis may reduce the risk of *N. meningitidis* that may occur despite adequate vaccination.

DISSEMINATED INTRAVASCULAR COAGULATION

1. What is DIC?

- DIC is an acquired systemic activation of intravascular coagulation, resulting in both micro- and macrovascular thrombi with associated consumption of platelets, coagulation factors. The clinical manifestations include bleeding and multiorgan dysfunction.

2. How is DIC diagnosed?

- The diagnosis of DIC is made clinically. Patients present with a range of symptoms but are frequently critically ill with fulminant sepsis and/or multiorgan dysfunction. Bleeding may be observed from mucocutaneous surfaces, GI tract, and even intravenous access sites.
- Laboratory studies typically include thrombocytopenia, prolonged prothrombin time (PT) and partial thromboplastin time (PTT), elevated D-dimer, and diminished fibrinogen.

3. How is DIC treated?

- First manage the underlying cause (e.g., sepsis, pancreatitis, malignancy, trauma) while providing aggressive supportive care, including circulatory support and airway management as indicated.
- Hematologic management is generally supportive with transfusion of blood products including packed red blood cells for symptomatic anemia, cryoprecipitate for hypofibrinogenemia, and FFP to correct coagulopathy if bleeding is present.
- In the setting of a thrombotic event, anticoagulation should be considered but weighed with the potential risk for hemorrhage.

THROMBOCYTOPENIA WITH MASSIVE TRANSFUSION

1. **What is thrombocytopenia with massive transfusion?**
   - Dilutional thrombocytopenia that can be observed following extensive blood product transfusion

2. **How is it treated?**
   - Replete coagulation proteins and platelets with massive RBC transfusions, in addition to aggressive supportive care
   - Most blood banks have massive transfusion protocols that account for this dilutional effect when dispensing blood products

THROMBOCYTOSIS

1. **What is thrombocytosis?**
   - Thrombocytosis (or thrombocythemia) refers to a platelet count of >450,000/microL

2. **What are the causes of thrombocytosis?**
   - Reactive or secondary thrombocytosis
     - Inflammation (such as inflammatory bowel disease, rheumatoid arthritis, infection): the most common cause of thrombocytosis, resulting from IL-6 and interferon-gamma-mediated megakaryocytopoiesis
     - Iron deficiency
     - Rebound following prior thrombocytopenia (i.e., following bone marrow suppression from chemotherapy-induced thrombocytopenia)
     - Surgical or functional asplenia, resulting in decreased physiologic clearance by phagocytes
     - Treatment directed at the underlying cause(s)
   - Clonal thrombocytosis: observed in several clonal hematopoietic disorders such as essential thrombocytosis, polycythemia vera, primary myelofibrosis, chronic myeloid leukemia, and in a subset of patients with myelodysplastic syndromes

Qualitative Platelet Disorders

CONGENITAL DISORDERS OF PLATELET FUNCTION

DISORDERS OF ADHESION

1. **What are the two most common disorders of platelet adhesions?**
   - von Willebrand disease (vWD)
   - Bernard–Soulier syndrome

2. **What is vWD?**
   - vWD is one of the most common congenital bleeding disorders, with an incidence of 1 in 10,000 (approximately 0.6%–1.3%).
   - It is characterized by deficiency or dysfunction of vWF causing impaired platelet adhesion to blood vessel subendothelium, leading to the reduced stability of factor VIII.
   - Symptoms vary by subtype, but include easy bruising, postoperative hemorrhage, and mucosal bleeding such as epistaxis and menorrhagia.

3. What are the different subtypes of vWD?

vWD is reviewed briefly in this section and is covered more extensively in Chapter 9.

- Type 1: mild quantitative deficiency of vWF; the most common form; autosomal dominant inheritance
- Type 2: qualitative defect of vWF; also autosomal dominant; further divided into several subcategories
  - Type 2A: autosomal dominant; decreased intermediate and large vWF multimers due to defective protein synthesis or increased susceptibility to ADAMTS13 proteolysis; ristocetin cofactor activity reduced
  - Type 2B: autosomal dominant; mutation of the large vWF multimer results in high affinity of vWF to GPIb receptor on platelets; ristocetin cofactor activity reduced; low-dose ristocetin-induced platelet aggregation (RIPA) increased; as in type 2A, vWF multimers also reduced
  - Type 2M: usually autosomal dominant; decreased affinity of vWF for platelet binding; ristocetin cofactor activity reduced
  - Type 2N: autosomal recessive; defective factor 8 binding site on vWF, resulting in clinical picture similar to hemophilia A; ristocetin cofactor activity normal
- Type 3: autosomal recessive; complete deficiency of vWF
- Platelet-type vWD: "gain-of-function" mutation of GPIba, resulting in similar phenotype to vWD type 2B, with increased clearance of platelet–vWF complexes; condition is autosomal dominant
- Acquired vWD: may be acquired in the setting of aortic stenosis with associated GI angiodysplasia (Heyde syndrome) or essential thrombocythemia (ET).

4. What is Bernard–Soulier syndrome?

- Bernard–Soulier syndrome is an autosomal recessive disorder characterized by defective GPIb/IX/V receptors (vWF receptor) resulting in defective platelet adhesion.
- Platelets tend to be large (increased mean platelet volume [MPV]) but decreased in number, commonly between 20 and 100,000/microL.
- Patients present with bleeding out of proportion to thrombocytopenia.
- Diagnosis may be confirmed with absent GPIb/IX/V receptor by flow cytometry.
- Ristocetin cofactor assay is normal because there is no vWF defect. In contrast, absence of aggregation is noted with RIPA, which tests the aggregation of the patient's platelets in the plasma with low concentrations of ristocetin. Absence of aggregation in RIPA test does not correct with addition of normal plasma, thereby differentiating it from vWD.
- Treatment is platelet transfusion.

STORAGE POOL DISORDERS

1. Name three storage pool disorders.

- Wiskott–Aldrich syndrome
- Chediak–Higashi syndrome
- Gray platelet syndrome

2. What is Wiskott–Aldrich syndrome?

- X-linked recessive disorder characterized by a mutated *WASp* gene, which is expressed in hematopoietic stem cells and is responsible for relaying cell surface signals to the actin cytoskeleton

3. **How do patients with Wiskott–Aldrich syndrome present?**
   - This syndrome manifests as storage pool-like disorder with platelets that cannot aggregate and with microthrombocytopenia, present in infancy, with a platelet count of <70,000/microL.
   - Patients present with immunodeficiency and susceptibility to infection with encapsulated organisms, with recurrent sinopulmonary infection, eczema, and lymphoproliferative disorders, including B-cell lymphoma.

4. **What is Chediak–Higashi syndrome?**
   - Autosomal recessive disorder due to mutations in the *LYST* and *CHS1* genes, characterized by abnormal microtubule function, disruption of the lysosomal granule secretory function, and absence of dense granules from platelets

5. **How does Chediak–Higashi syndrome present?**
   - The second wave of platelet aggregation is impaired due to deficient ADP-containing granules and serotonin on platelets.
   - Patients present with recurrent gram-positive infections due to defective degranulation and chemotaxis.
   - Oculocutaneous albinism is also a prominent feature.

6. **What is gray platelet syndrome?**
   - This condition is characterized by an absence in alpha granules, resulting in impaired release of vWF, fibrinogen, PF4, and PDGF.
   - Laboratory evaluation reveals normal platelet aggregation.
   - The constitutive secretion of PDGF results in splenomegaly and marrow fibrosis, the latter of which is found in up to 58% of patients.
   - Patients also present with mucocutaneous bleeding with trauma and thrombocytopenia with platelet count ~50,000/microL.
   - Platelets appear large and pale ("gray").

DISORDERS OF PLATELET AGGREGATION

1. **What is Glanzmann thrombasthenia?**
   - Glanzmann thrombasthenia is an autosomal recessive disorder characterized by abnormal integrin αIIbβ3 (also known as the fibrinogen receptor) resulting in defective platelet aggregation.
   - Patients will have a normal platelet count but will present with varying degrees of mucocutaneous bleeding and prolonged BT.
   - Platelet aggregation is normal with ristocetin but defective with agonists like thrombin, collagen, or ADP.
   - Treatment is platelet transfusions.

ACQUIRED FUNCTIONAL DISORDERS OF PLATELETS

1. **What are the common causes of acquired functional disorders of platelets?**
   - Antiplatelet drugs
     - Cyclooxygenase (COX) inhibitors
       - Inhibition of COX leads to impaired thromboxane formation, which results in defective intracellular signaling and ultimately platelet aggregation.
       - Aspirin is an irreversible inhibitor of COX1 at doses as low as 50 to 100 mg daily.

- Nonsteroidal anti-inflammatory drugs (NSAIDs) are reversible inhibitors of the COX enzymes but can still affect platelet aggregation and are generally avoided in platelet disorders accordingly.
  - P2Y12 inhibitors (ADP receptor agonists)
    - These inhibitors inhibit platelet activation.
    - They are commonly used in coronary artery disease following percutaneous coronary intervention; examples include clopidogrel and ticlopidine.
  - Integrin αIIbβ3 inhibitors
    - These inhibitors inhibit platelet aggregation.
    - Examples include abciximab, tirofiban, and eptifibatide.
- Other drugs: fibrinolytics and others
- Hematologic diseases
  - Myeloid neoplasms are associated with dysmegakaryopoiesis, resulting in dysfunctional platelets.
- Uremia
  - Retention of uremic toxins can inhibit all aspects of platelet function.
  - Dialysis will partially mitigate the associated bleeding risk.
  - DDAVP, or desmopressin, is an antidiuretic hormone (ADH) analogue which may also help improve platelet function in uremic patients who are taking antiplatelet agents. One of the proposed mechanisms for this effect is induction of platelet surface glycoprotein.

Platelet Disorders in Pregnancy

1. What are the common platelet disorders associated with thrombocytopenia during pregnancy?
- Gestational thrombocytopenia
- Immune thrombocytopenia
- Preeclampsia/eclampsia
- HELLP syndrome
- Acute fatty liver of pregnancy (AFLP)

2. What is gestational thrombocytopenia?
- Gestational thrombocytopenia is the most common cause of thrombocytopenia in pregnancy.
- It commonly presents in the third trimester (but could occur as early as in the mid-second trimester).
- Pathogenesis is unknown and this is a diagnosis of exclusion. Platelets are typically >80,000/microL; values in the 50,000–80,000 range should raise concern for ITP (see below).
- It is difficult to distinguish from ITP, although the latter is more likely if thrombocytopenia is severe and occurring in the first trimester.
- Patients are asymptomatic and the platelet count will normalize within 1 to 2 months of delivery.
- There are no known fetal risks and newborns do not have thrombocytopenia.
- There are no known maternal risks, although recurrence in subsequent pregnancies is common.
- Treatment is usually not required.

3. How does ITP manifest in pregnancy?

- ITP in pregnancy accounts for 4% to 5% of all pregnancy-associated thrombocytopenia.
- Patients often have a history of ITP.
- ITP in pregnancy can be difficult to distinguish from gestational thrombocytopenia, although again lower values (<80) are more common in ITP.
  - In ITP, the platelet count drops early in pregnancy (typically below 70) and will progressively decline throughout gestation.
  - Platelets may recover but do not typically normalize after pregnancy, unlike in gestational thrombocytopenia.
- Antiplatelet antibodies also cross the placenta, which can result in neonatal thrombocytopenia.
  - There is potential for newborn fetal hemorrhage, especially with vaginal birth due to neonatal thrombocytopenia.
  - There are no currently available methods to predict fetal platelet count at the time of delivery.
  - Cesarean section may be considered to reduce the theoretical risk of neonatal intracranial hemorrhage/other bleeding. There are, however, no firm guidelines here and the mode of delivery should ultimately be determined by the obstetricians.

4. What are the indications to treat ITP during pregnancy?

- The cutoff platelet count to treat and the timing of treatment should be discussed with the obstetrician.
- The platelet cutoff for epidural anesthesia should be discussed with the anesthesiologists (some consider a platelet count of >80,000/microL to be adequate for epidural/neuraxial anesthesia).

5. What are the treatment options for ITP during pregnancy?

- Glucocorticoids, IVIG
  - Can be used throughout pregnancy
  - Need to be cognizant of potential volume overload, gestational diabetes, and fetal adrenal suppression
- Splenectomy
  - Laparoscopic splenectomy: can be performed in the second trimester if there is failure to respond to IVIG and steroids.
- Anti-(Rh)D: can cause maternal and fetal hemolysis and is relatively contraindicated
- Rituximab and TPO mimetics: generally not recommended
  - Rituximab has been associated in the second trimester and beyond with risk of lymphopenia in the newborn, which also extends for several months postpartum.
- Newborn thrombocytopenia
  - Platelet count should be determined in neonates of mothers with ITP.
  - Further monitoring/management should be conducted in consultation with neonatology.

6. What is preeclampsia/eclampsia?

- Preeclampsia affects 5% to 8% of all pregnancies.

- Preeclampsia is defined as new hypertension after 20 weeks' gestation with either proteinuria or one of the following:
  - Thrombocytopenia (platelet count <100,000/microL)
  - Abnormal liver function tests (LFTs)
  - Acute kidney injury
  - Pulmonary edema
  - Cerebral/visual disturbances or new-onset headache
- Eclampsia is epileptic seizures in a patient with preeclampsia.

7. What is HELLP syndrome?

- This can occur in the setting of preeclampsia in 70% to 80% of patients, generally in the peripartum period.
- It has similar presentation as thrombocytopenic purpura (TTP), but abnormal aminotransferases are more common.

8. What is acute AFLP?

- AFLP is a rare rare condition characterized by microvascular fatty infiltration of the liver with subsequent liver failure and encephalopathy.
- Thrombocytopenia may be present, with or without other signs of DIC, the latter of which is common in AFLP.
- AFLP is usually diagnosed in the third trimester.
- Treatment and management of these disorders should be performed in collaboration with obstetricians.

QUESTIONS

1. A 35-year-old male presents to the clinic with a 3-month history of intermittent epistaxis and oral mucosal bleeding. He reports several episodes of unprotected sexual intercourse over the past 6 months. He does not take medications or supplements. Complete blood count demonstrated a hemoglobin of 13.2 g/dL, white blood cell (WBCs) of 16×10^9 cells/L and platelets of 13,000/microL. Prothrombin time (PT)/partial thromboplastin time (PTT) and bleeding time are all within normal limits. Peripheral blood smear examination reveals generalized thrombocytopenia without clumping. Platelet aggregation studies reveal normal ristocetin cofactor activity and aggregation in response to adenosine diphosphate and collagen. Transfusion of platelets resulted in a nonsustained increase in serum platelet up to 52,000/microL. What is the next most appropriate diagnostic step?
   A. Management with corticosteroids and intravenous immunoglobulin
   B. Viral serologic assessment
   C. Rotation thromboelastometry (ROTEM)
   D. Bone marrow aspirate and biopsy

2. A 56-year-old female presents to the ED with approximately 3 days of increasing bruising upon minor trauma, rash on her legs, and heavier-than-normal menstrual bleeding. She has an accompanying history of rheumatoid arthritis and hypothyroidism secondary to Hashimoto thyroiditis.

   Physical examination is remarkable for a palpable spleen tip approximately 3 cm below the left costal margin as well as bilateral lower extremity petechiae. Complete blood count confirms a hemoglobin of 10.5 g/dL, white count of 6 x 10^9 cells/L, and platelets of 6,000/microL; prothrombin time (PT) and partial thromboplastin time (PTT) are both normal. On peripheral smear, there is no evidence of platelet clumping or schistocytes. A secondary workup for nutritional deficiency (including folate, B_{12}, and iron studies) and viral infection (including cytomegalovirus, Epstein–Barr virus, HIV, hepatitis C) is negative; she is not taking any diseases-modifying antirheumatic drugs (DMARDs) and is only on home levothyroxine. One pack of platelets is transfused, which results in a modest elevation in platelets to 18,000/microL, but her value then returns to 10,000/microL. The patient is diagnosed with immune thrombocytopenia (ITP). What is the best initial management?

A. Discharge to hematology clinic with dexamethasone 40 mg for 4 days, followed by taper.
B. Discharge to hematology clinic with prednisone 1 mg/kg/day, followed by prednisone taper.
C. Admit to hospital for daily prednisone and intravenous immunoglobulin and in-person response assessment.
D. Admit to hospital for rituximab therapy.

3. A 68-year-old male is admitted to the hospital for an elective carotid endarterectomy, for which he is placed on heparin perioperatively on postoperative day (POD) 0; a preoperative complete blood count (CBC) revealed a hemoglobin of 14.2 g/dL, white count of 4.5 x 10^9 cells/L, and platelets of 275,000/microL. He remains heparinized postoperatively. On POD 8, the patient develops a painful, erythematous swelling of his left lower extremity, after which diagnostic vascular ultrasonography confirms a left proximal femoral deep venous thrombosis (DVT). A repeat CBC now reveals platelets of 55,000/microL; there is no liver or renal impairment. A review of his home medications continued on admission reveals no other apparent sources of thrombocytopenia. What are your diagnostic and management recommendations?

A. Stop all heparin products including flushes and transition to argatroban with IIa level-guided dosing. Send for a platelet factor 4 (PF4) assay.
B. Stop all heparin products including flushes and transition to coumadin with therapeutic international normalized ration (INR) dosing. Send for a PF4 assay.
C. Stop heparin infusion and transition to subcutaneous DVT prophylaxis in enoxaparin.
D. Continue heparin infusion and consult interventional radiology for inferior vena cava (IVC) filter placement.

4. A 46-year-old female presents to the hospital with several episodes of confusion over the past several days. She has scattered visual field defects, with generalized fatigue and lower extremity rash. She denies starting any new antibiotics or over-the-counter therapies. Her exam is remarkable for a temperature of 38.1°C, blood pressure (BP) of 100/65 mmHg, heart rate (HR) of 98, and respiratory rate (RR) of 12; she is ill-appearing, with generalized pallor and lower extremity purpuric lesions. Complete blood count is remarkable for hemoglobin of 8.5 g/dL (baseline

~12), white count of 11.6 × 10^9 cells/L, and platelets of 23,000/microL; additional labs include a creatinine of 1.75 mg/dL (baseline 0.7–1.3 mg/dL), lactate dehydrogenase (LDH) 568/L, and haptoglobin of <10 mg/dL. Coagulation studies are performed and demonstrate a normal partial thromboplastin time (PTT) of 30s, prothrombin time (PT) of 12s, and fibrinogen of 250 mg/dL. Review of peripheral smear demonstrates approximately 5 schistocytes/hpf. What are the next most appropriate steps?

A. Transfuse 2 units of platelets and 1 unit of packed red blood cells immediately.
B. Prepare cryoprecipitate and transfuse when available; repeat PTT/PT/international normalized ration and fibrinogen every 8 hours.
C. Send for an ADAMSTS13 level immediately; initiate corticosteroids and await results before considering plasma exchange.
D. Arrange immediately for urgent plasma exchange; send ADAMSTS13 level.

5. A 24-year-old female presents to your clinic for evaluation of recurrent menorrhagia. She underwent menarche at age 12 and experienced irregular bleeding initially but then normalized for the next several years. Her mother and maternal grandmother had similar bleeding histories and have each required multiple hospitalizations. Complete blood count demonstrates anemia with hemoglobin of 9 g/dL, with white blood cells of 7.5 × 10^9 cells/L and platelets of 15,000/microL. Prothrombin time, partial thromboplastin time, and fibrinogen are all within normal limits. Analysis of von Willebrand factor (vWF) multimers identifies large vWF multimers. Low-dose ristocetin-induced platelet aggregation (RIPA) demonstrates increased aggregation of platelets, which corrects following the addition of normal vWF to the patient's platelets. What is the most likely diagnosis?

A. Type 1 von Willebrand disease
B. Type 2A von Willebrand disease
C. Type 2B von Willebrand disease
D. Platelet-type von Willebrand disease

6. An 18-year-old male presents to a local ED with intractable epistaxis and gingival bleeding; he reports several similar episodes since childhood but cannot recall how they were treated nor ever having received a formal hematologic diagnosis. His two siblings are not impacted by these symptoms but he believes there is a similar bleeding history in various distant relatives on his father's side. He is hemodynamically stable but has some visible dried blood in the nares and oral mucosa. Complete blood count is remarkable for hemoglobin of 10.5 g/dL, white blood cells of 10 × 10^9 cells/L, and platelets of 210,000/microL. Prothrombin time, partial thromboplastin time, and fibrinogen are all normal, but bleeding time is mildly prolonged at 16 minutes. Ristocetin-induced platelet aggregation (RIPA) is normal, but platelet aggregation is impaired with adenosine diphosphate (ADP) and collagen. What is the most appropriate treatment for this patient?

A. Platelet transfusion
B. Recombinant factor VIII
C. DDAVP
D. Close observation

7. A 78-year-old male with chronic lymphocytic leukemia (CLL) presents to your clinic with worsening thrombocytopenia. His complete blood count (CBC) at diagnosis 2 years prior was notable for a hemoglobin of 9.0 g/dL, white blood cells (WBCs) of 160 × 10⁹ cells/L with absolute lymphocyte count (ALC) of 148,500/L and platelets of 95,000/microL; a *TP53* mutation was also present. He would begin treatment with ibrutinib and tolerate therapy well, with a most recent interim CBC 6 months ago demonstrating normalization of his hemoglobin to 14.2 g/dL, WBC to 12 × 10⁹ cells/L, and platelets to 150,000/microL. At present, however, his platelets have declined to 28,000/microL, with a hemoglobin of 15 and WBC of 10.6. He denies any weight loss, fevers, sweats, chills, skin lesions, or bleeding; there is no palpable splenomegaly on examination. Peripheral blood flow cytometry and bone marrow biopsy do not identify a population of clonal/infiltrative lymphocytes. What is the most appropriate next step in management?
A. Continue ibrutinib and observe interim CBC.
B. Continue ibrutinib and initiate corticosteroids.
C. Discontinue ibrutinib and transition to obinutuzumab + venetoclax.
D. Discontinue ibrutinib and initiate corticosteroids.

8. A 27-year-old G2P1 female at 37 weeks' gestation presents to the hospital with right upper quadrant pain and fatigue; she has also noticed some bleeding of the gums while brushing her teeth over the past 48 hours. She is hypertensive to 150/90 mmHg and has some discomfort in her right hemiabdomen with deep respiration; generalized pallor is also appreciable. Complete blood count is noteworthy for a hemoglobin of 7.6 g/dL, white blood cells of 12 × 10⁹ cells/L, and platelets of 17,000/microL. A comprehensive metabolic panel is significant for aspartate transaminase (AST) of 87 and alanine transaminase (ALT) of 80, with a normal serum creatinine; lactate dehydrogenase (LDH) is 480/L and haptoglobin is 20 mg/dL. Review of peripheral blood smear reveals approximately 4 schistocytes/hpf. What is the most likely diagnosis and most appropriate first step in management?
A. Preeclampsia; initiate antihypertensives and monitor closely.
B. Immune thrombocytopenic purpura; initiate corticosteroids.
C. Gestational thrombocytopenia; monitor carefully.
D. HELLP syndrome; consult with obstetricians and arrange for urgent delivery.

9. A 65-year-old female with chronic immune thrombocytopenic purpura (ITP) that is steroid-dependent comes to your office for a second opinion. Off of steroids, the platelet count is 12,000/microL. Which pharmacologic treatment is the best next step in ITP management?
A. Observation even if the platelet is as low as 12,000/microL
B. Thrombopoietin mimetic administration
C. Fostamatinib
D. Vincristine
E. Danazol

10. A 31-year-old man presents for a second opinion regarding immune thrombocytopenic purpura management. His platelet count has ranged around 40,000/microL for as long as he has had complete blood counts tested. The platelet count has not improved with prior steroid or intravenous immunoglobulin (IVIG) administration. His brother has a diagnosis of nephritis and sensorineural hearing loss. Peripheral smear evaluation shows blue-colored inclusions in leukocytes. Which of the following statements is correct?
    A. The patient should be managed with rituximab.
    B. The platelet size is expected to be small on peripheral smear evaluation.
    C. The patient has an X-linked disorder.
    D. The patient likely has a mutation in the *MYH9* gene.

11. Which of the following statement about hemolytic uremic syndrome (HUS) is correct?
    A. Atypical HUS is driven by increased von Willebrand factor (vWF) multimers.
    B. Eculizumab is the treatment of choice for patients presenting with HUS following gastrointestinal infection.
    C. Patients with atypical HUS have a lower risk of renal failure than patients with thrombotic thrombocytopenic purpura.
    D. Antibiotics are generally avoided in typical HUS.

ANSWERS

1. **B. Viral serologic assessment.** This patient's clinical history is most consistent with thrombocytopenia mediated by a viral infection he most likely contracted during unprotected sexual intercourse, such as hepatitis C or HIV, the latter of which is postulated to infect megakaryocytes through CXCR4 signaling. ROTEM may be considered if no other systemic cause of bleeding is identified, but impairment to clot formation is not at the top of the differential for this patient with normal PT, PTT, and bleeding time, and clinical history otherwise consistent with virally mediated thrombocytopenia. Bone marrow aspirate and biopsy are also considerations should an extensive serologic evaluation for thrombocytopenia return negative, but should not be offered prior to more routine workup. Empiric management for immune thrombocytopenic purpura would also be premature prior to viral serologies, given the potential immunosuppression and what may be an already-present immunodeficiency in HIV.

2. **C. Admit to hospital for daily prednisone and intravenous immunoglobulin and in-person response assessment.** The patient in the presented case has a diagnosis of ITP, which is likely related to her known autoimmune diseases in rheumatoid arthritis and/or Hashimoto thyroiditis. Adults with new diagnoses of ITP who are asymptomatic with platelet counts <20,000/microL and minor mucocutaneous bleeding should be admitted for corticosteroid therapy. Initial therapy in dexamethasone (generally given at 40 mg daily for 4 days) or prednisone (0.5–2.0 mg/kg/day) is advised, with in-person response assessment to determine the appropriate dose escalation/tapering strategy. Intravenous immunoglobulin is also frequently added for initial episodes, specifically when an immediate elevation in platelets are required. Outpatient management for newly diagnosed adults with minor bleeding may be offered for values >20,000/microL, but would not be appropriate for this patient given his persistent thrombocytopenia to below this level. Rituximab is not used for first-line treatment of ITP and is not expected to immediately raise the platelet count.

3. **A. Stop all heparin products including flushes and transition to argatroban with IIa level-guided dosing Send for a platelet factor 4 (PF4) assay.** The patient likely has developed type 2 heparin-induced thrombocytopenia (HIT). His calculated HIT score is 8 (>50% decline in platelets with nadir >20 [2 points], timing within 5–10 days of prior heparin exposure [2 points], new thrombosis [2 points], and no other apparent causes of thrombocytopenia [2 points]). Given this high pretest probability of HIT, all heparin products (including line flushes) should be discontinued immediately, with transition to a direct thrombin inhibitor in argatroban; a PF4 assay should also be sent as initial diagnostic testing. It would not be appropriate to continue any heparin products (options C and D). Warfarin, while a consideration in the long-term management of HIT if diagnosed, would not be initiated as empiric frontline therapy without an argatroban bridge or before the platelet count normalizes.

4. **D. Arrange immediately to for urgent plasma exchange; send ADAMSTS13 level.** The presented patient likely has thrombotic thrombocytopenia purpura (TTP), as evidenced by intravascular hemolysis secondary to microangiopathic hemolytic anemia (MAHA; with anemia, thrombocytopenia, elevated LDH, diminished haptoglobin). Other indicators of TTP in this patient include evidence of microvascular ischemia with fever, mental status changes, and renal insufficiency, as well as microscopic evidence of red blood cell shearing in schistocytes. If clinical and laboratory suspicion is highly suggestive of TTP, as in this case, plasma exchange should be urgently initiated for what is a potentially life-threatening ailment; therapy should not be withheld while awaiting an ADAMTS13 level (option C), which may take several days to result. Transfusion of platelets (option A) should be avoided as this may worsen the intravascular thrombotic microangiopathy. Disseminated intravascular coagulation (DIC) must always be excluded in cases of suspected TTP as there is clinical and laboratory study overlap (MAHA, schistocytes on smear), but the normal PT, PTT, and fibrinogen makes DIC unlikely.

5. **C. Type 2B von Willebrand disease.** Type 2B von Willebrand disease (vWD), an autosomal dominant condition that she likely inherited through her mother, is characterized by a spontaneous binding of vWF to platelets due to a high affinity of vWF to the GPIb platelet receptors, resulting in clearance of the vWF-platelet complex. Laboratory findings in type 2B vWD include thrombocytopenia and hyperactive agglutination by RIPA. One key laboratory finding in type 2B vWD is the correction of increased platelet aggregation with the addition of normal vWF to the patient's platelets, a correction which does not occur in platelet-type vWD (option D). Type 1 vWD (option A) is only a mild quantitative deficiency in vWF and would likely not result in thrombocytopenia. Type 2A (option B) is characterized by a decrease in large and intermediate vWF due to impaired protein synthesis and/or increased proteolysis by ADAMSTS13; large vWF multimers, like in type 2B, will be decreased, but hyperactive agglutination should not be visualized by RIPA.

6. **A. Platelet transfusion.** The presented patient likely has Glanzmann thrombasthenia, which in line with his provided clinical history is an autosomal recessive disorder characterized by abnormal integrin $\alpha IIb\beta 3$, leading to defective platelet aggregation. Clinicopathologic manifestations vary but do include prolonged bleeding time with mucocutaneous bleeding, all with a normal serum platelet count. RIPA, as in the presented patient, will be normal, but aggregation is notably defective with other agonists (e.g., thrombin and ADP). The mainstay of treatment is platelet transfusion. Recombinant factor VIII (B) is employed in various clinical scenarios in von Willebrand disease and DDAVP (option C) in uremic thrombocytopenia, but neither would be efficacious in Glanzmann. Observation alone would also be inappropriate given this patient's recurrent bleeding.

7. **B. Continue ibrutinib and initiate corticosteroids.** This patient was diagnosed with CLL and is under active therapy with a bruton tyrosine kinase (BTK) inhibitor in ibrutinib with an adequate therapeutic response, but his platelets are now declining. In this clinical scenario, the first priority is to ensure that his lymphocytic leukemia is not driving the thrombocytopenia, specifically that there is no bone marrow infiltration with resultant extramedullary hematopoiesis in the spleen, neither of which is clinically apparent here. The patient's clinical picture and peripheral flow cytometry are also not consistent with worsening of his known CLL. He has likely developed immune thrombocytopenic purpura, which is associated with CLL, and may be treated as an adult with new-onset immune thrombocytopenia with corticosteroids. His CLL-directed therapy should also be continued at this time.

8. **D. HELLP syndrome; consult with obstetricians and arrange for urgent delivery.** The patient is a pregnant female late into her third trimester and is notably hypertensive with microangiopathic hemolytic anemia (hemoglobin 7.6, LDH 480, haptoglobin 20, schistocytes of peripheral smear) and thrombocytopenia. Her liver function tests are also notably elevated and she is experiencing right upper quadrant pain, which is likely due to distension of the Glisson's capsule. These clinicopathologic features point to hemolysis, elevated liver enzymes, low platelets (HELLP) syndrome and warrant urgent delivery with trained obstetricians. Preeclampsia (option A) with severe features is possible here and may have even predisposed this patient to HELLP, but would not as its own diagnosis be accompanied by microangiopathic hemolytic anemia. Immune and gestational thrombocytopenia (options B and C) are also possible but are not associated with transaminitis and hemolytic anemia.

9. **B. Thrombopoietin mimetic administration.** Observation is not appropriate for a low platelet count of 12,000/microL. Fostamatinib, vincristine, and danazol are reserved for patients who fail (or cannot take) thrombopoietin mimetic or rituximab.

10. **D. The patient likely has a mutation in the *MYH9* gene.** The patient likely has a diagnosis of *MYH9*-related disorder, which is an autosomal dominant disease associated with macrothrombocytopenia and blue-colored inclusions (Döhle-like inclusions) in leukocytes. Nephritis, sensorineural hearing loss, and cataract may be seen. This disease does not respond to steroids, IVIG, or rituximab.

11. **D. Antibiotics are generally avoided in typical HUS.** Antibiotics should not be administered in typical HUS because they may worsen/ accelerate the disease process. Atypical HUS is driven by complement hyperactivation. Typical HUS is treated with supportive care. Eculizumab is the treatment of choice for patients presenting with atypical HUS. Renal failure is more common with atypical HUS compared with thrombocytopenic purpura.

Hemostasis

9

Jennifer E. Girard, Jordan K. Schaefer, and Suman L. Sood

MOLECULAR BASIS OF COAGULATION

1. **What are the main sequences of events in the process of primary hemostasis?**
   - Primary hemostasis has three phases:
     - Platelet adhesion:
       - Vessel injury leads to exposure of subendothelial matrix proteins, including collagen.
       - Platelets adhere to exposed subendothelial matrix, facilitated by interactions of the platelet GPIb complex (GPIb-GPV-GPIX) and von Willebrand factor (vWF).
     - Platelet activation:
       - Platelet GPVI and GPIa/IIa binding to collagen leads to platelet activation and calcium mobilization.
       - Platelet receptors interact with adenosine diphosphate (ADP), serotonin, platelet-activating factor, thromboxane A2, thrombin, and epinephrine originating from platelets or the surrounding cells at the site of vessel injury.
       - Platelet activation results in a cytoskeletal mediated shape change that facilitates subsequent platelet granule secretion.
     - Platelet aggregation:
       - The beta integrin αIIbβ3 (platelet GPIIb/IIIa receptor) is activated and binds soluble fibrinogen causing platelet aggregation and release of granules.

2. **Describe the contents of alpha granules and dense granules.**
   - Alpha granules contain fibrinogen, vWF, platelet factor 4 (PF4), P-selectin, clotting factors (FV, VII, XI, XIII), adhesion molecules, and growth factors.
   - Delta or dense granules provide ADP, adenosine triphosphate (ATP), calcium, histamine, and serotonin.

3. **What are integrins?**
   - Integrins are transmembrane receptors on cells that facilitate cell–extracellular matrix adhesion and activate cellular signal transduction.
   - Examples of integrins in platelet-related hemostasis are the beta-1 integrins (α2β1, α5β1) and the beta-3 integrin α2β3.

4. **What is secondary hemostasis?**
   - Secondary hemostasis occurs simultaneously with platelet adhesion and formation of the platelet plug. This is a series of enzymatic reactions mediated by coagulation factors to ultimately form fibrin to stabilize the platelet plug. This process occurs on the phospholipid membranes of cells through complexes.

5. **What is the sequence of procoagulant activation in secondary hemostasis?**
   - Exposed tissue factor (TF) in the damaged subendothelium binds to small amounts of circulating factor VII/VIIa, resulting in a complex (extrinsic Xase), which binds and activates factor X to Xa. The TF/factor VIIa/factor Xa complex converts a small amount of prothrombin to thrombin causing an initial small burst of thrombin.
   - An amplification loop is generated by thrombin activation of factors VIII, IX, and XI and this activates platelets leading to surface expression of platelet factor V. The TF/factor VIIa activation of factor IX is critical since the tissue factor pathway inhibitor (TFPI) inhibits the initial components of the extrinsic pathway.
   - Activated factors IXa and VIIIa form the intrinsic Xase complex resulting in conversion of large amounts of factor X to Xa.
   - Factor Xa complexed with platelet surface factor Va results in a burst of activation of prothrombin to thrombin and cleavage of factor I (fibrinogen) to fibrin monomers.
   - Fibrin monomers assemble into fibrils forming a clot, which is stabilized by covalent cross-linking of fibrin monomers by thrombin-activated factor XIIIa and incorporation of thrombin-activatable fibrinolysis inhibitor (TAFI). The cellular location of these reactions, in proximity to platelets at the damaged endothelium, helps mediate the formation of a fibrin clot to the required location.

6. **What is the role of vitamin K in clotting factor synthesis? What are the vitamin K-dependent clotting factors/cofactors?**
   - The cofactor vitamin K is necessary for terminal gamma-carboxylation in the synthesis of select clotting factor proteins to produce fully functional factors.
   - Vitamin K-dependent procoagulant factors are prothrombin (factor II) and factors VII, IX, and X.
   - Natural anticoagulant protein C and its cofactor, protein S, are also vitamin K-dependent.

7. **What are the clotting factor activation steps that comprise the intrinsic pathway?**
   - In sequential order, factor XII (contact factor) is activated by kallikrein, formed from the cleavage of prekallikrein with high-molecular-weight kininogen (HMWK) as a cofactor to generate factor XIIa.
   - Factor XIIa promotes coagulation by then activating factor XI to XIa and also activates fibrinolysis by converting plasminogen to plasmin.
   - Factor XIa converts factor IX to IXa with factor VIIIa and calcium as cofactors.
   - Factor IXa, with factor VIIIa as cofactor, converts factor X to Xa.
   - At factor X, the intrinsic pathway joins the final common pathway.

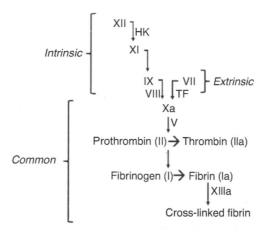

Simplified schematic of the classic model of the coagulation cascade. Cofactors (factor V, factor VIII, TF, HK) are shown in small font. For simplicity, the active and inactive factors of the extrinsic/intrinsic pathway have been condensed into one numeral representing both the active and inactive components; PK and inactive factors X and XIII are not shown.

HK, high-molecular-weight kininogen; PK, prekallikrein; TF, tissue factor.

8. **What are the clotting factor activation steps that comprise the extrinsic pathway?**
   - TF interacts with factor VIIa to activate factor X to Xa, joining the final common pathway.
   - Factor VIIa and TF also convert factor IX to IXa that then merges to the common pathway by converting factor X to Xa in the presence of factor VIIIa.

9. **What factors make up the final common pathway?**
   - Factor Xa binds to activated Va and forms the prothrombinase complex that converts prothrombin to thrombin (IIa). Thrombin cleaves fibrinogen into fibrin monomers. Fibrin monomers undergo polymerization. Factor XIIIa then cross-links the fibrin strands and stabilizes the thrombus.

10. **Where are the procoagulant factors synthesized?**
    - All procoagulant factors are made primarily in the liver hepatocytes, with the exception of factor VIII which is synthesized in endothelial cells. Factor VIII circulates with vWF. vWF is synthesized extrahepatically by megakaryocytes and endothelial cells.

11. **By what endogenous mechanisms is coagulation regulated or inhibited?**
    - Antithrombin (AT) inhibits thrombin (IIa), along with TF-VIIa, factors IXa, Xa, XIa, and XIIa, and kallikrein. AT activity is enhanced 1,000-fold by endogenous or exogenous heparins.
    - Thrombin is also inhibited by heparin cofactor II.
    - TFPI inhibits factor Xa and the TF-VIIa-Xa complex, thus inhibiting the extrinsic pathway.

- Natural anticoagulant protein C is activated by binding to the thrombin-activated thrombomodulin receptor on the endothelial cell surface. Protein Ca complexes with its cofactor protein S and inactivates factors Va and VIIIa.

12. What events occur during fibrinolysis?

- Tissue plasminogen activator (tPA) is released from the vessel wall at the site of injury. tPA activates plasminogen bound to fibrin to form plasmin. (Factors XIIa and XIa and kallikrein are also able to convert plasminogen to plasmin, but at a slower rate.)
- Plasmin then breaks down fibrin to soluble fibrin degradation products, most notably the D-dimer.
- Urokinase is a second enzyme released from select tissue beds, which also activates plasminogen to plasmin and is important in tissue repair and remodeling.

13. What factors regulate the activity of plasmin?

- Plasminogen activator inhibitor (PAI) and a2-antiplasmin regulate plasmin to terminate plasmin-mediated fibrinolysis.
- TAFI incorporated in fibrin clot limits binding sites for plasminogen on fibrin, delaying fibrinolysis.

LABORATORY EVALUATION

1. What should be considered when evaluating a new or unexpected reading of thrombocytopenia on a complete blood count (CBC) from an otherwise asymptomatic patient?

- Pseudothrombocytopenia should be excluded. A CBC is performed using ethylenediaminetetraacetic acid (EDTA) anticoagulated blood. EDTA can cause platelet clumping that may result in a spuriously low platelet count. Clumping is often evident on review of a peripheral blood smear. Redrawing the blood in an alternate anticoagulant, like sodium citrate, yields the correct platelet count.
- Exceptionally large platelets as seen in *MYH9*-related disorders or other macrothrombocytopenic conditions may not be counted due to the larger than normal size. This is recognized by a review of the blood smear.

2. What causes a prolongation of the prothrombin time (PT)?

- A prolonged PT reflects abnormalities of the extrinsic pathway or common pathway and is caused by reduced levels of factor VII, factor X, factor V, prothrombin, fibrinogen, or an inhibitor.
- Etiologies of an isolated prolonged PT include warfarin therapy (the assay is most sensitive to reductions in the vitamin K-dependent factor VII or X), mild vitamin K deficiency, liver disease, and hypofibrinogenemia.

3. What causes a prolongation of the partial thromboplastin time (PTT)?

- A prolonged PTT reflects abnormalities of the intrinsic pathway or common pathway.
- It can be caused by reduced levels of factor XII, prekallikrein, HMWK, factor XI, factor IX, factor VIII, factor X, factor V, prothrombin, or fibrinogen.
- Etiologies of an isolated prolonged PTT include heparin, bivalirudin, the presence of a lupus anticoagulant, all procoagulant factor deficiencies except factor XIII and factor VII, interference from a paraprotein, or an inhibitor.

4. What causes a prolongation of the thrombin time?

- The thrombin time is performed by adding thrombin and calcium to patient plasma and thus reflects the time to convert fibrinogen to fibrin. It can be prolonged by heparin, direct thrombin inhibitors, a quantitative deficiency, or a qualitative defect in fibrinogen.
- Prolongation of the thrombin time may also be due to interference in fibrin polymerization by high quantities of fibrin degradation products or paraproteins and some inhibitors.
- Some tumors produce heparin-like anticoagulants which interact with AT and prolong the thrombin time.

5. What is the reptilase time and how does the reptilase time differ from the thrombin time?

- The reptilase time is similar to the thrombin clotting time in that the time to fibrin polymerization and clot formation after addition of reptilase to plasma is measured. Reptilase specifically cleaves only fibrinopeptide (a) from fibrinogen.
- The reptilase time is not prolonged by heparin or direct thrombin inhibitors or tumor-related heparin-like substances, while the thrombin time is. Therefore, it can be used to detect heparin, argatroban, or dabigatran contamination. It is similarly prolonged with low fibrinogen levels, qualitative fibrinogen defects, or interference by fibrin degradation products.

6. How is an abnormal PT or PTT further investigated?

- A mixing study is based on the principle that the PT or PTT test only begins to prolong when there is a 50% reduction in any given clotting factor. Hence, the plasma mixing study combines dilutions of patient plasma with normal plasma, and the PT and/or PTT are repeated immediately and up to 2 hours after incubating the mixture at 37°C.

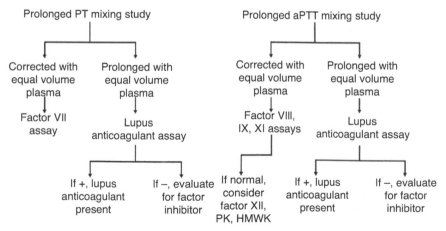

Evaluation of an isolated prolonged PT or activated aPTT. Note that if a prolonged clotting time fails to correct in the absence of a lupus anticoagulant, factor levels should be obtained to evaluate for a specific factor inhibitor.

aPTT, partial thromboplastin time; HMWK, high-molecular-weight kininogen; PK, prekallikrein; PT, prothrombin time; TF, tissue factor.

- An abnormal PT or PTT test that corrects in the mixing study suggests a factor deficiency, and specific factor levels are then checked for deficiency.
- A test that fails to correct with addition of normal plasma suggests an inhibitor (either lupus anticoagulant or specific factor inhibitor).
- Effects of some coagulation factor inhibitors are most evident after incubation of the test samples. A mixing study performed on plasma containing a specific factor inhibitor may initially show correction but subsequently fail to correct the abnormal clotting time in the presence of 50% normal plasma when measured after incubation for up to 2 hours later.

7. **How are specific procoagulant factor levels determined?**
   - Coagulation factors are assayed based on their activity levels. Coagulation factor assays can be performed either using chromogenic assays or more commonly using plasma clot-based methods.
   - Factors of the extrinsic and common pathway can be assessed using a PT-based assay in which the patient's plasma is mixed with plasma that is deficient in the specific factor being tested and the PT is determined. Similarly, the intrinsic pathway factors can be assayed with an aPTT-based assay using a similar method.
   - Chromogenic clotting assays can be used to assay some clotting factors. These methods are less likely to have interference by a lupus anticoagulant, heparin, or a direct thrombin inhibitor.
   - Screening for factor XIII deficiency relies on the fact that clots from factor FXIII–deficient patients are more soluble due to the lack of fibrin cross-linking. The urea clot solubility test is based on the time to dissolution of a patient's clot formed under controlled conditions compared with a control.

8. **How is fibrinogen measured?**
   - Fibrinogen is measured by a modification of the thrombin time such that fibrinogen, rather than thrombin, is rate-limiting in the reaction. Time to clot formation is calibrated against standard dilutions of fibrinogen.
   - Fibrinogen is also measured antigenically by immunologic methods.
   - Discrepancy between the fibrinogen activity level and fibrinogen antigen may indicate a dysfibrinogenemia.

9. **What tests are used to screen for the presence of a lupus anticoagulant?**
   - Common screening tests are the dilute Russell's viper venom time, hexagonal phase antiphospholipid assay, and the aPTT. In the presence of a lupus anticoagulant, the prolonged clotting time should not correct to normal range with the addition of normal plasma. If a phospholipid-dependent lupus anticoagulant is present, adding excess phospholipid or hexagonal-phase phospholipid should correct the prolonged clotting time to normal range.
   - These clot-based tests can be affected by anticoagulants, causing spurious results.
   - Anticardiolipin antibodies and anti-beta-2-glycoprotein I antibodies are enzyme-linked immunosorbent assay (ELISA)-based serologic tests used to detect specific antibody phospholipid reactivities in the diagnosis of antiphospholipid antibody syndrome.

10. How are coagulation factor inhibitors measured?

- Coagulation factor inhibitors are most commonly assessed using assays modeled on the Bethesda inhibitor assay for factor VIII that assesses the remaining factor VIII activity in dilutions of the patient's plasma mixed with normal plasma compared with that of a control. Bethesda units are calculated as the amount of inhibitor that can neutralize 50% of 1 unit of factor VIII in normal plasma. It is multiplied by the dilution to determine the inhibitor titer.

11. How is platelet aggregometry used to detect platelet disorders?

- Platelet aggregometry is one method to determine platelet function. It is performed using platelet-rich plasma from a citrated blood sample. Agonists are added to the blood sample and the change in light transmittance is measured using a photometric device. Patients must be off interfering medications prior to the test.
- Typical agonists include collagen, ADP, epinephrine, ristocetin, and arachidonic acid (see the following table).

Condition	Aggregometry Findings
Aspirin/Cox pathway defect	Aggregation reduced or absent for arachidonic acid and collagen; primary wave only with epinephrine; normal with thromboxane
Clopidogrel	Absent aggregation with ADP
Glanzmann thrombasthenia	Aggregation only with ristocetin (otherwise absent); not corrected with the addition of plasma
von Willebrand disease	Aggregation normal with agonists except for ristocetin; RIPA generally corresponds with the level of ristocetin cofactor assay; results normalize with the addition of plasma; type 2B von Willebrand disease shows aggregation with low-dose ristocetin
Bernard–Soulier syndrome	Aggregation normal with agonists except ristocetin, which is reduced; results do not normalize with the addition of plasma

ADP, adenosine diphosphate; RIPA, ristocetin-induced platelet aggregation.

12. What additional reference lab tests are used to help establish a diagnosis of Bernard–Soulier syndrome (BSS) or Glanzmann thrombasthenia?

- Flow cytometry for decreased glycoprotein 1b-alpha (CD42b) or GPIX (CD42a) in the case of BSS or decreased GPIIb/IIIa (CD41, CD61) for Glanzmann thrombasthenia can be useful.
- Genetic sequencing analysis of the GPIb-IX-V complex is available for confirmation of Bernard–Soulier mutations.

13. What is platelet transmission electron microscopy (PTEM)?

- PTEM is a transmission electron microscopy that assesses platelet ultrastructure in acquired and congenital platelet disorders. It quantifies the number of dense and alpha granules, thereby detecting platelet pool storage disorders.

14. **How is thromboelastography (TEG) used in the evaluation of bleeding disorders and assessment of hemostasis?**
    - TEG provides a global assessment of clot formation. A whole blood sample is added to a cup that rotates around a torsion wire (conventional TEG), or the pin rotates in the stationary cup of blood rotational thromboelastometry (ROTEM) measuring the force on the wire. This generates a real-time graphical display reflecting coagulation. Various additives to the blood can evaluate clotting through the extrinsic pathway, intrinsic pathway, the fibrinolytic system, and more. It can be used to guide blood product administration, assess anticoagulant drugs, and evaluate for disorders of hemostasis.

15. **What laboratory tests are used in the diagnosis of von Willebrand disease (vWD)?**
    - Diagnosis of vWD is based on abnormalities in vWF activity, antigen, factor VIII activity, and multimer analysis.
    - vWF platelet binding activity is measured by the use of a ristocetin cofactor or GPIb M assay.
        - Ristocetin induces glycoprotein 1b-mediated platelet agglutination to vWF detected by aggregometry. Impaired ristocetin-induced platelet agglutination (RIPA) can be seen with a deficiency of vWF or with an impaired GPIb or GPIX receptor, as in BSS. To eliminate the possibility of BSS, vWF activity is measured using patient plasma with ristocetin and normal control platelets. The slope of agglutination is compared with a reference standard of dilutions of vWF to estimate the relative vWF activity.
        - GPIb M assay uses a latex bead coated in GPIgb with gain-of-function mutation that binds spontaneously to vWF in the A1 domain and does not rely on ristocetin to induce aggregation.
    - vWF antigen levels are quantitated immunologically.
    - Factor VIII levels are typically checked when assessing for vWD due to the carrier function of vWF and to detect the abnormal vWF subtype type IIN or Normandy.
    - vWF multimeric analysis of plasma samples electrophoresed on agarose gel is helpful in subtyping vWD. Radiolabeled antibodies to vWF are used to determine the distribution of vWF multimer sizes on the gel. The patient sample is compared with a control.

Multimer Analysis in vWD

Type 1	Normal pattern, reduced concentration
Type 1 Vincenza	Ultralarge multimers
Type 2A	Absent/reduced intermediate–large multimers
Type 2B	Absent/reduced of large multimers
Type 2M	Normal pattern
Type 2N	Normal pattern
Type 3	Absent
Platelet vWD	Reduced large multimers

vWD, von Willebrand disease.

- vWF collagen binding tests are ELISA-based and can help differentiate vWD type 2A and 2B, which have abnormal collagen binding from vWD type 2N, which has normal collagen binding.
- Specific genetic sequencing is commercially available for confirmation of selected vWF subtypes such as type 2N, 2B, and 2M.

16. What pathologic states can alter vWF activity and antigen assay results?

- vWF is an acute phase reactant and levels are affected by inflammation, stress, trauma, hormones, pregnancy, blood type, thyroid disease, exercise, and infection. A single normal test does not exclude the diagnosis, and abnormal results must be assessed according to context in which the result was drawn.

17. Describe the implications of an abnormal euglobulin clot lysis time.

- The euglobulin protein fraction isolated from test plasma contains factor VIII, fibrinogen, factor XIII, plasminogen, and plasminogen activators. The euglobulin fraction is suspended, clotting is generated, and the time for clot dissolution is measured.
- Increased times reflect reduced fibrinolysis. Shortened times can be a result of increased fibrinolysis, as seen in disseminated intravascular coagulation (DIC), liver disease, with certain medications, or after thrombolysis.

HEREDITARY BLEEDING/VASCULAR DISORDERS

1. What are the inheritance characteristics of hemophilia A and B?

- Hemophilia A and B are X-linked disorders resulting in decreased synthesis of factors VIII and IX, respectively.
- Numerous point, frameshift, deletion, and two inversion genetic mutations (hemophilia A) have been described leading to hemophilias A and B.
- Thirty percent of factor VIII and IX mutations are de novo.
- All daughters of hemophilic men are obligate carriers. No sons of hemophilic men and normal women will inherit hemophilia. Sons of obligate carrier mothers have a 50% chance of inheriting hemophilia (see the following diagram).

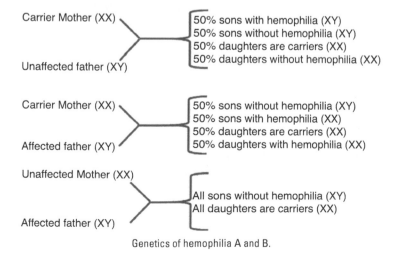

Genetics of hemophilia A and B.

2. **Are female carriers of hemophilia A or B symptomatic?**
   - Up to 20% of female carriers have levels less than 50% and are symptomatically affected due to situations of mosaicism, X chromosomal abnormalities, or imbalanced X chromosome inactivation (lyonization).

3. **What are the most frequent genetic mutations associated with severe hemophilia A?**
   - Nearly half of all severe hemophilia A cases result from two chromosomal inversions that involve introns 1 and 22 of the factor VIII gene, respectively. These inversions can be detected by specific polymerase chain reaction (PCR) testing and are useful for identifying carriers of severe hemophilia A.

4. **What are the clinical bleeding manifestations of hemophilia A and B?**
   - Delayed bleeding is the hallmark of a coagulation factor deficiency.
   - Spontaneous deep bruising, muscular hematomas, and intra-articular bleeding are characteristic of hemophilia. Spontaneous, nontraumatic intra-articular bleeding is not typically seen with factor VIII or IX levels of greater than 5% to 10%.

5. **How is the clinical severity of hemophilia A and B predicted?**
   - Severity of hemophilic bleeding is correlated with endogenous factor activity level.

Hemophilia Severity	Percent Factor Level (Factor VIII or IX)	Bleeding With...
Mild	5%–40%	Major trauma or surgery, rarely spontaneous
Moderate	1%–5%	Occasionally spontaneous, minor trauma or surgery
Severe	<1%	Spontaneous bleeding

6. **How are newborns born to known maternal carriers tested for hemophilia A or B?**
   - Inherited hemophilia can be established at birth by measuring factor VIII or IX levels on cord blood.
   - Results may be affected by inflammation, level of deficiency, and the normal decreased neonatal synthesis of vitamin K-dependent factors.

7. **What are the inheritance characteristics and clinical features of factor XI deficiency?**
   - Factor XI deficiency is most common in patients who are of Ashkenazi Jewish descent, where two specific mutations account for most of the deficiencies. However, the remaining reported cases are from all racial and ethnic groups.
   - Unlike hemophilia A or B, the factor XI activity level does not correlate with the degree of bleeding manifestations. Bleeding tendency is generally mild to moderate, with some patients not showing a bleeding phenotype despite a severe deficiency with levels less than 10%. When bleeding is present, it is often at sites of high fibrinolytic activity.
   - It is an autosomal recessive disease.

8. What are the inheritance characteristics and clinical features of the rarer inherited factor deficiencies?

■ Rare bleeding disorders due to other clotting factor deficiencies can be identified by clinical history and a laboratory workup guided by screening coagulation tests (PT, PTT, and thrombin time). This includes deficiencies of fibrinogen, factor II, factor V, combined factor V/factor VIII, factor VII, factor X, and factor XIII. Factor VII and XI deficiencies will be most common, making up nearly two-thirds of this group (see the following table).

Rare Bleeding Disorder	Frequency	Bleeding Sites	Other Features	Treatment
FVII deficiency	37.5%	Intracranial	Can have thrombosis	rFVIIa (R), factor VII concentrate* (PD)
FXI deficiency	26.5%	Surgery or trauma	–	FFP, FXI concentrate* (PD)
FV deficiency	9.0%	N/A	–	FFP, platelets
Fibrinogen deficiency	8.0%	N/A	Miscarriage, thrombosis, splenic rupture	Fibrinogen concentrate (PD), FFP, cryoprecipitate
FX deficiency	8.0%	Intracranial	–	Factor X concentrate (PD), PCC
FXIII deficiency	6.5%	Intracranial, umbilical stump, menorrhagia	Normal PT/ PTT, poor wound healing	Factor XIII A-subunit (R), factor XIII concentrate (PD), cryoprecipitate
FV + FVIII deficiency	3.0%	See FV and FVIII deficiency	–	FFP or platelets, factor VIII
FII	1.5%	N/A	–	PCC

*Available outside of the United States.

FFP, fresh plasma; N/A, not applicable; PCC, prothrombin complex concentrate, often contain factors II, IX, X, and sometimes VII; PD, plasma-derived; PT, prothrombin time; PTT, partial thromboplastin time; R, recombinant.

■ Inheritance is typically autosomal recessive.
■ Historical clues may include a history of parental consanguineous marriage or a socially or geographically restricted population.
■ Combined factor V and VIII deficiency is distinct from factor V and VIII deficiencies individually. This disorder is typically related to a mutation in the gene encoding a component involved in intracellular transport of these factors, the *LMAN1* gene, or the *MCFD2* gene that codes a cofactor for *LMAN1*.

- Factor XIII deficiency bleeding manifestations include delayed bleeding from the umbilical stump, recurrent abortion, poor wound healing, menorrhagia, intra-articular bleeding, and severe delayed bleeding. Coagulation screening tests (PT/PTT/fibrinogen) are normal in factor XIII deficiency.

9. **What factor deficiencies are not associated with bleeding?**
   - Factor XII, HMWK, and prekallikrein deficiencies are not generally associated with bleeding.

10. **What hereditary clotting disorders affect primary hemostasis?**
    - Hereditary disorders that affect platelet function or number (see Chapter 8) including Bernard–Soulier and Glanzmann thrombasthenia
    - vWD

11. **What process is defective in BSS and why?**
    - BSS is an autosomal recessive disorder characterized by thrombocytopenia, large platelets, and decrease in the number of GPIb receptors or a functionally defective GPIb complex.
    - Platelet adhesion is decreased.

12. **What process is defective in Glanzmann thrombasthenia and why?**
    - Glanzmann thrombasthenia is an autosomal recessive bleeding disorder with normal number and size of platelets.
    - The GPIIb/IIIa complex is required for binding fibrinogen.
    - Platelet aggregation is decreased or absent due to a deficiency or absence of the GPIIb/IIIa heterodimer complex caused by mutations in either IIb or IIIa.
    - Clot retraction may also be impaired by defects in the interaction of GPIIbIIIa with the platelet cytoskeleton.

13. **How is congenital afibrinogenemia distinguished from Glanzmann thrombasthenia?**
    - Both disorders result in decreased platelet aggregation to all agonists except ristocetin. Afibrinogenemia is associated with a prolonged PT, activated partial thromboplastin time (aPTT), and thrombin time, whereas those laboratory tests are normal in Glanzmann thrombasthenia.

14. **Describe the clinical features of vWD.**
    - vWD is the most common congenital bleeding disorder and is important for platelet adhesion.
    - Patients have mucocutaneous bleeding, menorrhagia, as well as immediate and delayed postoperative or posttraumatic bleeding.

15. **What are the three major types of vWD and the testing profile for each?**
    - Type 1 is the most common type, characterized by a reduced level of normally functioning vWF. It is generally autosomal dominant in inheritance with variable penetrance. Testing shows a reduced vWF antigen (<30), reduced ristocetin cofactor assay (<30), a ratio of ristocetin cofactor to antigen >0.5 to 0.7, and a normal or slightly decreased factor VIII. All vWF multimers are present but reduced in concentration. In the type I vWD Vincenza, patients have a rapid clearance of vWF.

- Type 2 vWD is characterized by a qualitative defect in vWF. There are four subtypes of type 2 vWD (see the following table). It is generally autosomal dominant (type 2A, 2B, 2M), but can be autosomal recessive (type 2N). Type 2N shows a normal vWF antigen, normal ristocetin cofactor activity, with a significant decrease in factor VIII; this may be confused with a diagnosis of hemophilia A.
- Type 3 vWD shows a marked quantitative deficiency in vWF with markedly reduced levels of vWF antigen, ristocetin cofactor activity, and factor VIII. It is inherited in an autosomal recessive fashion.

		vWF:RCo (IU/dL)	vWF:Ag (IU/dL)	FVIII	vWF:RCo/ vWF:Ag Ratio
Type 1	Partial reduction in vWF	<30	<30	Low or normal	>0.5–0.7
Type 2A	Decreased platelet adhesion	<30	<30–200	Low or normal	<0.5–0.7
Type 2B	Increased affinity for platelet GPIb	<30	30–200	Low or normal	<0.5–0.7
Type 2M	Decreased platelet adhesion	<30	30–200	Low or normal	<0.5–0.7
Type 2N	Decreased binding for FVIII	30–200	30–200	Very low	<0.5–0.7
Type 3	vWF deficiency	<3	<3	<10 IU/dL	–
Low vWF		30–50	30–50	Normal	>0.5–0.7
Normal		50–200	50–200	Normal	>0.5–0.7

vWF, von Willebrand factor.

16. How are the four qualitative defects representing type 2 vWD distinguished?

- Type 2A has an absence of high- and intermediate-molecular-weight multimers. RIPA is reduced.
- Type 2B results in vWF that binds platelets spontaneously, resulting in thrombocytopenia. High-molecular-weight multimers are decreased or absent. RIPA is increased and type 2B vWF can agglutinate platelets at lower ristocetin concentrations (0.5 mg/mL) compared with normal vWF.
- Type 2M, similar to type 2A, has reduced platelet adhesion. However, 2M has the full spectrum of multimers.
- Type 2N vWF has reduced binding of factor VIII, resulting in reduced factor VIII but normal vWF levels.

17. **What are inherited primary vascular disorders associated with bleeding manifestations?**
    - Hereditary hemorrhagic telangiectasia (Osler–Weber–Rendu or HHT) is one of the most notable, autosomal dominant, hereditary vascular disorders, with several identified mutations resulting in recurrent epistaxis, mucocutaneous telangiectasias, arteriovenous malformations (AVMs) of the lungs, liver, and cerebral vasculature, and intestinal bleeding.
    - Ehlers–Danlos syndrome (EDS) is a group of autosomal dominant connective tissue disorders that can affect joint mobility, tissue integrity, and wound healing. Skin and joint hypermobility with potential dislocations or subluxations are seen, along with poor wound healing and autonomic instability. In vascular EDS, vascular rupture or organ rupture is possible. Genetic testing is indicated.
    - Marfan syndrome is also a genetic connective tissue disorder that is associated with aortic root dilation (potentially manifesting as aortic aneurysms, aortic regurgitation, and aortic dissection), joint hypermobility, characteristic facial features and skeletal changes, tall stature, lens dislocation, and dural ectasia. Treatment consists of cardiac and vascular monitoring, can include cardiovascular pharmacotherapy, and may involve surgery for related complications.

18. **What is the management for HHT?**
    - Management involves assessing for sites of affected vasculature, local therapy for epistaxis, embolization of pulmonary or gastrointestinal (GI) tract AVMs, and ligation or coiling of brain AVMs. Experimental systemic therapy with agents like the antivascular endothelial growth factor A, monoclonal antibody, bevacizumab, or thalidomide may be considered for severe cases.

19. **Other vascular disorders:**
    - Several other hereditary vascular conditions can result in abnormal hemangiomas, small arteries, cutaneous vascular anomalies, cavernous malformations, capillary malformations, lymphedema from lymphatic malformations, and more. Treatment for these depends on the underlying condition and is often supportive. Large vascular hemangiomas as in Kasabach–Merritt syndrome are associated with chronic DIC.

ACQUIRED BLEEDING DISORDERS

1. **What situations are associated with acquired coagulation factor deficiencies?**
    - Acquired coagulation factor deficiencies can be seen with vitamin K deficiency (poor intake, malabsorption, altered gut flora, etc.), liver disease (reduced production), medications (warfarin, etc.), consumptive coagulopathies (DIC, fibrinolysis, etc.), nephrotic syndrome (loss of coagulation factors), massive transfusion (dilution), acquired von Willebrand syndrome (loss of vWF carrier function for factor VIII), amyloidosis, with acquired inhibitors of coagulation, and more.

2. **What disorders can cause an abnormal fibrinogen level?**
    - Decreased fibrinogen can occur with consumption (as in DIC) or the breakdown of a clot (as seen after therapeutic tPA-mediated fibrinolytic therapy), snake

venom, decreased production (as in liver disease or severe malnutrition), or a hereditary deficiency.

- Fibrinogen is an acute phase reactant and may be elevated in the setting of inflammation, tumors, vascular disease, or pregnancy.

3. **What are some conditions that are associated with acquired inhibitors of coagulation factors?**
   - Acquired coagulation factor inhibitors can be associated with pregnancy, autoimmune disorders (including systemic lupus erythematosus), malignancy, drugs, and can be idiopathic.

4. **What conditions are associated with acquired vWD?**
   - Acquired von Willebrand syndrome can be associated with a variety of conditions including lymphoproliferative disorders (lymphoma, multiple myeloma, chronic lymphocytic leukemia, Waldenstrom macroglobulinemia), myeloproliferative neoplasms, autoimmune disorders (systemic lupus erythematosus), cardiac conditions (ventricular septal defect, aortic stenosis, left ventricular assist device, extracorporeal membrane oxygenation), and drugs, among other conditions. The laboratory testing in acquired von Willebrand syndrome is similar to type 2A vWD.

5. **What factor deficiency is most commonly associated with amyloidosis?**
   - Factor X

6. **Describe the pathogenesis and clinical findings of DIC.**
   - DIC describes a consumptive coagulopathy characterized by dysregulated endogenous anticoagulant pathways and fibrinolysis with imbalanced coagulation. It is partially mediated by TF and cytokines. Clinically, this can manifest most commonly as bleeding but also with thrombosis.

7. **What conditions can lead to the development of DIC?**
   - Infection, sepsis, obstetric conditions (acute fatty liver of pregnancy, placenta abruption, amniotic fluid embolism, HELLP (hemolysis, elevated liver enzymes, low platelets) syndrome, fetal death, etc.), malignancy, trauma, transfusion reactions, liver disease, extremes of temperature, allergic reactions, snake bites, and vascular abnormalities (Kasabach–Merritt) are several entities that have been associated with DIC.

8. **What are characteristic laboratory features and management of DIC?**
   - DIC is associated with prolonged clotting times (PT/ PTT), reduced fibrinogen, elevated fibrin degradation products (D-dimer), and thrombocytopenia.
   - Therapy is directed at the underlying condition. Transfusion support is complex with judicious use of fresh frozen plasma (FFP), cryoprecipitate, and platelets. Prophylactic pharmacologic anticoagulation is selectively considered. Therapeutic anticoagulation (e.g., unfractionated heparin) is considered only in very select cases in the setting of thrombosis.
   - Antifibrinolytics should not be used.

HEMOSTATIC DRUGS

1. **Name two drugs that work to inhibit fibrinolysis and describe how they work.**
   - Aminocaproic acid and tranexamic acid compete for lysine binding sites on plasminogen and plasmin, thus preventing them from binding fibrin. They can be given intravenously (IV) or orally. Caution is needed in genitourinary bleeding due to the possibility of precipitating urinary retention due to obstructing ureteral clot.

2. **What are the therapeutic agents used for the treatment of hemophilia A and B?**
   - For hemophilia A and B, both recombinant and plasma-derived factor preparations are available. Cryoprecipitate contains factor VIII but is not typically used for primary treatment due to the risk of bloodborne pathogens and large volume required. Cryoprecipitate is not used for factor IX deficiency.
   - Factor VIII is dosed as ([desired factor VIII level – baseline level] multiplied by weight in kilograms), multiplied by 0.5; desired dosing level and frequency vary based on the bleed location/severity, the product being used, and patient-specific factors/pharmacokinetic data.
   - Emicizumab is a recombinant, humanized, bispecific antibody that binds to both activated coagulation factor IX and factor X, ultimately bypassing the function of factor VIIIa. It is used for bleeding prophylaxis for patients with hemophilia A with or without an inhibitor. Of note, emicizumab affects coagulation tests, including shortening the aPTT, and interferes with factor VIII activity assays that use human-derived coagulation factors. Factor VIII activity for patients on emicizumab is therefore measured with a chromogenic assay using bovine-derived coagulation factors.
   - Desmopressin (DDAVP) given IV or intranasally can also be considered for minor bleeding episodes as it causes the release of factor VIII and vWF from endothelial stores. It acts through type 2 vasopressin receptors. Adverse effects include flushing, headaches, hypotension, and antidiuretic effects. Free water should be restricted to reduce the risk of hyponatremia; caution is needed for patients with a history of seizures given this risk. Desmopressin is not advised for patients with cardiovascular disease.
   - For hemophilia B, recombinant factor IX or plasma-derived product replacements are available. Adult dosage is calculated as ([desired factor IX level – baseline level] multiplied by weight in kilograms) multiplied by approximately 1.2 depending on the product (desired dosing level and frequency vary based on the bleed location/severity, the product being used, and patient-specific factors/pharmacokinetic data).
   - Antifibrinolytic is a useful adjunctive therapy to improve clot integrity and reduce early degradation.

Hemophilia A Treatment Options

Type	Half-life
Recombinant	9–17 hours
Extended half-life	13–20 hours
DDAVP*	–

(continued)

Hemophilia B Treatment Options (*continued*)

Type	Half-life
Recombinant	16–26 hours
Recombinant, Fc fusion	54–90 hours
Recombinant, albumin fusion	104 hours

*DDAVP (desmopressin) not appropriate for severe hemophilia.

Note: Half-lives depend on the specific product and population; therapies may differ between adults and children.

3. How are coagulation factor inhibitors treated in patients with congenital hemophilia A?
- Long-term management can include inducing immune tolerance in appropriately selected hemophilia A patients through high-dose factor infusions. Drugs like intravenous immunoglobulin (IVIG), cyclophosphamide, and rituximab have also been used. In addition, emicizumab can be used as outlined above.
- For active bleeding or necessary surgical procedures, bypassing agents such as activated factor VII or factor VIII inhibitor bypassing activity (FEIBA, an activated prothrombin complex concentrate) are often used. Plasmapheresis and high-dose factor VIII infusion are also considerations depending on the clinical scenario and inhibitor titer.

4. How are rare factor deficiencies treated?
- Factor XII, HMWK, and prekallikrein do not lead to bleeding.
- Most rare factor deficiencies are managed with FFP, but this can be challenging due to excessive volume. For a 70-kg adult, 4 units of FFP raise a factor level by 10%.
- Plasma-derived concentrates of factors X, factor XI, and factor XIII are available.
- Cryoprecipitate and plasma-derived fibrinogen concentrates can be used for dysfibrinogenemias or fibrinogen deficiency.
- Recombinant concentrates of factor VIIa and factor XIII are available.

5. How is vWD treated?
- The subtype and bleeding event influence treatment options.
- Minor bleeding can often be managed with topical thrombin and local measures.
- Type 1 and some type 2 vWD patients who previously demonstrated a response to desmopressin can use IV DDAVP or intranasal DDAVP for minor procedures or bleeding.
- Desmopressin in type 2B vWD has the potential to lower platelet counts and potentially induce platelet aggregation. Therefore, its use in type 2B remains controversial and should probably be avoided. Patients with type 2M have a short duration of response.
- The mainstay of therapy for bleeding or bleeding prophylaxis in type 2 or type 3 vWD is vWF replacement therapy from plasma-derived or recombinant vWF products. Cryoprecipitate has been used in the past but is no longer the standard of care. Purified and recombinant factor VIII preparations do not contain sufficient vWF and are not used.
- Adjunctive measures may include oral contraceptives for menorrhagia and/or antifibrinolytic agents like tranexamic acid or aminocaproic acid.

QUESTIONS

1. A 34-year-old man with limited medical history presents with recurrent epistaxis and prolonged bleeding following a dental extraction. He notes a history of easy bruising. His nosebleeds last for up to an hour and he has required medical intervention on several occasions to control the bleeding. A complete blood count (CBC) shows normal platelet count (175 × 10^9/L) and is otherwise normal. Prothrombin time (PT) and partial thromboplastin time (PTT) are normal. Review of the peripheral blood smear shows normal-appearing platelets. Which of the following is least likely to support the diagnosis?
   A. von Willebrand factor activity, von Willebrand factor antigen, factor 8, multimer analysis
   B. Factor VIII, IX, XI testing
   C. Platelet function aggregation studies
   D. Platelet electron microscopy

2. A 65-year-old female, G2P2, is referred after screening labs performed prior to an elective cholecystectomy revealed a prolonged activated partial thromboplastin time (aPTT) of 67 seconds. The patient denies a history of easy bruising or menorrhagia. She has tolerated numerous operations, including a bowel resection and appendectomy, without any bleeding complications. She has never required a blood transfusion and denies mucocutaneous bleeding. Review of her medical records reveals her aPTT has been prolonged for many years, even before these operations. Physical exam is unremarkable. Complete blood count (CBC) and prothrombin time (PT) are normal. The aPTT corrects when mixed with an equal volume of normal plasma. Which is the most likely diagnosis?
   A. Factor V deficiency
   B. Factor VIII inhibitor
   C. Factor XI deficiency
   D. Factor XII deficiency

3. An 82-year-old man with moderate dementia is brought to the ED unresponsive with evidence of hematemesis after he was found down in his assisted living facility. His medications are unknown, but he has a reported history that includes hypertension, diabetes mellitus, transient ischemic attack (TIA), chronic back pain, coronary artery disease, and atrial fibrillation. The patient is afebrile, hypotensive, and has a rapid and irregular pulse. He is slow to respond. Physical exam is notable for small scattered ecchymoses and dried blood in the posterior oropharynx. Complete blood count (CBC) shows a hemoglobin of 6.8 g/dL and a normal platelet value. Prothrombin time (PT) is prolonged, corresponding to an international normalized ratio (INR) of 9.2. Activated partial thromboplastin time (aPTT) is prolonged at 52 seconds. The peripheral blood smear is normal. Aspartate aminotransferase (AST) is 76, alanine aminotransferase (ALT) is 64, and bilirubin and albumin are normal. CT of the head is negative. Laboratory testing is most likely to reveal which of the following?

A. Low fibrinogen related to hepatic synthetic dysfunction
B. Failure of the clotting times to correct by adding an equal volume of plasma
C. Low fibrinogen related to disseminated intravascular coagulation (DIC)
D. Reduced levels of factors II, VII, IX, and X

4. **A 64-year-old male who is currently receiving adjuvant chemotherapy for colon cancer was recently hospitalized for neutropenic fever. In addition to thrombocytopenia, he was found to have an abnormal activated partial thromboplastin time (aPTT) of 52 seconds. Prothrombin time in the hospital was 12 seconds. He is referred for further evaluation. He denies any recent or historic bleeding, but has had a blood transfusion during the course of his colon surgery and chemotherapy. He has no personal or family history of thrombosis. Hemoglobin is 9.6 g/dL, platelets 136 × 10⁹/L, and white blood cells (WBCs) 6.4 × 10⁹/L. His exam shows scattered small ecchymoses and no splenomegaly. What is the best next step for his evaluation?**
A. Mixing study
B. Thrombin time and reptilase time
C. Factor XII assay
D. Repeat the lab from a peripheral blood draw

5. **A 36-year-old woman with a long-standing history of menorrhagia, mucocutaneous bleeding, and easy bruising is referred for further evaluation. Hemoglobin is 9.8 g/dL, mean corpuscular volume (MCV) is 74 fL, platelets are 86,000 × 10⁹/L, and white blood cell (WBC) count is normal. Prothrombin time (PT) and partial thromboplastin time (PTT) are normal. Further workup shows von Willebrand factor (vWF) activity (ristocetin cofactor assay) is 26%, vWF antigen is 58%, and factor VIII is 96%. Multimer analysis reveals no high-molecular-weight multimers. Platelet aggregometry shows aggregation with 0.5 mg/mL of ristocetin. Which is the most likely diagnosis?**
A. Type 1 von Willebrand disease (vWD)
B. Type 2A vWD
C. Type 2B vWD
D. Type 2M vWD

6. **A 36-year-old female is admitted with a splenic laceration and intra-abdominal bleeding after being involved in a motor vehicle accident. She is unconscious on arrival and head CT shows a small subdural hematoma. Over the course of 6 hours, her hemoglobin dropped from 9.6 g/dL at presentation to 7.8 g/dL. Her platelet count is normal, as is the prothrombin time (PT) and activated partial thromboplastin time (aPTT). Lactate dehydrogenase (LDH), total bilirubin, and haptoglobin were normal. Reticulocytes are elevated and there are numerous polychromatophilic cells on peripheral smear. Her family reports and outside medical records confirm she has a history of factor XIII deficiency diagnosed after she had experienced menorrhagia. She has not required therapy since having a hysterectomy several years ago. She also had delayed umbilical cord bleeding and separation. The**

hospital has ordered recombinant factor XIII, but does not have any available. She has received 3 L of intravenous (IV) normal saline for low blood pressures and a blood transfusion has been initiated. What should be done for her factor deficiency?

A. Supportive care until the arrival of the recombinant factor XIII

B. Factor VIIa

C. Cryoprecipitate

D. Desmopressin

7. **Which of the following facts about von Willebrand factor (vWF) is correct?**

A. von Willebrand disease (vWD) is the second most common congenital bleeding disorder.

B. Thrombocytopenia is associated with type 2M vWD.

C. Type 2N vWD presents with normal vWF antigen, normal vWF ristocetin cofactor activity, and reduced factor VIII level.

D. vWF antigen and activity levels are higher in type 3 compared with type 1 vWD.

ANSWERS

1. **B. Factor VIII, IX, XI testing.** History supports a platelet function disorder and with normal PTT it would be unlikely to have an abnormal factor VIII, IX, or XI.

2. **D. Factor XII deficiency.** This patient has a long-standing abnormal clotting time without any bleeding history. Of the choices, only option D, factor XII deficiency, is not associated with bleeding and she can be cleared to proceed with surgery if the diagnosis is confirmed. Option A, factor V, would affect both the aPTT and PT given that factor V is part of the final common pathway. Option B, factor VIII inhibitor, would not be supported by the mixing study that suggests a factor deficiency. Factor XI deficiency, or hemophilia B, would be expected to be associated with bleeding, especially given the degree of prolongation of her aPTT.

3. **D. Reduced levels of factors II, VII, IX, and X.** The history is concerning for warfarin toxicity resulting in a gastrointestinal bleed. The patient has a history of atrial fibrillation and comorbidities that could indicate a need for warfarin. Warfarin results in a reduction in the vitamin K-dependent clotting factors. While the PT/INR is most sensitive to abnormalities in factor VII of the extrinsic pathway, reductions in the remaining vitamin K-dependent factors will impact the aPTT as well. For option A, albumin and bilirubin are normal and there is no history to suggest liver disease. The PT and aPTT are higher than would be anticipated for isolated liver disease. Option B describes a mixing study result that would implicate an inhibitor of a component of the common pathway or a lupus anticoagulant. Acquired spontaneous inhibitors of factors in the common pathway are rare. His known medical history does not include autoimmune disease, malignancy, or recent cardiac surgery in which bovine thrombin was used (associated with the development of a factor V inhibitor). A mixing study could be obtained but would be more likely to indicate a factor deficiency. There are insufficient physical findings or laboratory evidence to suggest DIC. His normal platelet count and blood smear make a consumptive coagulopathy.

4. **D. Repeat the lab from a peripheral blood draw.** An abnormal lab is a common indication for referral. In this case, the patient has no bleeding or clotting history. It could be assumed that the lab may have been drawn through a chemotherapy port and thus may be prolonged by heparin contamination. Repeating the lab through a peripheral blood draw or, if that is not possible, through the port after adequate flushing of the line would obviate the need for more extensive or costly workup. If the prolonged aPTT was still felt to be heparin contamination (in this clinical setting, this is a valid concern), option B could be a reasonable choice. Heparin contamination would be expected to prolong the thrombin time but not affect the reptilase time. If the patient had a significant bleeding history or heparin contamination was not suspected, a mixing study could be considered. Many mixing studies will include a thrombin time or use a heparinase to limit potential interference from heparin. Option C, factor XII, could be an explanation for an isolated prolonged aPTT in this clinical setting but would not be the next best test.

5. **C. Type 2B vWD.** The patient has a clinical history consistent with vWD and likely a concurrent iron deficiency anemia. Patients with type 2B vWD have a gain-of-function mutation in the platelet GPIb binding domain on vWF that allows for vWF to bind spontaneously with platelets in vivo and in the presence of low concentrations of ristocetin in platelet aggregation assays. Spontaneous binding of vWF in vivo and clearance of vWF–platelet complexes by the spleen can result in thrombocytopenia. vWF multimer analysis shows absence of high-molecular vWF multimers. The ratio of the vWF activity (ristocetin cofactor activity) to vWF antigen is less than 0.5, consistent with type 2 vWD. These labs are not consistent with the other choices.

6. **C. Cryoprecipitate.** A factor XIII level should be obtained, but the results would not be immediately available to guide management. A recombinant factor XIII A-subunit product is available in the United States that when administered combines with free factor XIII B-subunit to then function similar to endogenous factor XIII. However, given that it is not available, cryoprecipitate, based on weight, is the best option of the listed choices. Fresh frozen plasma could be considered but there would be concerns about the volume required in the setting of a severe bleed. Supportive care would not be appropriate given the critical nature of the bleed. Factor VIIa and desmopressin would not be the best choice in this situation. Animal studies showed thrombotic complications when factor VIIa and XIII A-subunit were given together at high doses. Desmopressin monotherapy would be insufficient for initial resuscitation.

7. **C. Type 2N vWD presents with normal vWF antigen, normal vWF ristocetin cofactor activity, and reduced factor VIII level.** vWD is the most common congenital bleeding disorder. Thrombocytopenia can be associated with type 2B vWD. vWF antigen and activity levels are lower in type 3 compared with type 1 vWD.

Thrombosis

Jordan K. Schaefer, Lauren Shevell, and Suman L. Sood

HEREDITARY THROMBOPHILIAS

1. **What are the five most common inherited thrombophilias and the mechanism by which they promote thrombosis?**
   - The five major inherited thrombophilias include factor V Leiden (FVL) gene mutation, prothrombin gene mutation, and deficiency of the natural anticoagulants, protein C, protein S, and antithrombin. Combinations of these thrombophilias are possible.

TABLE 10.1 ■ The Prevalence and Outcomes of Inherited Thrombophilias

	Population Prevalence	Prevalence With VTE	RR for Initial VTE	RR for Recurrent VTE
Factor V Leiden	2%–5%	12%–18%	4–5	1.4
Prothrombin 20210A mutation	0.7%–4%	5%–8%	3–4	1.4
Protein C deficiency	0.2–0.5%	2%–5%	7	1.4–1.8
Protein S deficiency	0.03%–0.13%	1%	5	1.0–1.4
Antithrombin deficiency	0.02%–0.2%	1%–7%	16	1.9–2.6

RR, relative risk; VTE, venous thromboembolism.

- The FVL polymorphism confers resistance of factor V (both activated and inactivated) to activated protein C, therefore relatively increasing the amount of activated factor V available to convert prothrombin to thrombin. It is the most common inherited thrombophilia in Caucasians but is less often seen in African American or Asian populations. It is most often seen in the heterozygous state (with four- to fivefold increase in thrombotic risk); homozygous individuals are at a significantly higher risk of venous thromboembolism (VTE). There are conflicting data on the effect of the mutation on arterial thrombosis; the vast majority of thrombosis will be venous.
- Prothrombin G20210A mutation is a gain-of-function mutation that leads to increased levels of prothrombin (factor II). As a result, there is more thrombin available to convert fibrinogen to fibrin and interact with other elements of the coagulation cascade. Similar to FVL, a heterozygous status confers a modestly

increased risk of venous thrombosis (three- to fourfold) and this risk is increased in homozygous individuals. The risk for VTE is higher in those who are heterozygous for both FVL and prothrombin gene mutations than in those with only one mutation.

- Protein C deficiency is usually an autosomal dominant condition, and most adults are diagnosed in the heterozygous state. Protein C levels for these patients are typically about half of normal. The reduction in the amount of this "natural anticoagulant" leads to increased thrombotic rates. Recall that protein C is activated by thrombin complexed with thrombomodulin, and it exerts an anticoagulant effect by inactivating coagulation factors Va and VIIIa through the activated protein C complex (see FVL in the preceding text). A quantitative defect (type I) or a qualitative/functional defect of protein C (type II) may exist. Adults most often experience recurrent VTE, but neonatal purpura fulminans has been described in homozygous children with a severe deficiency. Given that warfarin decreases protein C faster than other coagulation factors, warfarin can precipitate skin necrosis by disturbing the balance between pro- and anticoagulant factors. Venous thromboembolic events are more common with protein C deficiency, but rarely arterial events may occur.

- Protein S deficiency is an autosomal dominant condition. Protein S circulates bound to C4b-binding protein and as a free form. Deficiency can be a result of a quantitative disorder with proportionately reduced total protein S, free form, and activity (type I); a reduction in the activity, but with a normal total protein S and free form (type II); or a reduction in both the free protein S and the activity, but with a normal total protein S (type III). Clinically, it is similar to protein C deficiency. Neonatal purpura fulminans can occur in the homozygous state, and warfarin-induced skin necrosis can also occur.

- Antithrombin deficiency is an autosomal dominant condition with variable penetrance and can be either a quantitative defect (type 1) or a qualitative defect (type II) that is associated with recurrent venous thrombosis, both unprovoked and in association with other risk factors. The loss or impaired activity of antithrombin represents the loss of a "natural anticoagulant" and therefore disrupts the hemostatic balance. Recall that antithrombin inactivates several of the coagulation cascade enzymes, especially thrombin (factor IIa), factor IXa, and factor Xa, and that the activity of antithrombin is markedly increased by the activity of endogenous or exogenous heparins. Patients with antithrombin deficiency can demonstrate heparin resistance; this can be overcome by administering antithrombin. Pregnant patients with antithrombin deficiency are at an especially increased risk of thrombosis and can have adverse pregnancy outcomes. During pregnancy, antithrombin concentrates, along with low-molecular-weight heparin (LMWH), are often considered. When evaluating patients for antithrombin deficiency, as with protein C and S deficiencies, the timing of laboratory testing (discussed in the following text) is important, given that a variety of conditions can result in an acquired, rather than inherited, low antithrombin level.

2. **What are the general principles of evaluation and management for inherited thrombophilias?**
   - Family history is important in determining whom to screen for a thrombophilia as penetrance and clinical expression of inherited thrombophilias are quite variable.

- Management relies mostly on the clinical history of the particular patient and knowledge of a thrombophilia may not always change management. Asymptomatic individuals with a strong inherited thrombophilia (homozygous FVL, homozygous prothrombin gene mutation, heterozygous prothrombin gene mutation plus heterozygous FVL, or deficiency of antithrombin, protein C, or protein S) and no history of thrombosis should be considered for thrombosis prophylaxis during high-risk situations like prolonged periods of travel, pregnancy, or postoperatively. Females considering estrogen-containing oral contraceptives should consider alternative contraceptive options, given their increased risk of thrombosis.
- The presence of a strong thrombophilia (defined earlier) may influence decisions on length of anticoagulation in the setting of thrombosis (favoring long-term extended VTE prophylaxis). However, this is mostly based on expert opinion. See "Laboratory Testing and Imaging" section for indications of thrombophilia testing.
- As with any genetic condition, there are possible implications for children and family members when a diagnosis is made.

3. **What disorders of fibrinolysis can lead to increased rates of thrombosis?**
   - Deficient or defective plasminogen, tissue plasminogen activator, and increased levels of plasminogen activator inhibitor-1 can theoretically be associated with increased venous or arterial thrombosis. These are not widely tested clinically.
   - Dysfibrinogenemias are a group of generally autosomal dominant disorders in which an abnormal structure or function of fibrin impairs normal fibrinolysis and thus can be associated with thrombosis and/or bleeding.

ACQUIRED THROMBOTIC DISORDERS

1. **What situations are associated with an increased risk of venous thrombosis?**
   - Situational factors include recent surgery or trauma, hospitalization, long periods (generally greater than 4 hours) of travel, the presence of foreign material (like an intravascular device), pregnancy or exposure to estrogen, and immobility (e.g., using a cast).

2. **What diseases are associated with an increased risk of venous thrombosis?**
   - Generally, any systemic inflammatory process like malignancy, infection (including Covid-19), trauma, and many autoimmune disorders can increase the rate of thrombosis. Different malignancy subtypes are associated with a spectrum of thrombotic risk. Diseases associated with protein loss (nephrotic syndrome) may cause an acquired thrombophilia. Specific hematologic disorders, including antiphospholipid antibody syndrome (APLAS), myeloproliferative neoplasms, paroxysmal nocturnal hemoglobinuria (PNH), plasma cell dyscrasias, heparin-induced thrombocytopenia (HIT), and hemoglobinopathies are associated, to various degrees, with an increased risk of thrombosis through various mechanisms. There is conflicting evidence, but metabolic syndrome, chronic kidney disease, and vascular disease are also mildly associated with VTE.

3. **What medications are associated with an increased risk of venous thrombosis?**
   - Hormonal contraceptives (especially those containing estrogen), hormone replacement therapy, erythropoiesis-stimulating agents, thrombopoietin mimetics, testosterone, tamoxifen, bevacizumab, thalidomide or lenalidomide, L-asparaginase, various other chemotherapeutic agents, intravenous immunoglobulin (IVIG), and corticosteroids, among others, are associated with venous thrombosis.

4. **What anatomic variations are associated with venous thrombosis and how are they managed?**
   - Iliac vein compression syndrome (May–Thurner syndrome) generally results in a predisposition to left-sided venous thrombosis as a result of the right common iliac artery compressing the left common iliac vein against the lumbar spine. It most commonly occurs in young females and may require CT venous (CTV) or magnetic resonance venous (MRV) imaging to diagnose due to the anatomic location of the defect. Management of symptomatic disease often involves endovascular therapy with possible stenting.
   - "Effort-induced" upper extremity deep vein thrombosis (Paget–Schroetter syndrome) generally is the result of compression of the subclavian vein as it courses between the clavicle and the first rib in the setting of repeated, often overhead activity of the ipsilateral upper extremity (e.g., a tennis player). Cervical ribs, anomalous tendon insertions, anterior scalene, or subclavius hypertrophy may contribute to the compression. The inflammatory response to the compression ultimately leads to upper extremity thrombosis that tends to propagate distally to the axillary veins. The mechanical obstruction may limit the risk of large central embolic events. Ultrasound is often used in the diagnosis, but CT or magnetic resonance (MR) venography may be needed due to technical limitations with ultrasound. Therapy may include thrombolysis, systemic anticoagulation, and surgical thoracic outlet decompression.
   - Congenital abnormalities of the inferior vena cava (IVC) can also be associated with deep vein thrombosis. Anticoagulation is the mainstay of therapy for most abnormalities.

5. **What are other venous thrombosis risk factors?**
   - Modifiable factors include obesity and smoking.
   - Nonmodifiable risk factors include increasing age and male sex.

6. **What are causes of arterial thrombosis? What evaluation can be done?**
   - Arterial thrombosis can commonly result from a cardioembolic source as seen in atrial fibrillation or atrial flutter, endocarditis, cardiac tumors, and with a ventricular aneurysm, such as after myocardial infarction. A paradoxical embolism occurs when a venous thrombosis travels to the arterial side of circulation through a cardiac defect such as a patent foramen ovale. Arterial thromboemboli can also occur related to atherosclerotic plaque, typically at large-vessel bifurcations, or in association with vascular aneurysms. Other mechanical sources of arterial thrombosis include arterial dissection, fibromuscular dysplasia, vasculitis, arterial wall infection/arteritis, and from dislodgement of a thrombus after a procedure. Generally, any systemic inflammatory process like malignancy or inflammatory autoimmune disorders may also predispose to arterial

thrombosis. Some specific considerations include cocaine use, cold agglutinins, cryoglobulinemia, dysfibrinogenemia, hyperviscosity, APLAS, PNH, HIT, and myeloproliferative neoplasms, among others.

■ Testing for these conditions can be considered depending on the clinical situation. Inherited thrombophilias are rarely associated with arterial thrombosis and testing is generally of low yield.

7. **What is the difference between atheroembolism and thromboembolism? What are the risk factors for atherosclerosis?**

■ Atherosclerosis can be a source of emboli, either from thromboembolism of a thrombus associated with an atherosclerotic plaque, or less commonly atheroembolism from dislodgement of the material that makes up the plaque (cholesterol embolization syndrome). The latter (atheroembolism) is more commonly triggered by vascular intervention, such as a cardiac catheterization, but can rarely occur spontaneously. Aortic thromboembolism needs to be distinguished from atheroembolism (cholesterol embolization) as the treatment is different. Thromboembolism often presents as sudden occlusion of a medium-to-large vessel and is often treated with anticoagulation or antiplatelet therapy. Atheroembolism often affects multiple locations and small arterioles ("blue toe syndrome"). It may be associated with eosinophilia and livedo reticularis.

■ Risk factors for atherosclerosis include smoking, hypertension, hyperlipidemia, diabetes mellitus (metabolic syndrome), and age.

8. **What is HIT and when should HIT be suspected?**

■ HIT is an adverse reaction to heparin that paradoxically leads to thrombosis rather than bleeding, and thrombocytopenia. The mechanism is complex but results from platelet factor 4, released from the alpha granules of platelets, binding to heparin, which triggers an immune response, resulting in an immunoglobulin G (IgG) class antibody targeted against the heparin–platelet factor 4 complex. This culminates in platelet activation through cross-linking FcγIIA receptors that promotes thrombosis. Thrombocytopenia results from splenic clearance of the IgG complex. The mortality rate of HIT can be as high as 20% if left untreated. With early intervention, mortality rates drop below 2%.

■ There is a greater risk of HIT in patients receiving unfractionated heparin relative to LMWH, in those therapeutically anticoagulated relative to prophylactically, and in surgical patients over medical. Characteristically, it develops 5 to 10 days from exposure to heparin therapy. The platelets decrease in a characteristic pattern (typically an abrupt drop of 50%) and typically nadir at values above 20,000.

■ Patients with a history of heparin exposure within the past 3 months can have a rapid onset (within 24 hours) of HIT upon reexposure to the drug due to previously formed antibodies.

■ While overall incidence is rare, given the severe consequences of the condition, it should be suspected with a declining platelet count for any patient receiving, or having received, heparin-based therapy. A 50% drop in platelet count should prompt consideration of HIT, even if it has not reached the level of absolute thrombocytopenia. Additionally, it should be in the differential with any clinical manifestations consistent with HIT (see the following text).

9. What are some of the clinical manifestations of HIT?

■ New or worsening venous thrombosis is one of the most common, severe complications of HIT. Arterial thromboses can also occur, manifesting as limb ischemia or organ infarction. Heparin-induced skin necrosis, typically at the injection site, can occur. Some patients will also experience a systemic reaction (fevers, chills, vital sign changes, shortness of breath) after starting intravenous heparin. Despite the presence of thrombocytopenia and anticoagulation, bleeding is not common. Adrenal thrombosis and secondary hemorrhage have also been described.

10. What is the "4Ts score" and how is it applied to the evaluation of suspected HIT?

■ The 4Ts score (Table 10.2) is a risk prediction score for the diagnosis of HIT, which is composed of four elements, awarding 0 to 2 points based on clinical or laboratory parameters. The elements are thrombocytopenia, timing, thrombosis, and other causes of thrombocytopenia. Patients with ≤3 points are considered low risk, 4 to 5 points are intermediate risk, and ≥6 points are high risk (see Chapter 8).

TABLE 10.2 ■ 4T Score

Thrombocytopenia
- ■ Platelet count fall ≥50% and platelet count ≥20 (+2 points)
- ■ Platelet count fall 30%–50% or platelet nadir 10–19 (+1 point)
- ■ Platelet count fall <30% or platelet nadir <10 (0 points)

Timing of platelet fall
- ■ Clear onset between days 5 and 10 or platelet fall ≤1 day if prior heparin exposure within 30 days (+2 points)
- ■ Consistent with fall at 5–10 days but unclear, onset after day 10, or fall ≤1 day with prior heparin exposure 30–100 days (+1 point)
- ■ Platelet count fall at <4 days without recent heparin exposure (0 points)

Thrombosis or other sequelae
- ■ Confirmed new thrombosis, skin necrosis or acute systemic reaction after intravenous unfractionated bolus (+2 points)
- ■ Progressive or recurrent thrombosis, nonnecrotizing (erythematous) skin lesion, or suspected thrombosis that has not been proven (+1 point)
- ■ None (0 points)

Other causes for thrombocytopenia
- ■ None apparent (+2 points)
- ■ Possible (+1 point)
- ■ Definite (0 points)

■ Other scoring systems are available but have not shown superior performance.
■ While clinical judgment is important, some providers use the 4Ts score to guide initial management, with a low-risk score not requiring additional testing. Those with intermediate- or high-risk scores typically are tested with an antiplatelet factor 4 enzyme-linked immunosorbent assay (ELISA) and possibly a serotonin release assay. The ELISA assay is very sensitive but tends to produce more false positives than the serotonin release assay. Often an ELISA

is sent initially, and if positive the serotonin release is sent as a confirmatory test. During this time, there is strong consideration for stopping heparin anticoagulation and starting an alternative anticoagulant (direct thrombin inhibitor) while awaiting the result. Given the high risk of thrombosis in unrecognized HIT and the risk of bleeding with alternative anticoagulants in other causes of thrombocytopenia, initial management can be challenging, especially with intermediate-risk patients.

■ It is important to recognize that the diagnosis is based on clinical features in conjunction with laboratory findings. At times, the diagnosis can be made with an antiplatelet factor 4 ELISA in the right clinical setting, but the functional serotonin release assay is often required.

11. How is HIT managed?

■ Alternative, nonheparin anticoagulants (discussed in the following text) are used with diagnosed HIT or suspected HIT in patients at intermediate or higher risk. The choice of anticoagulant depends on the urgency of anticoagulation, possible need for reversal, and underlying comorbidities including kidney and liver disease. Patients requiring urgent anticoagulation should receive parenteral options such as argatroban, fondaparinux, or bivalirudin. Recent studies have also demonstrated the efficacy and safety of using direct oral anticoagulants (DOACs), although most data support their use after initial course of parenteral anticoagulation. Ultrasounds of the upper and lower extremities should be considered to rule out the presence of a clot, as it would affect the duration of anticoagulation. Heparin should be strictly avoided (heparin flushes, prophylaxis, etc.) in diagnosed HIT and in those with suspicion of HIT. Warfarin should be avoided until the platelet count has normalized (>150,000) given the risk of venous limb gangrene. Once started, it should be overlapped for at least 5 days with another anticoagulant. Anticoagulation should continue for at least 3 months in the presence of thrombosis and, while data are limited, at least 4 weeks in the absence of thrombosis.

■ Generally, after a diagnosis of HIT, patients should avoid any exposure to heparin in the future. However, patients with a remote history of HIT (>3 months in the past) and negative laboratory testing for HIT who require heparin, as with cardiopulmonary bypass, often can be briefly exposed to heparin for cardiac surgery and then use an alternative, nonheparin anticoagulant if needed postoperatively. For those who have positive HIT serologies or a more recent HIT diagnosis, when surgery cannot be delayed, performing the surgery using a direct thrombin inhibitor should be considered. Additionally, plasmapheresis can be considered.

12. When should APLAS be suspected?

■ Antiphospholipid syndrome can be a primary autoimmune disorder or secondary to another condition like systemic lupus erythematosus.

■ Clinical manifestations can range from asymptomatic to catastrophic antiphospholipid syndrome, which is characterized by diffuse thrombosis, affecting at least three organ systems simultaneously or within the course of a week. Catastrophic antiphospholipid syndrome can manifest similarly to thrombotic microangiopathies, HIT, and disseminated intravascular coagulation.

■ APLAS should be considered when a patient has venous, arterial, or small-vessel thrombosis, premature births related to preeclampsia or placental insufficiency, late miscarriages after 10 weeks, or recurrent embryonic losses (less than 10 weeks) without another explanation. Thromboses are most commonly venous. Some patients have associated neurologic symptoms like migraines, seizures, or strokes. Nonbacterial endocarditis has been reported and should be considered in the case of stroke. There is also an increased risk of myocardial infarction. Adrenal, cutaneous, ocular, osseous, and renal manifestations are also rarely associated.

■ Generally, laboratory clues can include a mild to moderate thrombocytopenia, a false positive test for syphilis, or an unexplained prolongation of the activated partial thromboplastin time (aPTT).

13. What are the Revised Sapporo Antiphospholipid Syndrome Classification Criteria?

■ The Sapporo classification criteria require at least one clinical criterion and one laboratory criterion. The laboratory criterion must be present on two occasions at least 12 weeks apart.

■ Clinical criteria can be a vascular thrombosis or pregnancy morbidity.

■ Vascular thromboses can be venous, arterial, or small vessel, in any tissue or organ. They should be confirmed on imaging, Doppler studies, or histopathology.

■ Pregnancy morbidity can be one or more unexplained fetal deaths after 10 weeks' gestation with a morphologically normal fetus; one or more premature births of a morphologically normal neonate (before 34 weeks' gestation) due to eclampsia, severe preeclampsia, or placental insufficiency; and finally three or more unexplained consecutive spontaneous abortions before the 10th week of gestation.

■ Laboratory criteria (reviewed in the "Laboratory Testing and Imaging" section) require high-titer IgG or immunoglobulin M (IgM) anti-beta-2 glycoprotein and/or anticardiolipin antibodies, and/or the presence of a lupus anticoagulant.

14. What is the management of antiphospholipid syndrome? What can be added for catastrophic antiphospholipid syndrome?

■ Treatment may vary depending on the clinical presentation and ongoing investigation. Initial management of thrombotic events is similar to that of other patients with thrombosis. Indefinite anticoagulation is recommended due to the high risk of recurrent thrombosis. Long-term warfarin (target international normalized ratio [INR] 2–3) is the treatment of choice among nonpregnant patients. A higher INR target has not shown superior outcomes in patients with an initial thrombotic event. Although limited data are available, recent studies have demonstrated inferiority of DOACs in preventing recurrent thrombosis, especially arterial, in patients with antiphospholipid syndrome. However, DOACs may be considered in patients who do not tolerate warfarin or have lower risk disease.

■ LMWH at therapeutic doses, as well as baby aspirin, is used in pregnancy for definite antiphospholipid syndrome and past thrombosis. Similar management is used for obstetric antiphospholipid syndrome during pregnancy (with the exception that prophylactic anticoagulation is often used in the absence of history of thrombosis). Some recent data suggest that women with obstetric

APLAS remain at increased long-term risk of developing thrombosis even outside of pregnancy.

■ There are conflicting data on the additional benefit of adding aspirin to warfarin in antiphospholipid syndrome following an arterial thrombosis, but it is used in pregnancy as already mentioned.

■ Antibody-positive patients who do not have a history of clinical events (thus not meeting the criteria for APLAS) are generally not anticoagulated. Treatment with hydroxychloroquine, often for a concurrent autoimmune condition, may lower thrombotic risk. Statins can also be considered in difficult-to-treat patients.

■ Laboratory monitoring of warfarin anticoagulation in antiphospholipid syndrome may be complicated by antibody interference with prothrombin times (PT) and activated prothrombin time. Chromogenic factor X assays or correlating factor II levels to the INR can be considered, among other strategies.

■ Catastrophic antiphospholipid syndrome has a high mortality rate. Therapy may include anticoagulation, steroids, plasma exchange, IVIG, and treating any potential provoking cause like infection. Some clinicians have added rituximab or eculizumab. Therapy should be administered in consultation and collaboration with rheumatology.

15. What diagnoses should be considered in splanchnic vein thrombosis?

■ Malignancy or other provoking factors (cirrhosis, pancreatitis, surgery, etc.) are the most common etiologies. These vascular territories can be associated with PNH and myeloproliferative neoplasms. Many clinicians consider testing for the *JAK2* V617F mutation and consider exon 12, or further evaluation for a myeloproliferative disorder like polycythemia vera. Antiphospholipid antibodies are also considered.

16. What diagnoses should be considered with cerebral vein thrombosis?

■ Pregnancy or other hormonal therapy is the most common provoking factor. Obesity, head trauma, and other medications including chemotherapeutic agents are also risk factors. Additionally, PNH, myeloproliferative disorders, and APLAS may be considered. There are some data to suggest that FVL and prothrombin gene mutation are seen with a higher incidence in cerebral vein thrombosis, especially in conjunction with hormonal contraception. Observational studies have also reported increased risk of cerebral vein thrombosis in patients hospitalized with Covid-19, associated with high mortality rates.

17. How does Covid-19 infection increase the risk for thrombosis?

■ The increased risk for arterial and venous thrombosis associated with Covid-19 is well-recognized, but the pathophysiology is not completely understood. It is partially attributed to the high degree of inflammation seen with severe Covid-19 infection, with laboratory values often revealing elevated platelet count, fibrinogen, D-dimer, factor VIII, and VWF antigen and activity. Some studies have also shown endothelial injury due to the Covid-19 virus. These factors are exacerbated by prolonged immobility in patients hospitalized with severe Covid-19 symptoms. Hospitalized patients should receive anticoagulation; the intensity of dosing should be individualized based on bleeding and thrombotic risk. Generally, nonhospitalized patients do not require prophylactic anticoagulation. Some evidence suggests that patients who are not critically ill and hospitalized with Covid-19 on low-flow oxygen should be placed on therapeutic anticoagulation, without needing a diagnosis of VTE. All other hospitalized Covid-19 patients (those in the ICU and those hospitalized for another reason and incidentally found to have Covid-19) should be on prophylactic anticoagulation. Patients with known thrombosis should be treated with therapeutic anticoagulation.

THROMBOSIS MANAGEMENT

1. **How long should a first, provoked, proximal deep vein thrombosis or pulmonary embolism be anticoagulated?**
   - These patients require a minimum of 3 months of anticoagulation, and extended anticoagulation should be considered for the duration of the provoking factor. Of note, thrombophilia workup is not indicated in these patients.

2. **How long should a first, unprovoked, proximal deep vein thrombosis or pulmonary embolism be anticoagulated?**
   - Indefinite anticoagulation should be considered in patients with acceptable bleeding risk. However, this may vary based on patient-specific recurrence risk, preferences, and comorbidities. Please note that after an initial period of 6 to 12 months, extended VTE prophylaxis may consist of either therapeutic or prophylactic dosing regimens, depending on the clinical situation.

3. **How long should a second, unprovoked, proximal deep vein thrombosis or pulmonary embolism be anticoagulated?**
   - Indefinite anticoagulation should, again, be considered depending on the particular circumstances.

4. **With what agent and for how long should a proximal deep vein thrombosis or pulmonary embolism be managed in the setting of active cancer?**
   - The efficacy of oral factor Xa inhibitors and LMWH are equal in terms of reducing risk of recurrent venous thrombosis in patients with cancer. Both are thought to be superior to warfarin, although the data comparing DOACs with warfarin are limited. Factor Xa inhibitors, including apixaban, rivaroxaban and edoxaban, may be chosen over LMWH to avoid daily injections. There are conflicting data regarding increased risk for bleeding with DOACs in patients with gastrointestinal (GI) or genitourinary (GU) cancers, and some providers avoid their use in these patients. At least 3 to 6 months of therapy is indicated, but many providers continue anticoagulation as long as patients have ongoing risk factors (active cancer, immobility, etc.).

5. **What are the treatment options for distal/calf deep vein thromboses?**
   - Deep vein thromboses of the anterior/posterior tibial, peroneal, or muscular veins of the calf (gastrocnemius or soleal veins), in the absence of popliteal or more proximal involvement, may be anticoagulated similar to a proximal deep vein thrombosis. This is often done if patients have significant symptoms or risk factors for propagation (immobility, active cancer, history of thrombosis, etc.). Alternatively, reliable patients can be monitored with serial ultrasounds and anticoagulated if thrombus extension is observed. The ultrasound is often repeated at 7 to 14 days.

6. **What are the treatment options for superficial deep vein thrombosis?**
   - Management depends on the clinical scenario and veins affected. For a superficial vein thrombosis under 5 cm in length, distant from the confluence with the deep veins (the saphenofemoral junction), supportive care is indicated. Surgical intervention or antibiotic therapy may be indicated in select situations.
   - For patients with superficial venous thrombosis that is close to the saphenofemoral junction, or longer than 5 cm, anticoagulation is indicated, typically for 45 days in duration. Fondaparinux and rivaroxaban are commonly considered agents at prophylactic doses, but other DOACs, unfractionated heparin, and LMWH are also likely effective.

7. **What considerations are needed for managing acute splanchnic vein thrombosis (hepatic vein, portal vein, mesenteric vein, splenic vein)?**
   - Treatment of the underlying predisposing condition (if possible) and starting anticoagulation, if safe to do so, are optimal to reduce the risk of developing bowel infarction and portal hypertension. Given the potential for esophageal varices from underlying portal hypertension, management of or screening for varices may be indicated before starting anticoagulation. However, some providers do not anticoagulate asymptomatic, incidentally detected thromboses. Many of these patients are at high risk for bleeding, given underlying cirrhosis, malignancy, and/or thrombocytopenia from splenomegaly. Data on the management of chronic thrombosis are controversial.

8. **What are absolute or relative contraindications to anticoagulation?**
   - Anticoagulation is often avoided or dose-adjusted in the setting of thrombocytopenia (platelets less than $30{,}000$–$50{,}000 \times 10^9$/L), around the time of surgery, in the setting of intracranial hemorrhage, in patients with a severe bleeding diathesis, or with recent or active bleeding.
   - The risks and benefits of anticoagulation must be carefully considered with esophageal varices, gastrointestinal telangiectasias, altered drug metabolism as a result of liver or renal impairment, trauma, active labor, large abdominal aortic aneurysms with uncontrolled hypertension, stable aortic dissections, peptic ulcer disease, poor follow-up or social support, substance abuse, central nervous system lesions, and those at risk for falls or trauma.

9. **What should be considered in a patient with a venous thrombosis that cannot be anticoagulated?**
   - A temporary IVC filter can be considered. This should be removed as soon as feasible to avoid long-term complications of IVC filters (perforation, increased lower extremity deep vein thrombosis, etc.).

10. **When should thrombolytic therapy be considered?**
    - The decision to pursue thrombolysis is very complex, patient-specific, and generally beyond the scope of this review. It can be considered in the care of patients who are hemodynamically unstable as a result of massive pulmonary embolism, in carefully selected patients without contraindications who experience an ischemic stroke, in select cases of myocardial infarction, and in select episodes of arterial thrombosis. Thrombolytic therapy can be administered systemically or catheter-directed.
    - Management decisions depend on the severity and clinical manifestations of the thrombotic event within the clinical context of the specific patient,

especially bleeding risk, given the potential for catastrophic bleeding complications. Mechanical thrombectomy alone may be used in some situations. Care is often multidisciplinary, influenced by institutional resources and expertise.

THROMBOSIS COMPLICATIONS

1. **What diagnosis should be considered if a patient is found to have pulmonary hypertension or unexplained exertional dyspnea? What imaging should be considered? What is the treatment?**
   - Chronic thromboembolic pulmonary hypertension (CTEPH) can be a complication of long-standing obstruction of the pulmonary arteries, eventually leading to pulmonary hypertension and right-sided heart failure. Ventilation perfusion scans and CT angiography are usually the initial diagnostic imaging tests. Echocardiography and right heart catheterization are often part of the evaluation. There are several other differential diagnoses that should be excluded in the workup. Treatment includes anticoagulation, consideration of surgical intervention, and pulmonary hypertension therapies. Patients may have other sequelae of pulmonary embolism (PE), including post-PE syndrome and chronic thromboembolic disease (CTED). Post-PE syndrome is due to changes in pulmonary artery flow, pulmonary gas exchange, or cardiac function after acute PE and usually presents as chronic dyspnea or decreased exercise capacity. CTED is persistent pulmonary vascular obstruction on imaging without evidence of pulmonary hypertension and also often causes symptoms of dyspnea.

2. **How is postthrombotic syndrome (PTS) diagnosed? What treatments are available?**
   - PTS is a complication of deep venous thrombosis that results from damage to the valves within the vein that normally help in returning blood back to the heart, culminating in aberrant venous flow, resulting in symptoms including extremity pain, skin color change, swelling, and when severe, ulceration.
   - The diagnosis is largely clinical and may utilize a clinical score like the Villalta score. Treatment can include compression garments, leg elevation, skin care, and when severe, endovascular or surgical intervention.

LABORATORY TESTING AND IMAGING

1. **What initial labs could be assessed with a patient experiencing venous or arterial thrombosis?**
   - For most patients, a laboratory evaluation will include a comprehensive blood count and a creatinine and liver function tests. Baseline coagulation tests (PT, aPTT) are also considerations. This is used less often to determine the cause of the thrombosis than to guide management.
   - Renal and hepatic function may have implications for anticoagulant choice. They also may suggest a primary or secondary renal or hepatic disease. Erythrocytosis or anemia, thrombocytosis or thrombocytopenia, or abnormal white blood cell values may require further investigation. As examples, thrombocytopenia may suggest portal hypertension or a marrow-replacing process and may influence bleeding risk when determining anticoagulation. Thrombocytosis may be indicative of iron deficiency, inflammation, or a myeloproliferative neoplasm.

Erythrocytosis can be seen with polycythemia vera or a variety of secondary causes like testosterone use. Anemia also has a broad differential but could suggest a hematologic malignancy, a marrow infiltrative disorder, blood loss, or a variety of other conditions; as with thrombocytopenia, severe anemia may be a consideration when considering anticoagulation risk.

- An elevated baseline PT/INR can be indicative of liver disease, vitamin K deficiency, and more. A prolonged aPTT, at baseline, can be associated with the presence of lupus anticoagulant. These tests can influence subsequent anticoagulation monitoring and diagnostic testing. Fibrinogen can be tested if there is a concern for disseminated intravascular coagulation or as part of an evaluation for dysfibrinogenemia.
- A peripheral blood smear can be considered to investigate abnormalities on the complete blood count (CBC) and may be informative of hemolysis (as in disseminated intravascular coagulation, PNH, thrombotic thrombocytopenic purpura [TTP]/hemolytic uremic syndrome [HUS], etc.), evidence of myelophthisis or marrow involvement, pseudothrombocytopenia, and more.
- Patients with recent heparin exposure may be tested for HIT, using an immunoassay (e.g., antiplatelet factor 4 assay) and/or a functional platelet activation assay (e.g., serotonin release assay) if indicated based on estimated clinical probability.
- A D-dimer is often considered for diagnostic purposes. Patients with a low pretest probability of deep vein thrombosis, as determined by a clinical decision rule like the Wells score, generally do not need further workup if the D-dimer is negative. Similarly, a negative high-sensitivity D-dimer can negate the need for further workup in a patient with a moderate pretest probability of deep vein thrombosis.
- Inflammation markers like an erythrocyte sedimentation rate and C-reactive protein can be useful when considering malignancy or inflammatory conditions like inflammatory bowel disease.
- A urinalysis can screen for proteinuria as is seen in nephrotic syndrome and can assess for hematuria, hemoglobinuria (as seen in PNH), or urine sediment.
- Depending on the clinical situation, serum or urine protein electrophoresis, tests for rheumatic conditions, and other laboratory studies or imaging may be entertained.
- In an otherwise asymptomatic individual, extensive screening for malignancy beyond what is indicated by age has been shown to be of low yield and is therefore discouraged.

2. What imaging is used in the diagnosis of VTE?

- Compression venous ultrasonography is the primary test for extremity venous thrombosis. Negative whole-leg compression ultrasonography does not require further investigation if a more proximal venous thrombosis is not suspected. If only a proximal ultrasound is performed, a repeat ultrasound at 1 week may be indicated based on patient risk and biomarker testing.
- Deep vein extremity thrombosis can also be assessed with CT venography or MR venography, and conventional contrast venography. The contrast agent or use of a magnet may be contraindicated in some patients. Conventional venography is invasive and can cause complications, including provoking thrombosis.

- MR venography and CT venography are the tests of choice for cerebral venous thrombosis.
- Splanchnic venous thrombosis can be diagnosed with CT, MR, or ultrasound with Doppler depending on the clinical situation and vascular bed of concern.
- Ventilation perfusion scans are considered to diagnose suspected pulmonary embolism when CT angiography is contraindicated, as with severe renal insufficiency. This is limited when patients have preexisting lung disease. MR pulmonary angiography, echocardiography, and conventional catheter-directed angiography are other imaging modalities considered for the diagnosis of pulmonary embolism.

3. **When is thrombophilia testing indicated?**
   - Thrombophilia testing is controversial. Generally, thrombophilia testing should only be considered when it would change management. Testing for inherited thrombophilias is discouraged by several organizations, including the Choosing Wisely initiative, for VTE that occurs around a major transient risk factor like surgery. Testing is low yield when an alternative explanation is present like an active malignancy, for women with pregnancy complications (pregnancy loss, abruption, preeclampsia, and intrauterine growth restriction), in the absence of a history of thrombosis (testing for antiphospholipid syndrome may be indicated), and in general for arterial thrombosis, especially at an older age.
   - Testing for an inherited thrombophilia is often considered with a strong family history of VTE. Some clinicians consider testing for thrombophilia in young patients, those with recurrent events, or when it is a nonextremity venous thrombosis (splanchnic vein or cerebral vein).
   - Protein C or S deficiency is commonly considered with warfarin-induced skin necrosis.

4. **What are the tests for the most common hereditary thrombophilias?**
   - FVL and prothrombin G20210A mutation can be tested directly with genetic testing and the tests are therefore not affected by anticoagulant therapy. Alternatively, to screen for FVL mutation, some clot-based tests for activated protein C resistance are used. A positive test shows a reduced anticoagulant effect in patient plasma from the addition of a standard amount of activated protein C, most often due to FVL mutation. Functional tests can be affected by the presence of a lupus anticoagulant or direct factor inhibitors. While most commonly due to FVL mutation, activated protein C resistance can result from protein S deficiency, high levels of factor VIII, in the setting of malignancy, and more.
   - Recall that protein C deficiency can be a quantitative defect (type 1) or a functional defect of protein C (type 2). Deficiency is most often evaluated using functional assays that can detect both types of disease, but immunoassays are also available. Furthermore, anticoagulation, vitamin K deficiency, liver disease, and consumption from acute thrombosis or acute illness can affect levels, making the diagnosis more challenging. Protein C activity is generally the initial test used to screen for protein C deficiency.
   - Protein S deficiency is challenging to diagnose. Recall that protein S circulates bound to C4b-binding protein and as a free form. Given that C4b-binding protein is an acute phase reactant and the potential for interference with functional assays due to activated protein C resistance and elevated factor VIII activity, the

diagnosis should not be made around an acute thrombosis. Immunoassays a
often used, given that they can detect both free protein S and total protein S
As with protein C deficiency, caution is needed when evaluating for this condition because vitamin K deficiency, pregnancy or estrogen hormones, liver disease, times of increased utilization, and anticoagulants can influence results.
Free protein S antigen is generally the initial test used for screening for protein
S deficiency.

- Antithrombin deficiency is commonly assessed using functional assays as they
can detect both types of disease (quantitative—type 1 and qualitative—type 2),
but immunoassays are also available. Caution is necessary given that anticoagulants can influence the results and a variety of conditions (nephrotic syndrome,
extracorporeal membrane oxygenation [ECMO], asparaginase, liver disease,
acute thrombosis, etc.) can cause an acquired antithrombin deficiency. While
ideally tested away outside from acute thrombosis, a rapid evaluation may be
needed, especially if considering heparin therapy, given the potential for heparin resistance. Antithrombin activity is often used for screening for antithrombin
deficiency.

5. **What is the cause and significance of an elevated serum homocysteine value? Is therapy indicated to reduce the risk of venous thrombosis?**
   - An elevated homocysteine level can be hereditary or acquired. Hereditary causes
   are most commonly due to mutations in the methylene tetrahydrofolate reductase (*MTHFR*) gene that result in reduced enzymatic activity. Acquired causes of
   hyperhomocysteinemia include folic acid, B_6, or B_{12} deficiencies.
   - Significantly elevated homocysteine levels have been suggested as a risk factor
   for cardiovascular, cerebrovascular, peripheral arterial, and venous thromboembolic disease; however, this is controversial and confounding may explain
   prior study results. Screening for elevated homocysteine is not routinely suggested for primary or secondary prevention of VTE based on trials not showing
   evidence of benefit for treating these patients with vitamin supplementation.
   MTHFR mutations are not associated with increased risk of thrombosis and
   should not be tested for in patients with thrombosis. Treatment of thromboses is the same as that in the general population. However, homocystinuria,
   which can present with high homocysteine levels, can be associated with an
   increased risk of thrombosis and should be evaluated when there is suspicion
   of this condition.

6. **What laboratory tests are used for the diagnosis of HIT?**
   - When testing is indicated, an immunoassay (e.g., antiplatelet factor 4 antibody
   testing by ELISA) is often used to screen for HIT due to the high sensitivity.
   However, it has a low specificity. A functional assay like platelet ^{14}C-serotonin
   release assay is considered the "gold standard" laboratory test for HIT due to
   the high sensitivity and specificity; when available, this test is suggested if an
   immunoassay is positive.

7. **What tests are used for the diagnosis of APLAS?**
   - While clinical correlation is necessary for a diagnosis of APLAS, laboratory
   abnormalities must be present on two occasions, at least 12 weeks apart.
   - The presence of a lupus anticoagulant is indicated by the prolongation of a phospholipid-dependent coagulation test (like the aPTT, dilute PT, dilute Russell's

viper venom time, or kaolin clotting time) plus failure of that prolonged clotting time to correct with normal plasma but correction with excess phospholipids. Exclusion of other coagulation defects is also required.

- A high-titer (>99th percentile) IgG or IgM isotype anticardiolipin antibodies by ELISA suggests diagnosis of antiphospholipid antibody syndrome.
- A high-titer (>99th percentile) test of IgG or IgM isotype β_2Gp1 antibodies by ELISA suggests diagnosis of antiphospholipid antibody syndrome.
- Positivity for all three tests and higher titers of antibodies predict a higher thrombotic risk.

8. **What tests can indicate the presence of a dysfibrinogenemia?**
- Elevated thrombin and reptilase times can be suggestive of a dysfibrinogenemia. Testing fibrinogen by an immunologic method often gives a higher value than a functional method; therefore, an elevated ratio of a fibrinogen antigen to activity can be suggestive. Genetic testing can be performed.

9. **What tests could suggest a diagnosis of PNH? What test confirms the diagnosis?**
- Labs in PNH will typically show findings consistent with a hemolytic anemia and pancytopenia. The urine is notable for hemosiderinuria and potentially hemoglobinuria. Urine dipstick will often be positive for blood, but microscopy will be negative for hematuria.
- The diagnosis is established with flow cytometry showing an absence or reduction in glycosylphosphatidylinositol (GPI)-linked proteins like CD59 or CD55. The presence of the GPI anchor is assessed using fluorescent aerolysin (FLAER).

ANTIPLATELET AND ANTICOAGULANT DRUGS

1. **What is the mechanism of action and half-life of aspirin? How can the effect of aspirin be reversed?**
- Aspirin acetylates and irreversibly inhibits cyclooxygenase, ultimately resulting in a reduction of thromboxane A_2, interfering with platelet aggregation. It has a half-life of about 20 minutes at low doses but has an irreversible effect on platelets.
- After about 7 to 10 days, new platelets will replace those acetylated by aspirin, giving the option of holding aspirin for 5 to 10 days before a nonemergent procedure. If it has been a short time since aspirin ingestion, platelet transfusion can be considered for urgent bleeding.

2. **What is the mechanism of action of clopidogrel, prasugrel, and ticagrelor? Can the effect be reversed?**
- These drugs act primarily on the adenosine diphosphate (ADP) receptor and thus reduce platelet activation and aggregation. They have a half-life of about 7 to 10 hours and the drugs can be held in nonurgent scenarios. In critical bleeding, platelet transfusion can be considered, but the antiplatelet drugs or their metabolites could inhibit the transfused platelets.

3. **What is the mechanism of action of abciximab, eptifibatide, or tirofiban?**
   - These intravenous drugs act on the GPIIb/IIIa receptor and can work to prevent platelet aggregation. Recall that this is the receptor that is defective in Glanzmann thrombasthenia.

4. **What is the mechanism of action of heparin or LMWH? Can the effect be reversed? How are these drugs monitored?**
   - Unfractionated heparin exerts an anticoagulant effect by binding antithrombin and potentiating its effects. This results in the inactivation of several clotting factors, in particular thrombin (factor IIa) and factor Xa. Heparin is processed in the reticuloendothelial system and ultimately degraded in the liver. It is a highly charged molecule and binds nonspecifically to plasma proteins and cells. It can be monitored by anti-Xa heparin levels or by following regular aPTT and adjusting the infusion by a standard nomogram. Reversal can be achieved by protamine sulfate; there is a small risk of anaphylaxis. Heparin resistance can be seen with antithrombin deficiency or by nonspecific binding of heparin to off-target cells or proteins (especially in an inflammatory state), with an inadequate amount left for therapy.
   - LMWHs also bind antithrombin, but their smaller size results in less inactivation of thrombin (factor IIa) relative to unfractionated heparin, thus resulting in greater activity against factor Xa relative to thrombin (factor IIa). Due to limited thrombin inhibition, the aPTT cannot be used to monitor therapy. However, anti-Xa levels can be used for this purpose and may be considered, such as in obese patients. LMWHs have a more predictable pharmacokinetic profile and clearance. Therefore, they can be given once or twice daily as a subcutaneous formulation. LMWH should be dose-adjusted or avoided in the setting of renal insufficiency. It can be partially reversed with protamine sulfate; andexanet could also be considered (studied, not Food and Drug Administration [FDA]-approved).

5. **What is the mechanism of fondaparinux? Can the effect be reversed? How can it be monitored?**
   - Fondaparinux similarly binds to antithrombin and primarily acts to facilitate the inactivation of factor Xa. It is administered subcutaneously once daily based on weight. It should be avoided in the setting of renal insufficiency. It can be monitored using anti-Xa levels and does not have a standardized reversal strategy at this time (theoretically andexanet could be considered).

6. **What is the mechanism of action of argatroban and bivalirudin? How can these drugs be monitored?**
   - These drugs are intravenous direct thrombin inhibitors, most commonly used for suspected or confirmed HIT. They have short half-lives and currently do not have a formal reversal agent. Argatroban is hepatically cleared, while bivalirudin is renally cleared. They can be monitored by the aPTT, but they also notably affect the PT, which must be considered when transitioning to warfarin. Some antifactor IIa assays can be used to monitor these drugs as well.

What is the mechanism of action of warfarin? What patient counseling is needed? How is warfarin monitored?

- Warfarin inhibits the enzymes necessary to reduce vitamin K, which is required for the gamma-carboxylation of coagulation factors II, VII, IX, and X and the anticoagulant proteins C and S. It has numerous drug interactions and dietary interactions with a relatively narrow therapeutic window. Monitoring of warfarin is done with the PT, which is standardized using the INR. An INR of 2 to 3 is targeted for most indications, but a higher target is used in some situations, like mechanical heart valves. When starting warfarin for an acute VTE, it is advised to have about 5 days of overlap with a parenteral anticoagulant, given the potential for a transient period of hypercoagulability, as the natural anticoagulant proteins C and S decrease prior to achieving therapeutic levels of the remaining vitamin K-dependent clotting factors. Warfarin can be effectively used in patients with renal disease; PT-/INR-based monitoring may be challenging in advanced hepatic disease.
- Warfarin is teratogenic and appropriate measures should be taken to prevent pregnancy for patients with childbearing potential. Patients should be educated on maintaining a consistent amount of dietary vitamin K and caution for interacting drugs. Given the long half-life, LMWH or intravenous (IV) heparin is considered for "bridging" anticoagulation in patients with high thrombotic risk when warfarin must be interrupted (surgery or procedures).
- Warfarin that needs to be reversed due to bleeding, supratherapeutic levels, or surgery can be managed by holding the drug, oral or IV vitamin K, fresh frozen plasma, or prothrombin complex concentrates. The intensity and method of reversal depend on the clinical situation, balancing bleeding and thrombotic risk.

8. **What are the DOACs and their mechanisms of action? What are their dosing schedules, toxicities, and general management?**
   - DOACs include apixaban, rivaroxaban, edoxaban, and dabigatran. Dabigatran is a direct thrombin inhibitor, while the first three inhibit factor Xa. They all have a rapid time (hours) to peak onset of action and a half-life around 10 to 14 hours. Dabigatran and apixaban are dosed twice daily, while the others are daily. Notable differences include dabigatran being associated with dyspepsia, rivaroxaban needs to be taken with food, and apixaban having the least renal clearance. Both dabigatran and edoxaban were studied with 5 days of bridging parenteral anticoagulation for acute VTE, while apixaban and rivaroxaban were given at higher initial doses in the beginning without parenteral anticoagulation bridging.
   - Patients on DOACs are generally not bridged for procedures or surgeries; instead medications are held.
   - Dabigatran is the most renally cleared. Reversal depends on the clinical situation but it could include idarucizumab (direct reversal agent), oral charcoal if recent ingestion, dialysis, or simply holding the medication. Reversal of the remaining DOACs can be managed by holding the drugs, giving prothrombin complex concentrates (limited data), or using a direct reversal agent for the anti-Xa medication in the setting of acute major bleeding (andexanet alfa; currently FDA-approved for apixaban and rivaroxaban reversal only, limited high quality data).

TABLE 10.3

Anticoagulant	Target	Dosing	Half-life*	Uses	Features
Apixaban	Xa	Oral BID	~12 hours	AF, VTE	Least renal clearance of DOACs
Edoxaban	Xa	Oral daily	~12 hours	AF, VTE	–
Rivaroxaban	Xa	Oral daily	~12 hours	AF, VTE	Need to take with food
Dabigatran	IIa	Oral BID	~15 hours	AF, VTE	Associated with dyspepsia
Argatroban	IIa	IV	~1 hour	HIT	Hepatic clearance
Bivalirudin	IIa	IV	~<1 hour	PCI (with HIT)	–
Heparin	IIa, Xa	IV	~1.5 hours	ACS, AF, VTE	Monitor aPTT or anti-Xa to dose
LMWH	Xa>IIa	SubQ daily—BID	~6 hours	ACS, VTE	Renal clearance, weight-based dosing
Fondaparinux	Xa	SubQ daily	~19 hours	VTE	Weight-based dosing, renally cleared
Warfarin	II, VII, IX, X, protein C + S	Oral daily	~40 hours, variable	AF, VTE	Drug/dietary interactions, monitor with INR
Aspirin (low dose)	COX	Oral daily	~20 minutes	AF, CAD, VTE, PAD, PP	Affects platelets for 7–10 days
Clopidogrel, prasugrel, ticagrelor	ADP	Oral daily to oral BID	~7–10 hours	ACS	–
Abciximab, eptifibatide, tirofiban	GPIIb/IIIa	IV	Minutes–hours	PCI	–

*Plasma half-life.

ACS, acute coronary syndrome; ADP, adenosine diphosphate; AF, atrial fibrillation; aPTT, activated partial thromboplastin time; CAD, coronary artery disease; COX, cyclooxygenase; DOAC, direct oral anticoagulant; GP, glycoprotein; HIT, heparin-induced thrombocytopenia; INR, international normalized ratio; LMWH, low-molecular-weight heparin; PCI, percutaneous coronary intervention; PP, primary prevention; SubQ, subcutaneously; VTE, venous thromboembolism.

QUESTIONS

1. A 27-year-old male with a history of an unprovoked right lower extremity proximal deep vein thrombosis 3 years ago is admitted with a severely symptomatic left lower extremity deep vein thrombosis. He is started on intravenous (IV) heparin with a bolus. He has consistently subtherapeutic anti-Xa lab values despite high doses of heparin administration and is ultimately discharged on warfarin. He does well until he experiences a recurrent event when bridging back to warfarin after an urgent appendectomy. He is referred for further evaluation. Which of the following is the most likely etiology of his thrombosis?
   A. May–Thurner syndrome (iliac vein compression syndrome)
   B. Antithrombin deficiency
   C. Factor V Leiden gene mutation
   D. Paroxysmal nocturnal hemoglobinuria

2. A 54-year-old male is admitted after a motor vehicle accident. He has a splenic laceration, a nondisplaced humerus fracture, and several fractured ribs. His admission labs show a hemoglobin of 13.6 g/dL, white blood cell count of 6.5×10^9/L, and platelets of 285×10^9/L. He receives supportive care with analgesics and immobilization of his arm. He is discharged to inpatient rehabilitation after 1 week of inpatient care. At this point, he complains of left lower extremity pain, and a lower extremity ultrasound confirms an acute deep vein thrombosis of the left lower extremity. Repeat complete blood count (CBC) shows a hemoglobin of 11.4 g/dL, white blood count of 8.2×10^9/L, and platelets of 141×10^9/L. Renal function, hepatic function, and a baseline set of coagulation tests are normal. He denies any bleeding and has had an otherwise uncomplicated hospital course. The patient is started on intravenous heparin. What would you suggest as the next step in management?
   A. Bridge to warfarin for 3 months for provoked deep vein thrombosis (DVT).
   B. Send a hypercoagulable workup.
   C. Change to a nonheparin anticoagulant and test for heparin-induced thrombocytopenia (HIT).
   D. Discharge on twice-daily low-molecular-weight heparin (LMWH).

3. A 65-year-old male with a history of obesity, nicotine dependence, obstructive sleep apnea, and coronary artery disease presents with a 3-day history of worsening abdominal pain. A CT of the abdomen shows an acute, occluding portal vein thrombosis but an otherwise normal-appearing liver. Labs show a hemoglobin of 17.6 g/dL, hematocrit of 50%, white blood cell count of 9.2×10^9/L, and platelets of 395×10^9/L. Renal and liver function tests are normal. Lactate dehydrogenase (LDH), haptoglobin, and a peripheral blood smear are normal. Urine dipstick and microscopy are also normal. Which of the following is the most likely to explain the cause of this patient's thrombosis?

A. Liver biopsy
B. Anticardiolipin antibodies, lupus anticoagulant, and anti-beta-2 glyco-
   protein antibodies
C. Flow cytometry for paroxysmal nocturnal hemoglobinuria (PNH)
D. *JAK2 V617F* mutation

4. A 62-year-old female was found to have bilateral segmental
   pulmonary emboli on a routine follow-up scan for stage IV, metastatic
   adenocarcinoma of the lung. Her chronic shortness of breath has been
   unchanged and she has recently been receiving palliative chemotherapy.
   A complete blood count (CBC) shows a hemoglobin of 9.2 g/dL, white
   blood cell count of 4.2×10^9/L, and platelets of 90×10^9/L. These values
   are consistent with her labs after past cycles of chemotherapy. Renal
   function and hepatic function are normal. Which of the following would
   you suggest?
   A. Warfarin with a goal international normalized ratio (INR) of 2 to 3
   B. Dabigatran
   C. Low-molecular-weight heparin
   D. No therapy given that it is asymptomatic

5. A 71-year-old male with a past medical history of hypertension, transient
   ischemic attack, coronary artery disease, type 2 diabetes mellitus, and
   gastroesophageal reflux disease presents for routine follow-up. He has
   been on warfarin for several years for his atrial fibrillation but would like
   to transition to a direct oral anticoagulant (DOAC). He travels frequently
   and does not eat regular or large meals. He has no liver disease or renal
   disease. He is on several medications that he takes twice daily but none
   has drug interactions with the DOACs. His international normalized
   ratios (INRs) have been stable in the range of 2 to 3. His body mass
   index (BMI) is 28 kg/m². Which anticoagulant would you suggest?
   A. Apixaban
   B. Dabigatran
   C. Rivaroxaban
   D. Continuation of warfarin

6. A 37-year-old female is admitted for a right segmental pulmonary
   embolism from which she had pleuritic chest pain and shortness of
   breath. She had delivered her second child about 9 months ago and
   recently drove 3 hours for her job in pharmaceutical sales. She has no
   significant medical history but does note that she had preeclampsia
   with both of her previous pregnancies. Additionally, she had one
   miscarriage at 11 weeks' gestation. Physical exam is normal. Labs show
   a normal complete blood count and comprehensive metabolic panel.
   Pregnancy test is negative. She is started on intravenous (IV) heparin
   and is planned to transition to warfarin. Homocysteine is elevated at 22
   mcmol/L, protein S antigen is 67%, and anticardiolipin antibodies and
   beta-2 glycoprotein 1 antibodies are strongly positive. Protein C and
   antithrombin activity are within the reference range, and no mutation

of factor V Leiden or the prothrombin gene is seen. The patient has no history of thrombosis. What is the best next step in management?

A. Suggest long-term warfarin for antiphospholipid syndrome.

B. Suggest warfarin for protein S deficiency for 3 months. Recheck protein S after holding anticoagulation at 3 months.

C. Test for the methylene tetrahydrofolate reductase (*MTHFR*) gene mutation for hyperhomocysteinemia.

D. Suggest warfarin therapy with repeat testing for anticardiolipin, beta-2 glycoprotein 1 antibodies, and a lupus anticoagulant in 3 months.

7. A 32-year-old, G1P0 woman with a history of obesity is at approximately 28 weeks' gestation with an uncomplicated pregnancy to date. She presents to the ED with a primary concern of shortness of breath and pleuritic chest discomfort. She endorses a 1-week history of left calf pain and swelling. She has no personal or family history of venous thromboembolism. Her heart rate is 105, with a normal blood pressure. Physical exam shows her chest to be clear but confirms left lower extremity pain and tenderness. Which is the best next step in management?

A. CT pulmonary angiography

B. Ventilation perfusion scan

C. D-dimer

D. Venous compression ultrasonography of the lower extremities

8. A 56-year-old male presents for a routine follow-up appointment 8 weeks after having a right knee arthroscopy. He notes an area of warmth, pain, and swelling on the inner aspect of his right calf. He has no history of venous thromboembolism. Exam shows swelling and warmth over the right calf but no varicose veins or evidence of infection. Labs include a normal complete blood count and liver function tests, and a normal creatinine. Lower extremity venous ultrasonography shows no evidence of deep vein thrombosis but does confirm a superficial vein thrombosis that is reported to be nearly 6 cm in length. It is not in close proximity to the saphenofemoral junction. You are asked for management recommendations. Which of the following would be the best next step in management?

A. Repeat ultrasound in 7 to 10 days

B. Enoxaparin bridge to warfarin, continue anticoagulation for at least 3 months

C. Enoxaparin bridge to warfarin, continue anticoagulation for at least 45 days

D. Fondaparinux, prophylactic dose for at least 45 days

ANSWERS

1. **B. Antithrombin deficiency.** The patient had a clot at a young age with no clear provoking factors. His labs suggested resistance to IV heparin. Of the choices listed, this would be most consistent with antithrombin deficiency. A heparin resistance phenomenon can also be observed with elevated heparin binding proteins (i.e., inflammation), increased heparin clearance, and when other coagulation factors are elevated. May–Thurner syndrome would be expected to cause left lower extremity clots, although would not expect to see heparin resistance. While factor V Leiden mutation is a common thrombophilia, it does not explain this patient's heparin response. Paroxysmal nocturnal hemoglobinuria is similarly not suggested in this scenario.

2. **C. Change to a nonheparin anticoagulant and test for heparin-induced thrombocytopenia (HIT).** The patient in this vignette has a presentation concerning for HIT. Over a course of 5 to 10 days, he experienced a 50% drop in his platelets and developed a new thrombosis. There are other possible explanations for the thrombocytopenia. The 4Ts score is therefore 7. Further evaluation and empiric management for HIT are indicated. Transitioning to warfarin in the setting of potential HIT would not be appropriate and risks complications of warfarin-induced skin necrosis. A hypercoagulable workup is not indicated as this DVT may be provoked by a hospitalization or potentially HIT. All forms of heparin including LMWH should be avoided in patients with a potential HIT diagnosis. Of note, increasing evidence supports the use of direct oral anticoagulants (DOACs) in HIT, but usually patients will have an initial course of parenteral anticoagulation before switching to a DOAC.

3. **D. *JAK2 V617F* mutation.** The patient presents with a portal vein thrombosis in the setting of an elevated hemoglobin and hematocrit. While the patient has risk factors for secondary erythrocytosis, this is concerning for a myeloproliferative disorder like polycythemia vera. Testing for the *JAK2* mutation would be appropriate to evaluate for this. PNH and antiphospholipid antibody syndrome could also be associated with a portal vein thrombosis. However, there is no evidence of hemolysis or suggestion of hemoglobinuria as could be seen with PNH. Antiphospholipid syndrome would not explain the elevated hemoglobin.

4. **C. Low-molecular-weight heparin.** The patient is diagnosed incidentally with a cancer-associated thrombosis (CAT). Low-molecular-weight heparin has been shown to be superior to warfarin for the treatment of CAT. Studies have shown that select direct oral anticoagulants are noninferior to low-molecular-weight heparin. However, there are currently no data to support the use of dabigatran. Therapy is indicated for this segmental pulmonary embolism, even in the absence of symptoms.

5. **A. Apixaban.** Of the listed DOACs, apixaban would be the most appropriate. Given the history of gastroesophageal reflux disease, dabigatran could be avoided as it is more likely to exacerbate this condition. Dabigatran is coated in tartaric acid to help adsorption, and gastrointestinal symptoms were a common reason for discontinuation in clinical trials. Rivaroxaban has to be taken with meals and should be dosed daily. Given that the patient does not eat regular meals, it may be best to use a medication that does not require consistent food intake. Apixaban is twice daily, but the patient is already taking twice-daily medications. The patient has expressed a preference to transition to a DOAC. As long as the patient understands the risks and benefits of the DOACs, transitioning from warfarin would be reasonable. However, with certain drug interactions, liver disease, renal impairment, compliance concerns, a history of a mechanical heart valve, or need for rapid reversal, continuing warfarin may be best. In the past, DOACs were avoided in patients with extreme body weights, but recent retrospective studies reveal DOACs appear safe in this patient population, but testing levels could be considered.

6. **D. Suggest warfarin therapy with repeat testing for anticardiolipin, beta-2 glycoprotein 1 antibodies, and a lupus anticoagulant in 3 months.** This patient could have antiphospholipid syndrome based on the strongly positive antibodies and the history of miscarriage. Furthermore, she had a pulmonary embolism without a strong provoking factor. However, the diagnosis requires the laboratory testing to be positive on two occasions, at least 12 weeks apart. Therefore, repeating the testing is indicated. Long-term warfarin would likely be suggested in the setting of antiphospholipid syndrome. In the setting of acute thrombosis, testing for protein S deficiency can be misleading and taking the patient off anticoagulation could be risky. This patient has another potential explanation for her pulmonary embolism and further evaluation of the low protein S level may not change management. If this patient was being considered for discontinuing anticoagulation, retesting could be considered either off of warfarin for 4 weeks (which lowers protein S) or on heparin/low-molecular-weight heparin therapy. If the protein S level was very low, warfarin may not be the best choice of anticoagulant, given some potential risk for warfarin-induced skin necrosis. This is unlikely, given the mild reduction in protein S here. *MTHFR* is the enzyme-involved folate metabolism that is commonly mutated and can result in hyperhomocysteinemia. However, *MTHFR* mutations are not associated with an increased risk of thrombosis.

7. **D. Venous compression ultrasonography of the lower extremities.** The patient is pregnant and has clinical symptoms suggestive of a lower extremity deep vein thrombosis and pulmonary embolism. To avoid the radiation associated with a CT scan or ventilation perfusion scan, many clinicians favor lower extremity ultrasound. If the diagnosis of venous thromboembolism is confirmed, anticoagulation can be initiated without additional diagnostic testing that may have risk. Given the higher pretest probability of venous thromboembolism in pregnancy, D-dimer screening is avoided in pregnant patients and this patient would be considered high risk based on presentation.

8. **D. Fondaparinux, prophylactic dose for at least 45 days.** Given the
   length of the superficial vein thrombosis, anticoagulation is generally
   pursued for symptomatic patients with an acceptable bleeding risk. Most
   often, prophylactic dosed anticoagulation can be given for approximately
   45 days with repeat clinical assessment. Monitoring with sequential repeat
   ultrasound can be considered in the case of patients with shorter segment
   superficial vein thromboses that remain away from the saphenofemoral
   junction and that do not have extensive risk factors for deep vein
   thrombosis, like active malignancy. While warfarin would likely be effective,
   studies have supported the use of prophylactic doses of anticoagulation
   for a short duration. Therefore, prophylactic fondaparinux would be the
   most appropriate choice of the listed options.

Chronic Myeloid Leukemia

11

Charles E. Foucar, Rami N. Khoriaty, and Dale L. Bixby

EPIDEMIOLOGY

1. **What is the median age at diagnosis of chronic myeloid leukemia (CML)?**
   - 67 years, with incidence increasing with age

ETIOLOGY AND RISK FACTORS

1. **What is one possible causative factor?**
   - High doses of ionizing radiation (therapeutic radiation or accidental exposures)

2. **What two genes are involved in the hallmark Philadelphia (Ph) chromosomal translocation of CML and what chromosomes are they on?**
   - *ABL1* proto-oncogene on chromosome 9 and *breakpoint cluster region (BCR)* on chromosome 22

3. **What is the protein product of balanced translocation between the long arms of chromosomes 9 and 22?**
   - The BCR-ABL1 oncoprotein

DIAGNOSTIC CRITERIA

1. **What is required to make a diagnosis of CML?**
   - Bone marrow assessment demonstrating features consistent with CML. These **can include** granulocytic hyperplasia with a shift to immaturity and an elevated blast percentage. Small megakaryocytes with hypolobulated nuclei (the so-called "dwarf megakaryocytes") are also often present. Elevated eosinophils and basophils are also a hallmark of CML.
   - Identification of the Philadelphia chromosome:
     - Identification of t(9;22) in cytogenetic analysis, *or*
     - Identification of the *BCR-ABL1* fusion gene by fluorescence in situ hybridization (FISH), *or*
     - Identification of the BCR-ABL1 transcript with quantitative reverse transcription polymerase chain reaction (RT-PCR)

2. **Name two other hematologic malignancies that can harbor t(9;22).**
   - Ph+ acute lymphoblastic leukemia
   - Ph+ acute myeloid leukemia (AML)

STAGING

1. **What are the phases of CML and what characterizes each phase?**
   - There are several diagnostic criteria for CML, including the World Health Organization (WHO), International Bone Marrow Transplant Registry (IBMTR), European LeukemiaNet (ELN), and MD Anderson criteria. We will focus on the WHO criteria since this is the most frequently referenced. Additionally, there is a significant change between the 2016 WHO and 2022 WHO criteria, where accelerated-phase disease has been removed and replaced with an acknowledgment of the factors associated with higher risk chronic phase disease. Key features are highlighted in Table 11.1.

TABLE 11.1

WHO Criteria	Chronic Phase	Accelerated Phase	Blast Phase
2016 WHO	■ No features of accelerated- or blast-phase disease	■ Persistent or worsening leukocytosis, splenomegaly, thrombocytosis, or thrombocytopenia despite therapy ■ 10%–19% myeloblasts in the peripheral blood and/or bone marrow ■ Basophils ≥20% ■ New additional clonal cytogenetic abnormalities in Ph+ cells after therapy initiation ■ Major route additional chromosome abnormalities in Ph+ cells at the time of diagnosis including second Ph, trisomy 8, isochromosome 17q, trisomy 19, complex karyotype, or abnormalities of 3q26.2	■ Peripheral blood or bone marrow blasts ≥20% (no difference was emphasized for myeloid or lymphoid blasts) ■ Extramedullary infiltrates of leukemic blasts in extramedullary tissues or large clusters of blasts in the bone marrow core biopsy

(continued)

TABLE 11.1 (continued)

WHO Criteria	Chronic Phase	Accelerated Phase	Blast Phase
2022 WHO	■ No features of accelerated- or blast-phase disease ■ Emphasis on identifying and monitoring for high-risk features associated with disease progression including major route additional chromosome abnormalities in Ph+ cells at the time of diagnosis, including second Ph, trisomy 8, isochromosome 17q, trisomy 19, complex karyotype, or abnormalities of 3q26.2	■ Removed as a phase of disease	■ ≥20% myeloid blasts in the blood or bone marrow ■ Presence of an extramedullary proliferation of blasts ■ Presence of increased lymphoblasts in peripheral blood or bone marrow

Ph, Philadelphia; WHO, World Health Organization.

SIGNS AND SYMPTOMS

1. **What is the classic presentation of CML?**
   - Neutrophilia with a left shift, thrombocytosis, eosinophilia, and basophilia on a routine complete blood count (CBC)
   - Clinically, gradual onset of fatigue, night sweats, splenomegaly, early satiety, and weight loss

2. **Are infections rare or common at presentation?**
   - Rare, because neutrophil function is preserved

3. **What is a typical CBC on presentation?**
   - Leukocytosis (>10,000 to greater than 1,000,000) with circulating myeloblasts, myelocytes, metamyelocytes, and band forms
   - Basophilia and eosinophilia
   - Mild normochromic, normocytic anemia
   - Normal or elevated platelet count

PROGNOSTIC FACTORS

1. **What are two important poor prognostic factors?**
   - Disease status at diagnosis, with accelerated (according to 2016 WHO or with adverse prognostic features according to 2022 WHO; see Table 11.1) and blast phases having poorer prognosis compared with chronic-phase disease
   - Failure to achieve (or loss of) hematologic, cytogenetic, and molecular responses (see the table 11.2 found below)

2. **What prognostic factors at diagnosis are associated with worse outcomes in CML?**
   - Age, spleen size, platelet count, and blast percentage in the peripheral blood (all included in the Sokal risk assessment score); additionally, peripheral blood basophil and eosinophil percentages with prognostic values in the Hasford scoring system.

TREATMENT

1. **How is newly diagnosed CML in chronic phase treated?**
   - Tyrosine kinase inhibitor (TKI) therapy should be initiated as quickly as possible: Nilotinib (300 mg BID), dasatinib (100 mg daily), imatinib (400 mg daily), and bosutinib (400 mg daily) are the four Food and Drug Administration (FDA)-approved TKIs for first-line treatment of chronic phase CML.
   - Consider hydroxyurea in patients with white blood cell (WBC) count greater than 100,000 (only temporarily until WBC goes down) while awaiting the introduction of the TKI to prevent leukostasis.
   - Addition of allopurinol 300 mg daily until blood counts normalize minimizes the risk of gout during cytoreduction.

2. **What should be taken into consideration when selecting one of the four TKIs (dasatinib, nilotinib, imatinib, or bosutinib) in the first-line treatment of chronic-phase CML?**
   - Sokal and Hasford prognostic scores: a second-generation TKI (nilotinib, dasatinib, or bosutinib) rather than imatinib recommended in patients with intermediate- or high-risk scores; in patients with a low-risk score, imatinib or one of the three second-generation TKIs are acceptable options
   - Side effects of the different TKIs
   - Patient comorbidities
   - Patient preference and cost/insurance coverage

3. **What are some characteristic toxicities associated with nilotinib?**
   - QT prolongation, gastrointestinal (GI) upset, pancreatitis, hyperglycemia, hypercholesterolemia, and liver toxicity are associated with nilotinib.
   - Patients taking nilotinib also have an increased risk of arterial adverse vascular events such as peripheral arterial occlusive disease.
   - Nilotinib is the only TKI that needs to be taken twice a day. Patients cannot have food intake for 2 hours before or 1 hour after each dose of nilotinib.

4. **What are some characteristic toxicities associated with dasatinib?**
   - QT prolongation, thrombocytopenia, gastroesophageal reflux disease (GERD), pleural or pericardial effusion, bleeding from platelet dysfunction, and pulmonary hypertension are associated with dasatinib.

5. **What are some characteristic toxicities associated with imatinib?**
   - Skin rash, muscle cramps, diarrhea, periorbital swelling, edema, liver function test abnormalities, and QT prolongation are associated with imatinib.

6. **What are some characteristic toxicities associated with bosutinib?**
   - Diarrhea, nausea/vomiting, hepatotoxicity, rash, fluid retention, cardiovascular events including heart failure and ischemic events, and renal insufficiency are associated with bosutinib.

7. **Based on the toxicities of the different TKIs, which of the four TKIs approved in the first-line treatment setting (imatinib, dasatinib, nilotinib, bosutinib) should be avoided in the following conditions?**
   - History of pancreatitis: Avoid nilotinib.
   - History of pericardial/pleural effusions: Avoid dasatinib.
   - History of (or significant risk factors for) arterial thrombotic events: Avoid nilotinib.
   - Patient with pulmonary hypertension: Avoid dasatinib.
   - Patients who are not able to fast for 3 hours twice a day (2 hours before and 1 hour after each dose of medication): Avoid nilotinib.
   - History of irritable bowel syndrome or inflammatory bowel disease: Consider alternative to bosutinib (due to diarrhea), although not a strict contraindication.

8. **What are the treatment response goals and treatment failure criteria for CML patients treated with first-line TKIs?**
   - The current National Comprehensive Cancer Network (NCCN) criteria focus on the use of a quantitative polymerase chain reaction (qPCR) for Bcr-Abl on peripheral blood for assessment of milestones for response. They also emphasize the use of the International Standardization (IS) scale for normalizing results to minimize lab-to-lab variation.

TABLE 11.2 ■ Molecular Response Milestones for Patients Treated With TKIs

qPCR (% IS)	3 months	6 months	12 months	15 months
>10% IS	⚠️	STOP	STOP	STOP
1%–10% IS	GO	GO	⚠️	STOP

(*continued*)

TABLE 11.2 ■ Molecular Response Milestones for Patients Treated With TKIs (*continued*)

qPCR (% IS)	3 months	6 months	12 months	15 months
0.1%–1% IS	GO	GO	GO	GO

STOP = Evaluate patient compliance and drug interactions. Assess a Bcr-Abl domain mutational analysis.

⚠ = Evaluate patient compliance and drug interactions. Consider Bcr-Abl kinase domain mutational analysis. Consider performing a bone marrow biopsy and sending a cytogenetic analysis to assess for major cytogenetic response (<35% Ph+ metaphases) at 3 months or a complete cytogenetic response at 12 months.

IS, International Standardization; Ph, Philadelphia; qPCR, quantitative polymerase chain reaction.

9. **What is a practical approach to monitor chronic-phase CML after first-line TKI therapy?**
Perform CBCs with platelet count and differential (CBCPDs) every 1 to 2 weeks until the risk of therapy-induced myelosuppression is complete. Then perform CBCPDs every 1 to 3 months to assess for hematologic toxicity and loss of a hematologic response.
 ■ At 3 months: Perform qPCR for Bcr-Abl using the IS scale.

   • **GO** If the qPCR is ≤10% (IS scale), this is an optimal response and therapy should be continued with ongoing monitoring.

   • ⚠ If the qPCR is >10% (IS scale), therapy adjustments are not indicated, but the NCCN recommends evaluating patient compliance and drug interactions. They also indicate considering Bcr-Abl kinase domain mutational analysis. They also ask to consider performing a bone marrow biopsy and sending a cytogenetic analysis to assess for major cytogenetic response (< 35% Ph+ metaphases).
 ■ At 6 months: Perform qPCR for Bcr-Abl.

   • **GO** If the Bcr-Abl transcripts are ≤10% (IS scale), this constitutes an optimal response and therapy should be continued with ongoing monitoring.

   • **STOP** If the BCR-ABL transcripts are >10% (IS scale), this is treatment failure. Recommendations are to assess for compliance and possible drug–drug interactions. If no issues can be identified, switch to an alternate TKI based on the side effect profile and Abl kinase domain mutation assessment if a mutation exists.
 ■ At 12 months: Perform a qPCR for Bcr-Abl.

   • **GO** If the Bcr-Abl transcripts are ≤1% (IS scale), continue the same treatment.

- ⚠️ If the BCR-ABL transcripts are >1% (IS scale), this represents a suboptimal response but not a treatment failure. Again, evaluate for patient compliance and possible drug–drug interactions. Additionally, consider a Bcr-Abl kinase domain mutation assessment.

- 🛑 If the BCR-ABL transcripts are >10% (IS scale), this is treatment failure. Recommendations are to assess for compliance and possible drug–drug interactions. If no issues can be identified, switch to an alternate TKI based on the side effect profile and Abl kinase domain mutation assessment if a mutation exists.
■ At 15 months: Perform a qPCR for Bcr-Abl.

- 🟢 If the qPCR is < 1% (IS scale), this is an optimal response and treatment should continue with ongoing monitoring.

- 🛑 If the Bcr-Abl transcripts are ≥1% (IS scale), this is treatment failure. Recommendations are to assess for compliance and possible drug–drug interactions. If no issues can be identified, switch to an alternate TKI based on the side effect profile and Abl kinase domain mutation assessment if a mutation exists.
■ For patients on TKI therapy, the NCCN recommends monitoring the qPCR for Bcr-Abl every 3 months for 2 years after the patient obtains a qPCR of < 1% (IS scale) and then every 3 to 6 months thereafter.

10. **What are the management options for patients with TKI intolerance?**
   ■ Patients with intolerance to one TKI can be switched to one of the other TKIs approved for first-line or later treatment. An additional option is ponatinib, a third-generation TKI, FDA-approved for patients with a T315I *ABL* kinase mutation or for patients with resistance or intolerance to at least two prior kinase inhibitors. If the patient is intolerant to two or more TKIs, then asciminib, a first in-class allosteric inhibitor of BCR-ABL, can also be considered.

11. **What are the management options for patients with failure to first-line TKI therapy?**
   ■ Evaluate for compliance and drug–drug interactions.
   ■ Test for *Abl* kinase domain mutations to help guide the choice of the second-line TKI. Approximately 50% of patients with chronic phase disease with treatment failure have mutations in the *Abl* kinase.
   ■ If no mutations that guide therapy are identified, in patients who received imatinib in the first line, switching to any second-generation TKI is appropriate (bosutinib, dasatinib, or nilotinib) based on an assessment of the side effect profile of the medication and the patient's comorbidities. For those who received a second-generation TKI as initial therapy, another second-generation TKI can be considered. Patients who initially received a second-generation TKI should not be switched to imatinib.

12. **What are the management options for patients failing multiple TKIs?**
   - Third-line treatment options include any of the remaining second-generation TKIs, ponatinib, asciminib, or omacetaxine, the only non-oral therapy for CML.
   - Allogeneic transplant is an appropriate treatment option for the very rare patients presenting with blast-phase CML at diagnosis, patients with disease that is resistant to all TKIs, patients with progression to accelerated-phase (AP) (according to WHO 2016) or blast-phase (BP) CML while on TKI therapy, or patients intolerant to all TKIs.

13. **What ABL kinase mutation confers resistance to all first- and second-generation TKIs: imatinib, nilotinib, dasatinib, and bosutinib?**
   - *T315I* mutation
     - Patients with treatment failure due to *T315I* mutation should be treated with either ponatinib of asciminib. Note that the dosing of asciminib is different for patients with the *T315I* mutation (200 mg BID) compared with that used in patients with non–*T315I*-mediated resistance (40 mg BID or 80 mg once daily). Allogeneic transplant should be considered based on clinical context. Omacetaxine can be considered as a less favorable alternative to ponatinib or asciminib, but only in the third-line or later setting.

14. **What ABL kinase mutations help decide the choice of the second-line TKI therapy?**
   - Mutations associated with resistance to nilotinib include Y253H, E255K/V, F359C/V/I, and G250E.
   - Mutations associated with resistance to dasatinib include F315A, F317L/V/I/C, and V299L.
   - ABL kinase mutations conferring resistance to bosutinib include V299L, G250E, or F317L.

15. **What are some characteristic toxicities associated with ponatinib?**
   - Arterial and venous thrombotic events, pancreatitis, rash, and hypertension

16. **What is the role of allogeneic transplant in CML?**
   - Allogeneic transplant is reserved for patients with chronic-phase CML that is resistant to at least a second- and a third-generation TKIs or who are intolerant of all TKIs.
   - It is also indicated for AP or BP after best response to TKI is achieved (regardless of the depth of response), including those who progress to AP or BP from chronic phase.
   NOTE: *As the new WHO classification system no long recognizes AP disease, it remains to be seen how allogeneic transplant will be utilized in patients with historically defined AP disease in the future.*

17. **How successful is allogeneic transplant for CML?**
   - Allogeneic transplant has a long-term cure rate of approximately 65% in patients transplanted in chronic phase.
   - Transplant-related mortality and relapse are higher in patients transplanted for AP or BP CML.

18. **How should AP-CML (according to 2016 WHO) be treated?**
   - Note that many TKI recommendations for AP disease are based on clinical trial experience and the current label indications for treatments differ from clinical

practice. There are currently no TKIs that are FDA-approved as frontline therapy for AP-CML.

■ Patients in AP-CML should be treated with dasatinib 140 mg daily, nilotinib 400 mg BID, bosutinib 500 mg daily, ponatinib 45mg daily, or less favorably omacetaxine or 1.25 mg/m² BID for 14 days or imatinib 600 mg PO daily. This should be followed by allogeneic transplant (if eligible) after best response is achieved with the TKI. Patients with optimal/deep response to the TKI might choose to be monitored very carefully and defer allogeneic transplant until the first sign of disease progression, but progression can occur without much lead time and patients may lose their window for transplant if they do not obtain the necessary level of response to become transplant-eligible.

19. How are patients with BP-CML treated?

■ As noted above, there are no TKIs that are FDA-approved for initial therapy in a patient presenting with de novo BP-CML. Additionally, only imatinib, dasatinib, bosutinib, and ponatinib are approved for use in BP disease. Nilotinib, asciminib, and omacetaxine are not approved for this indication.

■ All patients should be evaluated for allogeneic transplant while receiving TKI-based therapies.

■ The therapy recommendations for BP-CML may depend on whether the patient presents with myeloid BP disease or lymphoid BP disease.

● Patients with lymphoid blast crisis (defined as ≥5% lymphoblast in blood or bone marrow) are treated with combination cytotoxic chemotherapy (regimen often used to treat acute lymphoblastic leukemia) with a TKI, followed by allogeneic transplant.

● Myeloid blast crisis does not typically respond well to AML induction regimens. Patients with de novo myeloid blast crisis CML are treated with a TKI without chemotherapy until best response, followed by an allogeneic transplant.

QUESTIONS

1. A 70-year-old woman with a past medical history notable for hypertension, diabetes, and stroke is found to have leukocytosis (white blood cell [WBC] count of 25,000) on routine labs. Hemoglobin is mildly reduced at 11.5 g/dL and platelet count is mildly elevated at 500,000. She notes some mild fatigue but is otherwise asymptomatic. Examination is notable for a spleen tip palpable 3 cm below the left costal margin. Further testing reveals BCR-ABL by fluorescence in situ hybridization (FISH) to be positive, and cytogenetics performed on her bone marrow show no additional chromosomal abnormalities.
She had an echocardiogram that showed a normal ejection fraction and no evidence of a pericardial effusion. Her Sokal score is calculated and she is found to be high risk. What is the next best step in management?
A. Initiation of ponatinib
B. Initiation of imatinib
C. Initiation of nilotinib
D. Initiation of dasatinib

2. A 63-year-old male with a history of chronic myeloid leukemia (CML) on imatinib presents to the clinic for routine follow-up. Labs are notable for a white blood cell (WBC) count of 50,000 (10,000 6 months ago) and platelet count of 650,000 (normal 6 months ago). Quantitative polymerase chain reaction (PCR) for BCR-ABL returns elevated at 5% (International Standardization [IS]; previously undetectable), and this result was confirmed by repeat testing. The patient confirms that he is compliant with imatinib and has not been prescribed any new medications in the last year. What is the next best step in management?
   A. Increase imatinib dose and repeat PCR again in 1 month.
   B. Transition to a second-generation tyrosine kinase inhibitor.
   C. Perform an ABL1 kinase domain mutation analysis.
   D. Switch to ponatinib.

3. A 67-year-old woman with a past medical history notable for hypertension, glaucoma, and diabetes presents to the clinic for evaluation of 2 months of progressive fatigue, early satiety, and weight loss. Labs are obtained and complete blood count (CBC) shows a white blood cell (WBC) count of 95,000 with basophilia (22%). Hemoglobin is 9.5 and platelets are 650,000. Differential reveals 12% blasts. Fluorescence in situ hybridization (FISH) for BCR-ABL is positive. Bone marrow biopsy shows 15% blasts, with cytogenetics revealing the Philadelphia chromosome in 20 out of 20 cells examined. What is the next best step in management?
   A. Admit to hospital for cytotoxic chemotherapy.
   B. Initiate second-generation tyrosine kinase inhibitor (TKI).
   C. Refer for consideration of allogeneic stem cell transplant (ASCT).
   D. B and C.

4. Which tyrosine kinase inhibitor should be avoided in a patient with chronic-phase chronic myeloid leukemia who has a bleeding disorder?
   A. Imatinib
   B. Dasatinib
   C. Nilotinib
   D. Bosutinib

5. Which of the following is not a side effect of dasatinib?
   A. Pulmonary hypertension
   B. QT prolongation
   C. Platelet dysfunction
   D. Pleural effusions
   E. Pericardial effusions
   F. None of the above (i.e., all the above are side effects of dasatinib)

6. Which of the following tyrosine kinase inhibitors should be avoided in a patient with chronic-phase chronic myeloid leukemia who has history of arterial vascular disease (coronary artery disease or stroke)?
   A. Nilotinib
   B. Dasatinib
   C. Bosutinib
   D. Imatinib

7. **Which tyrosine kinase inhibitor (TKI) is taken twice daily with no food for 2 hours before and 1 hour after each dose?**
   A. Dasatinib
   B. Imatinib
   C. Bosutinib
   D. Nilotinib

ANSWERS

1. **D. Initiation of dasatinib.** The patient is high risk based on her Sokal score; therefore, outcomes are improved with a second-generation tyrosine kinase inhibitor (TKI) (nilotinib, dasatinib, or bosutinib) compared with imatinib. She has a history of arterial events (as well as multiple risk factors for arterial thrombosis), making nilotinib a less desirable option. Ponatinib is also not considered a first-line therapy in the absence of intolerance or failure of other TKIs. Her history of hypertension and stroke would also be a concern in considering her for ponatinib as arterial thrombosis is a potential side effect. Therefore, the best option for this patient is dasatinib.

2. **C. Perform an ABL1 kinase domain mutation analysis.** Patients who show resistance to imatinib should be evaluated for mutations in the *ABL* kinase domain. Certain mutations may guide therapy and therefore this test should be done instead of empirically transitioning to second-generation tyrosine kinase inhibitor (TKI). For example, the patient could have acquired a *T315I* mutation, which would render his disease resistant to second-generation TKIs. Increasing the imatinib dose is only considered in patients with a suboptimal response after initiation of therapy and not in those with a loss of response (in this case hematologic relapse as well as >1-log increase in BCR-ABL1 transcripts and loss of Major Molecular Response [MMR]). Empirically switching to ponatinib would not be considered in this setting unless a *T315I* mutation in the ABL kinase domain was identified or unless the anticipated side effect profile or patient tolerance precluded the use of a second-generation TKI.

3. **D. B and C.** This patient is in an accelerated phase of chronic myelogenous leukemia (CML). Cytotoxic chemotherapy is not indicated. Patients in accelerated-phase CML should be treated with a second-generation TKI, and ASCT should strongly be considered at best response. However, as we noted in the chapter, this treatment paradigm may shift as accelerated-phase CML is no longer a recognized entity by one of two main classification systems published in 2022.

4. **B. Dasatinib.** Dasatinib can cause bleeding due to platelet dysfunction.

5. **F. None of the above (i.e., all the above are side effects of dasatinib).** Pulmonary hypertension, QT prolongation, platelet dysfunction, pleural and pericardial effusions, gastroesophageal reflux disease, and thrombocytopenia are all side effects of dasatinib.

6. **A. Nilotinib.** Patients taking nilotinib have an increased risk of arterial adverse vascular events.

7. **D. Nilotinib.** Nilotinib is the only TKI that needs to be taken twice a day. Patients cannot have food intake for 2 hours before or 1 hour after each dose of nilotinib.

Myeloproliferative Neoplasms

12

Charles E. Foucar and Rami N. Khoriaty

1. **What characterizes a myeloproliferative neoplasm (MPN)?**
   - Clonal hematopoietic stem cell disease with overproduction of one or more blood cell lines
   - Normal maturation with effective hematopoiesis and extramedullary hematopoiesis
   - Risk for leukemic transformation

2. **What are the eight MPNs recognized by the World Health Organization (WHO) in 2022?**
   - BCR-ABL1-positive chronic myeloid leukemia (CML)
   - Polycythemia vera (PV)
   - Essential thrombocythemia (ET)
   - Primary myelofibrosis (PMF)
   - Chronic neutrophilic leukemia
   - Chronic eosinophilic leukemia
   - Juvenile myelomonocytic leukemia
   - MPN, Not otherwise specified (NOS)

3. **What is the most common gene mutated in PV, ET, and PMF?**
   - *JAK2*

4. **What is *JAK2*'s normal function?**
   - Tyrosine kinase, which is critical in intracellular signaling for the erythropoietin, thrombopoietin, interleukin-3, granulocyte colony-stimulating factor (G-CSF), and granulocyte/macrophage colony-stimulating factor (GM-CSF) receptors

5. **What *JAK2* mutations are tested for in MPN?**
   - *JAK2* V617F (most common) and *JAK2* exon 12 mutations
   - *JAK2* V617F mutation: causes constitutive activation of downstream messengers through the JAK–STAT, PI3K, and AKT pathways

6. **In which MPN is *JAK2* mutation most prevalent?**
   - PV (98%–99%), ET (~60%), and PMF (~55%)

7. **Name two additional frequently mutated genes in ET and PMF.**
   - *MPL* (mutation in the transmembrane domain of the thrombopoietin receptor)
   - *CALR*
   - *JAK2*, *CALR*, and *MPL* mutations generally mutually exclusive

8. **What thrombophilic conditions should raise the suspicion of a *JAK2* mutation?**
   - Budd–Chiari syndrome
   - Mesenteric venous thrombosis

9. **Which gene is characteristically mutated in chronic neutrophilic leukemia?**
   - *CSF3R*

Polycythemia Vera

EPIDEMIOLOGY

1. **What is the median age at diagnosis of PV?**
   - Approximately 60 years old, but occurs in all age groups

2. **What is the median survival of PV patients?**
   - Median survival approximately 14 years (and ~24 years in patients <60 years)

3. **What are the prognostic factors for worse survival in PV?**
   - Risk factors predicting worsening survival in PV: age >57 (with age >67 being even higher risk), leukocytosis (white blood cell [WBC] >15,000), venous thrombosis, and abnormal karyotype

4. **What are the risks of transformation to myelofibrosis and risk of leukemic transformation in PV?**
   - Transformation to myelofibrosis occurs in 12% to 21% of PV patients.
   - Risk of transformation to acute myeloid leukemia (AML) is ~8% at 20 years.

5. **What characterizes PV pathophysiologically?**
   - Growth factor (EPO)-independent proliferation of erythroid cells, producing an elevated red cell mass

DIAGNOSTIC CRITERIA

1. **What are the WHO diagnostic criteria for PV?**

TABLE 12.1 ■ WHO 2022 Diagnostic Criteria for Polycythemia Vera

	2022 WHO Criteria*
Major	■ Hgb >16.5 g/dL (men) or Hgb >16.0 g/dL (women), OR Hct >49% in men or >48% in women, OR increased red cell mass
	■ Bone marrow biopsy showing trilineage hyperplasia (panmyelosis) with pleomorphic mature megakaryocytes
	■ Presence of *JAK2* V617F or *JAK2* exon 12 mutation
Minor	■ Subnormal Erythropoetin (EPO) level

*Diagnosis requires all three major criteria or the first two major criteria and the minor criterion. Bone marrow biopsy may not be necessary if Hgb >18.5 (or Hct >55.5) in men or if Hgb >16.5 (or Hct >49.5) in women, if all other major and minor criteria are met.

Note: A competing classification system, International Consensus Criteria (ICC), exists.

Hct, hematocrit; Hgb, hemoglobin; WHO, World Health Organization.

2. **What are the features of PV that help distinguish it from secondary polycythemia?**
   - Splenomegaly
   - Leukocytosis
   - Thrombocytosis
   - Low epo level
   - Panhyperplasia in bone marrow (BM)
   - Normal arterial oxygen saturation
   - Increased vitamin B_{12} level

SIGNS AND SYMPTOMS

1. **What are the common presenting signs/symptoms in patients with PV?**
   - Incidental polycythemia (± thrombocytosis ± leukocytosis) on complete blood count, pruritus aggravated by hot shower, erythromelalgia, gout, kidney stones, palpable splenomegaly (50%–70%), early satiety, joint pain, thrombosis symptoms (arterial or venous), and neurologic symptoms such as headache and confusion

TREATMENT

1. **Which patients should be treated with aspirin?**
   - All patients with PV who do not have a contraindication should be treated with aspirin 81 mg daily.
   - Additionally, all patients should have their cardiovascular risk factors strictly controlled.
2. **In addition to aspirin, what are the treatment options for patients with PV in the first-line setting?**
   - Phlebotomy and cytoreduction with either hydroxyurea or peginterferon alfa-2a
3. **What is the goal hematocrit when the patient is getting phlebotomies or cytoreduction?**
   - The target hematocrit is always less than 45% in PV (some consider goal of <42% in women), regardless of treatment modality.
4. **How do we choose between phlebotomy alone and a cytoreductive agent to achieve the hematocrit goal of <45%?**
   - Hydroxyurea or peginterferon alfa-2a should be used in the following situations:
     - Hydroxyurea or peginterferon alfa-2a can be used in patients ≥60 years of age.
     - Hydroxyurea or peginterferon alfa-2a can be used in patients with history of thromboembolism (consider in patients with strong risk factors for thromboembolic disease).
     - Patients with acquired von Willebrand disease (vWD) should also be considered for cytoreduction. Always check von Willebrand factor (vWF) activity if platelets are >1 million before administering aspirin (see the "Essential Thrombocythemia" section).
     - Additional potential indications for cytoreductive therapy include frequent need for phlebotomy with poor tolerance of phlebotomy, symptomatic or progressive splenomegaly, symptomatic thrombocytosis, progressive leukocytosis, progressive disease-related symptoms (e.g., pruritis, night sweats, fatigue), and disease-related major bleeding.
   - Patients who do not have any of these criteria should be treated with aspirin and phlebotomies as needed (to keep hematocrit <45%).

5. **When is peginterferon alfa-2a considered instead of hydroxyurea?**
   - Hydroxyurea is the most commonly used (and generally preferred) cytoreductive agent in first-line therapy for PV.
   - Peginterferon alfa-2a should be considered in younger patients in whom long-term exposure to hydroxyurea may confer a risk of secondary malignancy, in pregnant patients in need of cytoreductive therapy (risk category C), or in patients who defer hydroxyurea. Of note, it is debatable whether hydroxyurea is leukemogenic with recent data suggesting that the leukemia risk does not appear to be increased when hydroxyurea is used as a single agent.

6. **In addition to aspirin, which therapy in PV has demonstrated the greatest reduction in thrombotic events?**
   - Hydroxyurea

7. **What are the indications to change the cytoreductive agent to a second-line agent?**
   - Intolerance or resistance for first-line cytoreductive agent
   - New thrombosis or disease-related major bleeding
   - Frequent need for phlebotomy with poor tolerance of phlebotomy
   - Symptomatic or progressive splenomegaly
   - Symptomatic thrombocytosis
   - Progressive leukocytosis
   - Progressive disease-related symptoms (e.g., pruritis, night sweats, fatigue)

8. **What are second-line treatment options for PV?**
   - Ruxolitinib (particularly if significant splenomegaly or constitutional symptoms)
   - Interferon alpha or peginterferon alpha (if not previously used)
   - Hydroxyurea (if not previously used)
   - Clinical trial
   - Busulfan (least favorable option)

9. **Is allogeneic stem cell transplantation indicated for PV?**
   - Allogeneic stem cell transplantation is the only curative option, but is almost never indicated in PV, unless the disease progresses to myelofibrosis or acute leukemia (for treatment of post-PV myelofibrosis, please refer to the "Primary Myelofibrosis" section).

Essential Thrombocythemia

EPIDEMIOLOGY

1. **What is the typical age at presentation for ET?**
   - Age of presentation has bimodal distribution: one peak around age 30, with a second (larger) peak at 50 to 60 years of age.
   - Women to men ratio is 1.5 to 2:1 in the early peak.

2. **What is the median survival in ET patients?**
   - Median survival is approximately 20 years (and ~33 years in patients <60 years of age); in some reports, survival is comparable to that of the age-matched population.

3. **What percent of ET patients have mutations in *JAK2, CALR*, or *MPL*?**
   - *JAK2* mutation (~60% of patients)
   - *CALR* mutation (~22% of patients)
   - *MPL* mutation (~3% of patients)

4. **What are prognostic factors for worse survival in ET?**
   - Risk factors predicting worse survival in ET: age >60 years, leukocytosis (WBC >11,000), and history of thrombosis

5. **What percent of ET patients transform to myelofibrosis of acute leukemia?**
   - Risk of transformation to myelofibrosis: ~5% to 10% at 15 years
   - Risk of transformation to AML: ~5% at 20 years

6. **Does *CALR* mutation result in a similar risk compared with *JAK2* mutations in ET?**
   - Patients with *CALR* mutations have a lower risk of thrombosis compared with patients with *JAK2*-mutated ET.
   - Patients with *CALR* mutations appear to have a comparable risk of transformation to myelofibrosis (MF) or AML compared with patients with *JAK2*-mutated ET.

DIAGNOSTIC CRITERIA

1. **What are the WHO diagnostic criteria for ET?**

TABLE 12.2 ■ 2022 WHO Criteria for the Diagnosis of ET

	2022 WHO Criteria*
Major	1. Platelet count >450,000
	2. Bone marrow showing proliferation mainly of the megakaryocyte lineage with increased numbers of enlarged megakaryocytes with hyperlobulated nuclei; no significant increase in granulopoiesis or erythropoiesis and no left shift; very rarely, minor (grade 1) increase in reticulin fibers can be found
	3. Not meeting WHO criteria for CML, PV, PMF, MDS, or other myeloid neoplasms
	4. Presence of *JAK2, CALR*, or *MPL* mutation
Minor	Presence of a clonal marker or absence of evidence for reactive thrombocytosis

*Diagnosis requires four major criteria or the first three major criteria and minor criterion.

CML, chronic myelogenous leukemia; MDS, myelodysplastic syndrome; PMF, primary myelofibrosis; PV, polycythemia vera; WHO, World Health Organization.

SIGNS AND SYMPTOMS

1. **What are the most common presenting signs/symptoms in ET?**
   - Asymptomatic (50%)

- Vasomotor symptoms: visual changes, lightheadedness, headaches, palpitations, typical/atypical chest pain, erythromelalgia, livedo reticularis, and acral paresthesias
- Palpable splenomegaly and related symptoms: early satiety or left upper quadrant abdominal pain
- Thrombosis (~15% at presentation)

2. **In addition to the thrombosis risk and the risk of transformation to myelofibrosis and AML, what are other complications of ET?**
   - Major hemorrhage (5%–10%) from acquired vWD
   - Recurrent first-trimester abortions

TREATMENT

1. **How are patients in the different risk categories treated?**
   - Patients with very-low-risk disease (age ≤60, no *JAK2* mutation, and no prior history of thrombosis) and patients with low-risk disease (age ≤60 with *JAK2* mutation and no prior history of thrombosis) are treated with aspirin 81 mg PO daily or observation. Of note, in one report, aspirin use did not affect the risk of thrombosis in patients with *CALR*-mutated low-risk ET but was associated with higher bleeding risk. The latter has not been confirmed in a prospective clinical trial. Therefore, the risks/benefits of aspirin in low-risk disease are considered on a case-by-case basis and informed by cardiac risk factors of the patient.
   - Patients with intermediate-risk disease (age >60 with no *JAK2* mutation and no prior history of thrombosis) are treated with aspirin 81 mg PO daily.
   - Patients with high-risk disease (age >60 with *JAK2* mutation or history of thrombosis at any age) are treated with aspirin 81 mg PO daily + cytoreduction.
   - All patients should have their cardiovascular risk factors monitored and strictly managed.
   - Potential additional indications for cytoreductive therapy regardless of the ET risk group include symptomatic or progressive splenomegaly, symptomatic thrombocytosis, progressive leukocytosis, progressive disease-related symptoms (e.g., pruritis, night sweats, fatigue), disease-related major bleeding, and vasomotor/microvascular disturbances not responsive to aspirin (e.g., headaches, chest pain, erythromelalgia).

2. **In what situations should aspirin be avoided in ET?**
   - Aspirin should be avoided in patients with acquired vWD.
   - In patients with platelets ≥1 million/microL, check vWD ristocetin cofactor activity before starting aspirin. Patients with vWD ristocetin activity ≤30% are at increased risk of bleeding and should undergo platelet cytoreduction to result in vWD ristocetin activity ≥30% prior to starting aspirin.

3. **What are the first-line cytoreductive options in ET?**
   - Hydroxyurea is the most commonly used and preferred first-line treatment in ET.
   - Interferon alpha (or peginterferon alpha) could be considered in younger patients, or in pregnant patients who require cytoreductive therapy (risk category C), or in patients who defer hydroxyurea.
   - Anagrelide is also an option.

4. **When is plateletpheresis indicated in ET?**
   - Plateletpheresis is indicated in patients with significantly elevated platelet counts in the setting of acute and serious thrombotic or hemorrhagic events (such as stroke, ischemic limb, significant hemorrhagic event due to acquired vWD).
   - The effect of plateletpheresis on reducing platelet count is transient and the patient should be started at the same time on a cytoreductive agent.
   - It should also be noted that the benefits of plateletpheresis have never been demonstrated in a prospective clinical trial.

5. **What are the indications to change the cytoreductive agent to a second-line agent?**
   - Intolerance or resistance to first-line cytoreductive agent
   - New thrombosis, acquired vWD, or disease-related major bleeding
   - Symptomatic or progressive splenomegaly
   - Symptomatic thrombocytosis
   - Progressive leukocytosis
   - Progressive disease-related symptoms (e.g., pruritis, night sweats, fatigue)
   - Vasomotor/microvascular disturbances not responsive to aspirin (e.g., headaches, chest pain, erythromelalgia)

6. **What are second-line cytoreductive agents in ET?**
   - Hydroxyurea (if not previously used)
   - Interferon alpha (if not previously used)
   - Anagrelide (if not previously used)
   - Clinical trial
   - Could consider ruxolitinib or busulfan (less favorable options than the ones above)

7. **What is the mechanism of action of anagrelide?**
   - Interferes with terminal differentiation of megakaryocytes

8. **In what group of patients should anagrelide therapy be avoided and why?**
   - In those with cardiovascular comorbidities because it can cause fluid retention, palpitations, and pulmonary hypertension

9. **Is allogeneic stem cell transplantation indicated for ET?**
   - Allogeneic stem cell transplantation is almost never indicated in ET, unless the disease progresses to myelofibrosis or acute leukemia (for treatment of post-ET myelofibrosis, please refer to the "Primary Myelofibrosis" section).

Primary Myelofibrosis

EPIDEMIOLOGY

1. **In addition to PMF, which two hematologic disorders most commonly lead to secondary myelofibrosis?**
   - Myelofibrosis could be a primary disease (PMF) or secondary to ET or PV.
   - Fibrosis in the BM could result from other etiologies such as hairy cell leukemia, metastatic solid tumor to the BM, and autoimmune or chronic inflammatory conditions.

2. What is the median survival of patients with PMF?

- Median survival: ~6 years (but highly variable)

DIAGNOSTIC CRITERIA

1. What are the WHO 2022 diagnostic criteria for PMF?

TABLE 12.3 ■ 2022 WHO Criteria for Diagnosis of Myelofibrosis

		Prefibrotic PMF*	PMF†
Major*	1.	Megakaryocyte proliferation and atypia without reticulin fibrosis > grade 1; increased age-adjusted BM cellularity, granulocytic proliferation, and decreased erythropoiesis	1. Megakaryocyte proliferation and atypia accompanied by either reticulin and/or collagen fibrosis (grades 2–3 on 0–3 scale).
	2.	Not meeting the WHO criteria for CML, PV, MDS, or other myeloid neoplasms	2. Not meeting WHO criteria for CML, PV, ET, MDS, or other myeloid neoplasms
	3.	Demonstration of *JAK2*, *CALR*, or *MPL* mutation or presence of another clonal marker or absence of minor reactive reticulin fibrosis	3. Demonstration of *JAK2*, *CALR*, or *MPL* mutation or another clonal marker or no evidence of reactive myelofibrosis
Minor‡	1.	Anemia unrelated to medical comorbidities	1. Leukoerythroblastosis (absent in prefibrotic PMF)
	2.	Leukocytosis ≥11 × 10⁹/L	2. Increased serum LDH
	3.	LDH above upper limit of normal	3. Anemia
	4.	Palpable splenomegaly	4. Palpable splenomegaly
			5. Leukocytosis ≥11 × 10⁹/L

*Diagnosis requires all three major criteria and one minor criterion.

†Diagnosis requires three major criteria and at least one minor criterion.

‡Confirmed on two sequential measurements.

BM, bone marrow; CML, chronic myelogenous leukemia; ET, essential thrombocythemia; LDH, lactate dehydrogenase; MDS, myelodysplastic syndrome; PMF, primary myelofibrosis; PV, polycythemia vera; WHO, World Health Organization.

2. What are the three most commonly mutated genes in PMF?

- *JAK2* (~55% of patients)
- *CALR* (~27% of patients)
- *MPL* W515L (~7% of patients)
- ~10% of patients with PMF do not have any of the above mutations.

3. What are the diagnostic criteria for post-PV and post-ET myelofibrosis?

TABLE 12.4 ■ 2022 WHO Criteria for the Diagnosis of Post-PV Myelofibrosis and Post-ET Myelofibrosis

	Post-PV Myelofibrosis*	Post-ET Myelofibrosis†
Major*	1. Documentation of a prior diagnosis of PV 2. Bone marrow fibrosis (grade 2–3 on 0–3 scale or grade 3–4 on 0–4 scale)	1. Documentation of a prior diagnosis of ET 2. Bone marrow fibrosis (grade 2–3 on 0–3 scale or grade 3–4 on 0–4 scale)
Minor	1. Anemia or lack of requirement of phlebotomies in the absence of cytoreductive therapy 2. Leukoerythroblastosis 3. New splenomegaly or increase in palpable splenomegaly of ≥5 cm 4. One or more of these constitutional symptoms: unexplained fever (>37.5°C), night sweats, or >10% weight loss in 6 months	1. Anemia and ≥2 g/dL decrease from baseline hemoglobin 2. Leukoerythroblastosis 3. New splenomegaly or increase in palpable splenomegaly of ≥5 cm 4. One or more of these constitutional symptoms: unexplained fever (>37.5°C), night sweats, or >10% weight loss in 6 months 5. Increased LDH

*For diagnosis of post-PV myelofibrosis: two major and two minor criteria are required.

†For diagnosis of post-ET myelofibrosis: two major and two minor criteria are required.

ET, essential thrombocythemia; LDH, lactate dehydrogenase; PV, polycythemia vera.

SIGNS AND SYMPTOMS

1. Name several common presenting symptoms of PMF.
- Fatigue, anemia, abdominal discomfort and early satiety (from splenomegaly), fever, night sweats, weight loss, bone pain, pruritus, and complications of portal hypertension (such as variceal bleed, ascites)

2. What are the two most common physical exam findings in patients with PMF?
- Palpable splenomegaly and hepatomegaly

3. What does the classic peripheral blood smear of PMF show?
- Leukoerythroblastosis (immature cells of the granulocytic series and nucleated red blood cells) and teardrop-shaped red blood cells (seen in fibrotic PMF)

PROGNOSTIC FACTORS

1. What are the factors associated with decreased survival in PMF based on the Dynamic International Prognostic Scoring System-Plus (DIPSS-Plus)?

- Age >65 years
- Presence of constitutional symptoms
- Anemia, hemoglobin ≤10 g/dL
- Leukocytosis, WBC greater than 25,000 × 10⁶/L
- Presence of ≥1% circulating peripheral blasts
- Presence of unfavorable karyotype (complex karyotype, +8, −7/7q−, i(17q), inv(3), −5/5q, 12p−, or 11q23 rearrangement)
- Platelet count <100,000/microL
- Red blood cell transfusion need (patients with red blood cell transfusion need will automatically get 2 points because their hemoglobin would be <10 g/dL)

2. **How are patients with PMF divided into risk groups? What is the median survival in each risk group?**
   - Risk factors from the prior questions are added up.
     - Low risk: zero risk factors; median survival approximately 15.4 years
     - Intermediate-1 risk: one risk factor; median survival approximately 6.5 years
     - Intermediate-2 risk: two or three risk factors; median survival approximately 2.9 years
     - High risk: at least four of the aforementioned risk factors; median survival approximately 1.3 years

TREATMENT

1. **What is the goal of treatment in PMF?**
   - Palliation in most cases, except in patients who are candidates for autologous stem cell transplant (ASCT), where cure might be attained (see the following text)

2. **How do you treat patients with low- and intermediate-1-risk PMF?**
   - The mainstay of therapy is supportive care, symptom control, and improving quality of life.
   - Assess symptom burden using Myeloproliferative Neoplasm Symptom Assessment Form Total Symptom Score (MPN-SAF TSS).
     - In asymptomatic patients, observation is reasonable.
     - The treatment of symptomatic patients is highly individualized. Treatment options include ruxolitinib, interferon (or peginterferon) alpha, hydroxyurea, or a clinical trial. ASCT could be considered in patients with intermediate-1 risk PMF who have low platelet count, complex karyotype, or high-risk mutations.
     - Symptomatic splenomegaly:
       - Hydroxyurea and ruxolitinib are reasonable first-line therapies for symptomatic splenomegaly. The response of splenomegaly to ruxolitinib is superior to the response to hydroxyurea. Other less favorable options include splenectomy and splenic irradiation. Splenectomy is associated with significant risks, and the decision to proceed with splenectomy should be individualized. The risks of splenic irradiation include profound cytopenias and the benefit of this modality is only transient.
     - Cytoreduction in patients without significant/symptomatic splenomegaly:
       - Hydroxyurea is often considered first-line for cytoreduction in these patients if cytoreduction is felt to be beneficial.
     - Patients with symptomatic anemia have generally higher risk disease (because symptomatic anemia is generally an indication for RBC transfusion,

and transfusion requirement by itself puts patients immediately in at least the intermediate-2 risk group). See treatment for symptomatic anemia in the following question.

3. **How do you treat patients with intermediate-2 or high-risk PMF?**
   - Transplant candidates should undergo allogeneic stem cell transplantation.
   - Nontransplant candidates with platelets ≥50,000 can be treated with ruxolitinib (certainly if symptomatic) or a clinical trial. Fedratinib is generally reserved for patients who fail to respond or lose response to ruxolitinib, although it can also be considered as frontline therapy. For patients with platelets <50, pacritinib can be considered.
   - Nontransplant candidates with symptomatic anemia only should be worked up for other etiologies of anemia. If no other cause is identified, erythropoietin levels should be obtained.
     - If epo is <500 mU/mL, patients can be treated with an erythropoiesis-stimulating agent or a clinical trial. Avoid erythropoiesis-stimulating agents in patients with significant splenomegaly because they might worsen the splenomegaly.
     - If epo is ≥500 mU/mL, options include danazol, lenalidomide, or thalidomide ± prednisone, or a clinical trial. Use lenalidomide particularly in the presence of del 5q. Splenectomy can be considered in refractory cases with significant splenomegaly; however, this decision should not be taken lightly due to the morbidity and mortality associated with the procedure (~10% perisurgical mortality) and because a subset of patients develop compensatory hepatomegaly, some of whom might die of liver failure.

4. **What is a contraindication to treatment with fedratinib or ruxolitinib?**
   - Platelet count <50 × 10^8/L is a contraindication for both ruxolitinib and fedratinib. Pacritinib can be used in patients with intermediate- or high-risk disease with a platelet count <50 × 10^8/L.
   - For platelet counts between 50 and 200 × 10^8/L, ruxolitinib (but not fedratinib) requires dose reduction.
   - Fedratinib has been associated with serious and fatal encephalopathy (Wernicke encephalopathy). Thiamine (vitamin B_1) and nutritional status should be assessed in all patients before starting fedratinib and periodically. If a patient is deficient in thiamine, thiamine repletion should be confirmed before starting fedratinib.

5. **What are some notable complications of ruxolitinib and fedratinib?**
   - Ruxolitinib toxicities include cytopenias; lipid elevation; infections including tuberculosis (TB), increase in hepatitis B viral load, progressive multifocal leukoencephalopathy (PML), and herpes zoster; and nonmelanoma skin cancer.
   - Fedratinib toxicities include Wernicke encephalopathy (as above) cytopenias, nausea and vomiting, hepatic toxicity, and amylase and lipase elevation.
   - Both medications can result in a cytokine storm if stopped immediately without a taper. Therefore, a slow taper is recommended when these medications need to be stopped.

6. **What are some notable complications of pacritinib?**
   - Pacritinib is contraindicated in patients taking other CYP3A4 inducers or inhibitors.

- Diarrhea, lower platelet counts, nausea, anemia, and leg swelling can occur. There is also a risk of major bleeding and thus patients with active bleeding should avoid pacritinib, and pacritinib should be stopped 7 days before any planned surgery.

7. **How is myelofibrosis-associated pulmonary hypertension diagnosed and treated?**
   - Diagnosis is confirmed by a technetium 99m sulfur colloid scintigraphy.
   - Single-fraction whole lung radiation (100 cGy) has been shown to be effective.

QUESTIONS

1. **A 55-year-old woman is referred to hematology for evaluation of a hemoglobin of 16.8/hematocrit of 51% found on routine labs. White blood cell (WBC) and platelet counts are normal. Upon further questioning, she reports minimal pruritus following hot baths, but denies burning and erythema of her hands. Her past medical history is otherwise notable for mild hypertension and tobacco dependency. She denies any family history of hematologic disorders. There is no personal or family history of thrombosis. Physical examination is unremarkable. What is the next best step in management?**
   A. Initiate *JAK2* inhibitor therapy.
   B. Immediately phlebotomize.
   C. Evaluate for causes of secondary polycythemia.
   D. Initiate hydroxyurea.

2. **A 46-year-old man presents with polycythemia (hemoglobin 18.7, hematocrit 56%). He does not have a history of prior thromboembolic events. Workup demonstrated negative *JAK2* V617F mutation. Bone marrow biopsy demonstrated increased cellularity with panmyelosis and pleomorphic mature megakaryocytes. Epo level is below the normal reference range. How should this patient be managed?**
   A. Initiation of *JAK2* inhibitor therapy
   B. Aspirin and phlebotomy
   C. Aspirin only
   D. Observation and optimizing risk factors for thrombosis
   E. Aspirin and hydroxyurea

3. **A 68-year-old woman is found to have a platelet count of 800,000 on routine labs. She is asymptomatic. She has no history of arterial or venous thrombotic events. Physical examination is notable for a palpable spleen tip 2 cm below the costal margin. Testing for *JAK2* V617F is positive. Bone marrow biopsy demonstrates findings consistent with essential thrombocythemia (ET) and rules out other possible disorders. What is the next best step in management?**
   A. Hydroxyurea and aspirin
   B. Interferon alpha and aspirin
   C. Aspirin monotherapy
   D. Check von Willebrand factor (vWF) activity; no therapy needed because she is asymptomatic

4. A 78-year-old man with a past medical history of diabetes, coronary artery disease, heart failure (ejection fraction 35%), and hypertension presents for evaluation of fatigue, night sweats, unintentional weight loss, left upper quadrant abdominal pain, and early satiety. The patient developed these symptoms gradually over the past 6 months. Physical exam is notable for splenomegaly (spleen tip palpated about 15 cm below the left costal margin). Labs revealed a white blood cell (WBC) count of 14,000 (2% circulating blasts), hemoglobin of 9 g/dL, and platelet count of 75,000. These are similar to labs drawn in his primary care physician's (PCP's) office 2 months ago. Peripheral smear is notable for teardrop cells. A bone marrow biopsy reveals megakaryocytic proliferation and atypia, with grade 2 fibrosis and cytogenetics demonstrating 46,XY, inv(3) in 20/20 analyzed cells. *JAK2* V617F and exon 12 mutations are negative, as is *MPL* mutation. The patient has a *CALR* mutation identified. Infections are ruled out. The patient reports that fatigue and abdominal pain are limiting his ability to perform his activities of daily living. What is the best management option for this patient?
   A. Supportive care with transfusions as needed
   B. Hydroxyurea
   C. Ruxolitinib
   D. Cytotoxic chemotherapy followed by allogeneic bone marrow transplantation

5. Which gene is characteristically mutated in chronic neutrophilic leukemia?
   A. *JAK2*
   B. *CALR*
   C. *MPL*
   D. *CSF3R*
   E. *ELANE*

6. What percentage of patients with essential thrombocythemia (ET) do not have a mutation in *JAK2, CALR,* or *MPL*?
   A. 1%
   B. 10%–15%
   C. 40%–40%
   D. 50%–60%

7. A 64-year-old male patient with *JAK2*-positive essential thrombocythemia (ET) is referred to you for a second opinion for management. He has never had a thromboembolic event in the past. He takes no medications and has no other medical problems. Review of complete blood counts shows platelet count of 1.5 million/microL, with normal white blood cells and hemoglobin. What is the next step in management?
   A. Start aspirin.
   B. Start aspirin and cytoreduction.
   C. No additional tests or therapy are needed.
   D. Obtain von Willebrand factor (vWF) activity.

8. **Which of the following is incorrect regarding pulmonary hypertension associated with myelofibrosis?**
   A. Diagnosis of pulmonary hypertension associated with myelofibrosis is confirmed by a technetium 99m sulfur colloid scintigraphy.
   B. Pulmonary hypertension associated with myelofibrosis is treated with single-fraction whole lung radiation.
   C. Pulmonary hypertension has never been associated with myelofibrosis.
   D. Hydroxyurea is the treatment of choice for pulmonary hypertension associated with myelofibrosis.

ANSWERS

1. **C. Evaluate for causes of secondary polycythemia.** Patients who are relatively asymptomatic and present with elevated hematocrit in the outpatient setting should be evaluated for the etiology prior to initiation of therapy directed at lowering the hemoglobin. Secondary polycythemia is much more common than myeloproliferative neoplasms (MPNs), and smoking is a very common cause of secondary polycythemia. A history, physical exam, and sometimes lab work such as erythropoietin (EPO) can help distinguish between the two. If concern for an MPN persists despite this evaluation, then usually molecular testing for mutations such as *JAK2 V617F* is pursued. There is no established role for cytoreduction with Hydrea in secondary polycythemia and therefore empiric treatment would not be pursued. In addition, there are no data to support phlebotomy in secondary polycythemia outside of acute symptoms thought to be related to elevated hemoglobin. Therefore, phlebotomy would not be pursued unless a diagnosis of polycythemia vera (PV) was established in the patient. Lastly, Jak inhibitors such as ruxolitinib are not first-line therapy for PV and have no role in secondary polycythemia and would therefore not be considered empirically.

2. **B. Aspirin and phlebotomy.** Patients who present with polycythemia and exhibit typical bone marrow abnormalities for polycythemia vera (PV), as well as low epo level, have a diagnosis of PV. *JAK2* V617F mutation is present in most patients with PV, but approximately 5% to 7% of patients with PV have the *JAK2* exon 12 mutation instead, while ~1% of patients with PV do not have either *JAK2* V617F or *JAK2* exon 12 mutations. In these patients, the typical bone marrow findings coupled with a low epo level establish the diagnosis. This patient is <60 years of age and has no prior history of thromboembolic events; therefore, he is categorized as low-risk and should be treated with aspirin and PRN phlebotomy (goal hematocrit <45%), instead of aspirin and hydroxyurea.

3. **A. Hydroxyurea and aspirin.** This is a patient with high-risk ET given her age (>60 years) and the presence of a *JAK2* mutation. She therefore has an indication for low-dose aspirin (no contraindication described) and cytoreductive therapy. Hydroxyurea is the preferred first-line option for cytoreduction in high-risk ET. Hydroxyurea is theorized to have potential teratogenicity, but this is less of a concern given the patient's age and the reduced likelihood of long-term side effects. Patients of childbearing age who desire to become pregnant should be counseled about pregnancy while on hydroxyurea and should employ safe contraception methods that do not increase risk of thrombosis and hydroxyurea should be stopped before pregnancy. Interferon therapy can be considered in certain clinical situations, including in younger patients, in pregnant patients who require cytoreductive therapy (risk category C), or in patients who defer hydroxyurea. However, interferon would not be recommended over hydroxyurea in this clinical scenario. vWF activity should be checked in patients with a very high platelet count (>1 million) prior to aspirin administration to rule out acquired von Willebrand disease. This would be less of a concern in this patient.

4. **C. Ruxolitinib.** This patient meets the criteria for higher risk (intermediate-2/high risk) primary myelofibrosis according to the DIPSS-PLUS (Dynamic International Prognostic Scoring System-Plus) risk calculator. He is not a candidate for allogeneic stem cell transplantation given his age and comorbidities. He has symptomatic splenomegaly and fatigue, as well as a platelet count >50,000; therefore, he would benefit from ruxolitinib therapy (or fedratinib as less favorable first-line option) as opposed to supportive care alone or Hydrea. The patient does not require a transfusion based on his complete blood count and supportive transfusions would not help with symptoms or shrink his spleen.

5. **D. *CSF3R*.** *CSF3R* is the gene that is characteristically mutated in chronic neutrophilic leukemia.

6. **B. 10%–15%.** 10%–15% of patients with ET do not have a mutation in *JAK2, CALR,* or *MPL.*

7. **D. Obtain von Willebrand factor (vWF) activity.** In patients with platelets >1 million/microL, ristocetin cofactor activity needs to be checked before starting aspirin. Patients with activity level <30% are at increased risk of bleeding and should undergo platelet cytoreduction to result in vWF ristocetin activity >30% prior to starting aspirin.

8. **D. Hydroxyurea is the treatment of choice for pulmonary hypertension associated with myelofibrosis.** Pulmonary hypertension has been associated with myelofibrosis. The diagnosis of pulmonary hypertension associated with myelofibrosis is confirmed by a technetium 99m sulfur colloid scintigraphy and is treated with single-fraction whole lung radiation.

Acute Leukemias and Hairy Cell Leukemia

13

Morgan A. Jones and Dale Bixby

Acute Myeloid Leukemia

EPIDEMIOLOGY

1. **What is the median age at diagnosis of acute myeloid leukemia (AML)?**
   - 68 years, with an exponential increase beginning in an individual's fifth and sixth decades of life.

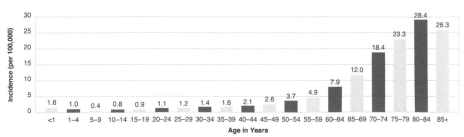

FIGURE 13.1 ■ Age-specific incidence rates for acute myeloid leukemia (AML), 2013–2017.

Source: Derived from Leukemia and Lymphoma Society Facts 2020–2021.
(https://www.lls.org/sites/default/files/2021-08/PS80%20FactsBook_2020_2021_FINAL.pdf).

2. **What is the incidence of AML?**
   - 20,000 new cases seen in the United States in 2022

ETIOLOGY AND RISK FACTORS

1. **What are the common risk factors for AML?**
   - Older age
   - Exposure to chemotherapeutic agents
     - Topoisomerase II inhibitors: latency of 1 to 3 years, associated with rearrangement of the histone-lysine N-methyltransferase 2A (*KMT2A*) gene (previously known as the mixed lineage leukemia [*MLL*] gene) positioned at chromosome 11q23
     - Alkylating agents: latency period of 3 to 7 years, associated with del 5q/-5 and/or del 7q/-7 chromosomal abnormalities, as well as complex cytogenetic changes; patients often with an antecedent myelodysplastic syndrome (MDS) that precedes the development of the AML
   - Bone marrow failure disorders like MDS or aplastic anemia (AA)
   - Myeloproliferative neoplasms

- Exposure to chemicals: benzene, pesticides, and petroleum products
- Radiation exposure
- Congenital disorders: Down syndrome, Bloom syndrome, Fanconi anemia, dyskeratosis congenita (Zinsser–Cole–Engman syndrome), *GATA2 deficiency*, Shwachman–Diamond syndrome, Diamond–Blackfan anemia, and others

PATHOLOGY—CLASSIFICATION

1. **Define the subtypes of AML according to the 2022 World Health Organization (WHO) classification.**
   - AML with defining genetic abnormalities
     - Acute promyelocytic leukemia (APL) with *PML-RARA*
     - AML with *RUNX1-RUNX1T1*
     - AML with *CBFB-MYH11*
     - AML with *DEK-NUP214*
     - AML with *RBM15-MRTFA*
     - AML with *BCR-ABL1*
     - AML with *KMT2A* rearrangement
     - AML with *MECOM* rearrangement
     - AML with *NUP98* rearrangement
     - AML with *NPM1* mutation
     - AML with *CEBPA* mutation
     - AML, myelodysplasia-related
     - AML with other genetic alterations
   - AML, defined by differentiation
     - AML with minimal differentiation
     - AML without maturation
     - AML with maturation
     - Acute basophilic leukemia
     - Acute myelomonocytic leukemia
     - Acute monocytic leukemia
     - Acute erythroid leukemia
     - Acute megakaryoblastic leukemia
   - Myeloid sarcoma

2. **What are the cytogenetic and molecular abnormalities that define myelodysplasia-related AML (AML-MR)?**
   - Cytogenetic abnormalities include the following:
     - Complex karyotype (≥3 abnormalities)
     - Chromosome 5q changes (deletion or loss through an unbalanced translocation)
     - Chromosome 7 alterations (monosomy, 7q deletion, loss of 7q through an unbalanced translocation)
     - 11q deletion
     - 12p alterations (deletion or loss through an unbalanced translocation)
     - Monosomy 13 or 13q deletion
     - 17p alterations (deletion or loss through an unbalanced translocation)
     - Isochromosome 17q
     - idic(X)(q13)

- Defining molecular mutations involve *ASXL1, BCOR, EZH2, SF3B1, SRSF* *STAG2, U2AF1*, and *ZRSR2*.
- Note that an antecedent history of MDS that preceded the diagnosis of AML is also compatible with the diagnosis of AML with myelodysplastic-related changes, but significant (>50%) dysplasia in one or more hematopoietic lineages is no longer diagnostic of this subtype of AML.

3. **How are secondary leukemias defined?**
   - The 2022 WHO defines secondary leukemia as a leukemia arising in the setting of prior chemotherapy or within the context of a germline predisposition.
   - Note that an AML transformation of an antecedent myeloproliferative neoplasm is retained in the MPN category, while an AML transformation of MDS or MDS/MPN is kept under the AML-MR category.

SIGNS AND SYMPTOMS

1. **What are the common signs and symptoms of AML?**
   - Fever and other constitutional symptoms of infections
   - Bruising or bleeding (due to thrombocytopenia)
   - Fatigue and other symptoms of anemia
   - Leukostasis: central nervous system (CNS) manifestations, cardiopulmonary symptoms, retinal hemorrhage, and priapism
   - Disseminated intravascular coagulation (DIC)
   - Tumor lysis syndrome

DIAGNOSTIC WORKUP

1. **Define the diagnostic criteria for AML.**
   - In the absence of a leukemia-defining genetic lesion, ≥20% myeloid blasts in the bone marrow or peripheral blood are found.
   - Of the genetic events listed under the "AML with defining genetic abnormalities" in the 2022 WHO criteria, only AML with *BCR-ABL* and AML with *CEBPA* mutations require 20% blasts. In the case of any other listed event, the genetic lesion is sufficient to establish the diagnosis irrespective of blast percentage.
   - The myeloid lineage is established if *any* of the following are identified:
     - Auer rods
     - Blasts myeloperoxidase-positive (by flow cytometry, immunohistochemistry, or cytochemistry)
     - Blasts expressing two or more myeloid antigens (CD13, CD33, CD117)
     - Monocytic differentiation (with at least two of the following: nonspecific esterase, CD11c, CD14, CD36, CD64)

PROGNOSTIC FACTORS

1. **How are patients with AML stratified into different risk groups?**
   - The National Comprehensive Cancer Network (NCCN) and European LeukemiaNet (ELN) uses cytogenetics and single-gene mutations as prognostic factors. We also recognized that older age is often a poor prognostic factor often due to the presence of increased high-risk genetic changes and poor tolerance to available therapies.

TABLE 13.1 ■ Risk Stratification System: NCCN and ELN

Risk Status	Cytogenetics/Molecular Abnormalities
Favorable risk	■ t(8;21)(q22;q22.1) ■ inv(16)(p13.1;q22) or t(16;16)(p13.1;q22) ■ Normal cytogenetics with *NPM1* mutation without *FLT3-ITD* or with *FLT3-ITD* (low variant allele frequency) ■ Biallelic *CEBPA* mutation
Intermediate risk	■ Normal cytogenetics without favorable risk or poor risk gene mutations ■ Mutated *NPM1* and *FLT3-ITD* (high variant allele frequency) ■ Normal cytogenetics with wild-type *NPM1* without *FLT3-ITD* mutation or with *FLT3-ITD* (low variant allele frequency) ■ t(9;11)(p21.3;q11.2)(*MLLT3-KMT2A*)
Poor risk*	■ Complex cytogenetics† ■ Monosomal karyotype‡ ■ −5 or del(5q) ■ −7 ■ −17 or abnormal 17(p) ■ t(v;11q23.3); *KMT2A* rearranged ■ inv(3)(q21.3q26.2) or t(3;3)(q21.3q26.2);*GATA2,MECOM(EVI1)* ■ t(6;9)(p23;q34.1);*DEK-NUP214* ■ t(9;22)(q34;q11.2); *BCR-ABL1* ■ Normal cytogenetics with wild-type *NPM1* and *FLT3-ITD* (high variant allele frequency) ■ *TP53* mutation ■ *RUNX1* mutation ■ *ASXL1* mutation

*Poor-risk AML also includes patients with secondary AML—antecedent hematologic disease or treatment-related AML.

†Complex cytogenetics is defined as three or more chromosomal abnormalities.

‡Monosomal karyotype is defined as the presence of at least two autosomal monosomies or a single autosomal monosomy associated with at least one structural abnormality.

AML, acute myeloid leukemia.

2. How are patients with APL risk-stratified?
■ Sanz criteria

TABLE 13.2 ■ Risk Stratification: Sanz Criteria

Low-risk APL	WBC <10,000 and platelet >40,000
Intermediate-risk APL	WBC <10,000 and platelet <40,000
High-risk APL	WBC ≥10,000

APL, acute promyelocytic leukemia; WBC, white blood cell.

■ In most clinical circumstances, low-risk APL and intermediate-risk APL are treated similarly, so the clinical distinction of these two diagnostic subgroups is limited and thus often combined into low/intermediate-risk disease.

TREATMENT

NON-ACUTE PROMYELOCYTIC LEUKEMIA-ACUTE MYELOID LEUKEMIA

1. **What are the induction treatment options for younger, fit patients with non-APL AML?**
   - In many publications, there are statements made about treatment algorithms based on age alone. However, one must consider age, organ function, and performance status when deciding on fitness for chemotherapy.
   - In general, for those aged ≤75 with a suitable overall performance status and organ function, curative intent therapy is often considered. The NCCN guidelines currently list the following therapies in no ranked order within the subgroups.

TABLE 13.3 ■ Candidate for Intensive Induction Chemotherapy

Risk Category	Regimen
Favorable risk	■ Anthracycline (daunorubicin or idarubicin or mitoxantrone) + cytarabine
	■ Daunorubicin + cytarabine + gemtuzumab ozogamicin
Intermediate risk	■ If *FLT3*-mutated: daunorubicin + cytarabine + midostaurin
	■ Anthracycline (daunorubicin or idarubicin or mitoxantrone) + cytarabine
	■ Daunorubicin + cytarabine + gemtuzumab ozogamicin
Poor risk	■ Anthracycline (daunorubicin or idarubicin or mitoxantrone) + cytarabine
	■ Venetoclax + a hypomethylating agent (azacitidine or decitabine)
	■ Hypomethylating agent (azacitidine or decitabine)
	■ High-dose cytarabine with an anthracycline or fludarabine
	■ If therapy-related or antecedent myelodysplastic syndrome, one can consider liposomal cytarabine and daunorubicin

Note: All patients should be considered for clinical trial enrolment.

2. **How do we evaluate the efficacy of induction therapy?**
   - Obtain a bone marrow biopsy 7 to 14 days after completion of induction therapy (14–21 days after start) if providing an anthracycline and cytarabine combination treatment. Otherwise, most bone marrow assessments occur on/around day 28 from the start of chemotherapy.
     - Aplastic marrow (<5% cellular and <5% blasts): Await count recovery and consider growth factor support.
     - Significant cytoreduction and a low percentage of blasts: Consider repeating the marrow in 7 to 10 days.
     - Significant residual blasts: high-dose cytarabine-based regimen or standard-dose cytarabine + an anthracycline or venetoclax + a hypomethylating agent

■ Obtain the next marrow at count recovery (absolute neutrophil count [ANC] ≥1, platelet count ≥100, and no transfusion needs for red blood cells; see Question 5) to determine remission status.

3. **What are the induction treatment options for older or frail patients with non-APL AML?**

   ■ These therapy considerations are often made for patients aged >75, those with poor cardiac, renal, hepatic or pulmonary function, those with resistant infections, or those with long-term poor performance status.

   ■ Some patients with AML may not be candidates for any disease-directed therapy depending on the severity of these comorbidities.

TABLE 13.4 ■ Candidate for Less-Intensive Induction Chemotherapy

Scenario	Regimen
No actionable mutations	■ Venetoclax + a hypomethylating agent (azacitidine or decitabine) ■ Hypomethylating agent (azacitidine or decitabine) ■ Venetoclax + low-dose cytarabine ■ Glasdegib + low-dose cytarabine ■ Gemtuzumab ozogamicin ■ Low-dose cytarabine ■ Best supportive care
IDH1 mutation	■ Ivosidenib ± a hypomethylating agent ■ Hypomethylating agent (azacitidine or decitabine) ± venetoclax
IDH2 mutation	■ Enasidenib ■ Hypomethylating agent (azacitidine or decitabine) ■ Venetoclax + a hypomethylating agent (azacitidine or decitabine)
FLT3 mutation	■ Sorafenib + azacitidine or decitabine ■ Venetoclax + a hypomethylating agent (azacitidine or decitabine)

4. **When is complete remission (CR) evaluated for and how is it defined?**

   ■ Evaluation of CR requires that a bone marrow biopsy be performed after count recovery: ANC ≥1,000, platelets ≥100,000 (independent of transfusions), and a hemoglobin value high enough to be independent from red cell transfusions.

   ● *Morphologic CR:* marrow blasts less than 5%, no Auer rods, no persistence of extramedullary disease

   ● *Cytogenetic CR:* morphologic CR as well as normal cytogenetics in patients who had abnormal cytogenetics at the time of diagnosis

   ● *Complete remission with incomplete count recovery (CRi):* CR with persistence of a single cytopenia

5. **What is the postremission treatment of choice for fit patients with non-APL AML in CR?**
   - Favorable-risk AML:
     - High-dose cytarabine
     - Clinical trial
   - Intermediate-risk AML:
     - Allogeneic hematopoietic stem cell transplant (patients may receive high-dose intermittent ARA-C [HIDAC] consolidation until donor is found)
     - High-dose cytarabine
     - The specific consolidation built into the treatment scheme of the induction therapy utilized
     - Clinical trial
   - Poor-risk AML:
     - Allogeneic hematopoietic stem cell transplant (ASCT; patients may receive HIDAC consolidation until donor is found)
     - The specific consolidation built into the treatment scheme of the induction therapy utilized
     - Clinical trial

6. **What is the postremission treatment of choice for unfit or older patients with non-APL AML in CR?**
   - ASCT (patients may receive HIDAC consolidation until donor is found) if their performance status improves
   - Intermediate/high-dose cytarabine patients with favorable- or intermediate-risk AML with good performance status and organ function
   - Standard-dose cytarabine ± anthracycline for one or two cycles
   - For patients who received a hypomethylating agent ± venetoclax for induction: continuation of therapy until toxicity or disease progression
   - For those receiving an IDH inhibitor: continuation of therapy until toxicity or disease progression
   - Clinical trial
   - Observation

7. **What is the surveillance strategy for patients with AML in CR postconsolidation therapy?**
   - Complete blood count (CBC) every 1 to 3 months for 2 to 3 years, then every 3 to 6 months until 5 years
   - Bone marrow aspirate and biopsy only if cytopenias or abnormalities are identified on peripheral smear

8. **What is the treatment strategy for relapsed non-APL AML patients?**
   - The only chance for a cure is with ASCT, ideally in the second CR.
     - Clinical trial followed by ASCT
     - Salvage chemotherapy followed by ASCT
   - If a patient is not eligible for an allogeneic hematopoietic stem cell transplant, one can offer consolidation based on the induction strategy used, but curative percentages are very low.
   - Provide best supportive care.

Acute Promyelocytic Leukemia

1. **What are the induction and consolidation treatment options for patients with *high-risk* APL?**
   - High-risk APL is defined as a presenting white blood cell count >10,000 cells/microL
   - Strategy is dependent on the presence or absence of cardiac issues, defined as decreased ejection fraction or prolonged QTc.

TABLE 13.5 ■ Induction and Consolidation Treatment Options for High-Risk APL

PRESERVED EJECTION FRACTION AND NORMAL QTc		
APML-4	Induction	■ ATRA ■ Age-adjusted idarubicin ■ Arsenic trioxide
	Consolidation/maintenance	■ ATRA ■ Arsenic trioxide
C9710	Induction	■ ATRA ■ Daunorubicin ■ Cytarabine
	Consolidation	■ Arsenic ■ ATRA ■ Daunorubicin
LPA-99	Induction	■ ATRA ■ Idarubicin ■ Cytarabine
	Consolidation	■ Daunorubicin ■ Cytarabine
LPA-2005	Induction	■ ATRA ■ Idarubicin
	Consolidation	■ ATRA ■ Idarubicin ■ Cytarabine ■ Mitoxantrone
REDUCED EJECTION FRACTION		
MD Anderson	Induction	■ ATRA ■ Arsenic trioxide ■ Gemtuzumab ozogamicin
	Consolidation/maintenance	■ ATRA ■ Arsenic trioxide

(continued)

TABLE 13.5 ■ *(continued)*

AML-17	Induction	■ ATRA ■ Arsenic trioxide ■ Gemtuzumab ozogamicin
	Consolidation/maintenance	■ ATRA ■ Arsenic trioxide

PROLONGED QTc

MD Anderson	Induction	■ ATRA ■ Gemtuzumab ozogamicin
	Consolidation	■ ATRA ■ Gemtuzumab ozogamicin
LPA-99 and APL 2000	Induction	■ ATRA ■ Daunorubicin ■ Cytarabine
	Consolidation	■ Daunorubicin ■ Cytarabine
LPA-2005	Induction	■ ATRA ■ Idarubicin
	Consolidation	■ ATRA ■ Idarubicin ■ Cytarabine ■ Mitoxantrone

ATRA, all-trans retinoic acid.

- Note that each regimen may have unique timing and dosing of the agents listed. Additionally, the regimens may contain maintenance therapy as indicated in the manuscript.
- Current NCCN guidelines also call for consideration for four to six doses of intrathecal prophylaxis in patients with high-risk APL.

2. **What is the treatment of choice for patients *with low/intermediate-risk* APL?**
   - Low-risk APL is defined as a presenting white blood cell count of ≤10,000 cells/microL and a platelet count of >40,000/microL.
   - Intermediate-risk APL is defined as a presenting white blood cell count of ≤10,000 cells/microL and a platelet count of <40,000/microL.
   - Clinically, the therapies for both low- and intermediate-risk APL overlap, so the therapeutic significance of this prognostic distinction is limited.

TABLE 13.6 ■ Treatment of Choice for Low/Intermediate-Risk APL

APL-0406	Induction	■ ATRA
		■ Arsenic trioxide
	Consolidation	■ ATRA
		■ Arsenic trioxide
AML-17	Induction	■ ATRA
		■ Arsenic trioxide
	Consolidation	■ ATRA
		■ Arsenic trioxide
LPA-2005	Induction	■ ATRA
		■ Idarubicin
	Consolidation	■ ATRA
		■ Idarubicin
		■ Cytarabine
		■ Mitoxantrone
MD Anderson	Induction	■ ATRA
		■ Gemtuzumab ozogamicin
	Consolidation	■ ATRA
		■ Gemtuzumab ozogamicin

ATRA, all-trans retinoic acid.

- Note that each regimen may have unique timing and dosing of the agents listed. Additionally, the regimens may contain maintenance therapy as indicated in the manuscript.
- Patients started on an induction regimen according to one treatment protocol should receive consolidation and maintenance following the same protocol. Switching from one protocol to another should not be done.

3. **How are patients with APL monitored during and after consolidation and what is the postconsolidation therapy if the polymerase chain reaction (PCR) is negative?**
   - Bone marrow biopsy should be performed to document cytogenetic and molecular (PCR) remission during or at the completion of consolidation if not achieving these milestones after induction.
   - If PCR is negative, patients should receive maintenance therapy as per the initial treatment protocol if indicated. Not all regimens employ maintenance therapy.
   - PCR monitoring should be performed for up to 2 years after the completion of all therapies.

4. **How should patients with PCR-positive disease (after consolidation or if PCR turns positive during postconsolidation therapy) be treated?**
   - PCR should be repeated in 2 to 4 weeks for confirmation and to rule out a false positive result. If it is confirmed positive, patients are considered in first relapse.
     - No prior exposure to arsenic trioxide or late relapse (≥6 months) after arsenic trioxide containing regimen: arsenic trioxide ± all-trans retinoic acid (ATRA) until count recovery with marrow confirmation of remission

- Early relapse (<6 months) after ATRA or arsenic trioxide only (no anthracy-cline): ATRA + idarubicin + arsenic trioxide until count recovery with marrow confirmation of remission
- Early relapse (<6 months) after arsenic trioxide/anthracycline containing regimen: arsenic trioxide ± ATRA until count recovery with marrow confirmation of remission
- Those who achieve second morphologic remission should be strongly considered for CNS prophylaxis.
- If the PCR turns negative, patients should be consolidated with an autologous stem cell transplantation. Those who are not transplant candidates should undergo up to six cycles of arsenic consolidation.
- If the PCR stays positive, patients should be treated with an allogeneic hematopoietic stem cell transplant (or on a clinical trial if not transplant candidates).
- Patients who do not achieve a second morphologic remission should be considered for a clinical trial or treated with an allogeneic hematopoietic stem cell transplant.

Acute Lymphoblastic Leukemia

EPIDEMIOLOGY

1. What is the median age at diagnosis of acute lymphoblastic leukemia (ALL)?
- 15 years
  - There is a bimodal age distribution in ALL, with peaks in children aged 1 to 4 and then again in older adults in their sixth and seventh decades of life.

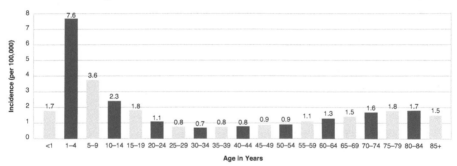

FIGURE 13.2 ■ Age-specific incidence rates for acute lymphoblastic leukemia (ALL), 2013–2017
Source: Derived from Leukemia and Lymphoma Society Facts 2020–2021
(https://www.lls.org/sites/default/files/2021-08/PS80%20FactsBook_2020_2021_FINAL.pdf).

- 57% of patients diagnosed at less than 20 years of age, and 27% diagnosed at 45 years or older

2. What is the incidence of ALL?
- 6,500 new cases per year in the United States

ETIOLOGY AND RISK FACTORS

1. What are the common risk factors for ALL?
- Hispanics > Whites > African Americans
- Men > women

- Intrauterine exposure to radiation
- Environmental exposure: nuclear radiation
- Chemical exposure: benzene
- Congenital disorders: Down syndrome, ataxia telangiectasia, and Bloom syndrome

PATHOLOGY—CLASSIFICATION

1. **What is the current WHO classification of ALL?**
   - B-lymphoblastic leukemia/lymphoma
     - B-lymphoblastic leukemia/lymphoma, not otherwise specified (NOS)
     - B-lymphoblastic leukemia/lymphoma with high hyperdiploidy
     - B-lymphoblastic leukemia/lymphoma with hypodiploidy
     - B-lymphoblastic leukemia/lymphoma with *BCR-ABL1* fusion
     - B-lymphoblastic leukemia/lymphoma with *BCR-ABL1*-like features
     - B-lymphoblastic leukemia/lymphoma with *KMT2A* rearrangement
     - B-lymphoblastic leukemia/lymphoma with *ETV6-RUNX1* fusion
     - B-lymphoblastic leukemia/lymphoma with *ETV6-RUNX1* like features
     - B-lymphoblastic leukemia/lymphoma with *IGH-IL3* fusion
     - B-lymphoblastic leukemia/lymphoma with *TCF3-PBX1* fusion
     - B-lymphoblastic leukemia/lymphoma with *TCF3-HLF* fusion
     - B-lymphoblastic leukemia/lymphoma with iAMP21
     - B-lymphoblastic leukemia/lymphoma with other defined genetic abnormalities
   - T-lymphoblastic leukemia/lymphoma
     - T-lymphoblastic leukemia/lymphoma, NOS
     - Early T-cell precursor lymphoblastic leukemia/lymphoma

SIGNS AND SYMPTOMS

1. **What are the common signs and symptoms of ALL?**
   - Lymphadenopathy and/or hepatosplenomegaly
   - Painless testicular swelling
   - Fever and other constitutional symptoms of infections
   - Bruising or bleeding from thrombocytopenia
   - Fatigue and other symptoms of anemia
   - Infections (due to neutropenia)
   - Leukostasis: CNS manifestations, cardiopulmonary symptoms, retinal hemorrhage, and priapism
   - Tumor lysis syndrome
   - Mediastinal mass
   - Musculoskeletal pain

DIAGNOSTIC WORKUP

1. **Define the diagnostic criteria for ALL.**
   - Marrow and/or peripheral blood and/or lymph node involvement with lymphoid blasts
     - Typically, there will be ≥20% lymphoblasts in the marrow at the time of diagnosis, but no absolute cutoff is actually needed.

■ Immunophenotypic and genetic determination of the lymphoblasts to allow for appropriate subclassification as outlined earlier

PROGNOSTIC FACTORS

1. How are patients with ALL stratified into different risk groups?

TABLE 13.7 ■ ALL Risk Stratification

	Adverse Risk	Standard Risk
Age	■ <1 year or >35 years	■ >1 year but <35 years
Immunophenotype	■ ETP ■ Pro-B (especially CD20+)	■ T-cell ■ Pre-B
WBC count	■ >100,000 for T-cell ■ >30,000 for B-cell	■ <100,000 for T-cell ■ <30,000 for B-cell
Genetic aberrations	■ Complex (≥5 changes) ■ Hypodiploidy (<44 chromosomes) ■ t(9;22) or *BCR-ABL* ■ *KMT2A* (*MLL*) rearranged ■ Ph-like ALL	■ High hyperdiploidy (51–65 chromosomes) ■ t(12;21)(*ETV6-RUNX1*)
CNS involvement	■ Present	■ Absent
Response to therapy	■ Minimal residual disease present after induction	■ Minimal residual disease negative after induction

ALL, acute lymphoblastic leukemia; CNS, central nervous system; ETP, early T precursor; WBC, white blood cell.

TREATMENT

1. How are adult patients with Philadelphia chromosome-positive (Ph+) ALL treated?

■ Patients who are less than 75 years old without major comorbidities: induction cytotoxic chemotherapy (often age-adjusted R-hyper-CVAD) + a tyrosine kinase inhibitor (TKI).
   ● If CR is achieved, patients should undergo an allogeneic hematopoietic stem cell transplant in first remission, followed by consideration for use of a maintenance TKI for a period of time following the allogeneic transplant.
   ● If no donor is available, they should be continued on consolidation multiagent chemotherapy + TKI, followed by maintenance therapy + TKI.
   ● Examples of cytotoxic regimens include the following:
      ▪ TKIs + (R)hyper-CVAD
      ▪ TKI + COG AALL-0031
      ▪ TKI + EsPhALL
■ Patients who are 75 years old or older, or with significant comorbidities: induction therapy with TKI + steroids or TKI + low-dose chemotherapy. If they achieve CR, they should be continued on TKI as consolidation.

- Examples of regimens include the following:
  - LAL1205 protocol: TKI + corticosteroid
  - TKI + vincristine + dexamethasone
  - EWALL-PH-01 or EWALL-PH-02 protocol

2. **How are adult patients with Ph– ALL treated?**
   - Patients less than 70 years old without major comorbidities: induction with multiagent chemotherapy (multiple regimens available—the backbone of these therapies is steroids + anthracycline + vincristine)
     - For fit patients under age 39, strong consideration should be given for a pediatric-inspired asparaginase-based regimen.
     - If CR is achieved, patients should continue multiagent chemotherapy as consolidation, followed by maintenance therapy, or undergo an allogeneic hematopoietic stem cell transplant if a donor is available (typically in patients with high-risk cytogenetic features or those with persistent morphologic or minimal residual disease).
     - Examples of regimens include the following:
       - CALGB 10403
       - COG AALL0232
       - CALGB 8811
       - Linker regimen
       - Hyper-CVAD
       - MRC UKALLXII/ECOG2993
   - Patients who are 70 years old or older, or with significant comorbidities: induction with dose-limited chemotherapy and steroids
     - If they achieve CR, they should receive consolidation with chemotherapy followed by maintenance therapy.

3. **How are patients with relapsed/refractory ALL treated?**
   - Ph+ ALL: Consider *ABL* kinase domain mutation testing to determine optimal TKI as a portion of the patient's therapy.
     - Treatment options include clinical trial, chemotherapy ± TKI, and TKI ± steroids. Blinatumomab or inotuzumab ozogamicin can also be considered.
     - Patients who are refractory or in second or later relapse may also be considered for treatment with chimeric antigen receptor-T cell therapy (tisagenlecleucel).
     - Allogeneic hematopoietic stem cell transplant is considered if a morphologic remission is obtained.
   - Ph (–) ALL:
     - Treatment options include clinical trial or multiagent chemotherapy. Blinatumomab and inotuzumab ozogamicin are considered for B-ALL and nelarabine for T-ALL.
       - For patients treated with an asparaginase-based regimen upfront, one often considers a high-dose methotrexate and high-dose cytarabine-based regimen like the B-arm of hyper-CVAD.
       - For patients treated with hyper-CVAD, one often considers an asparaginase-based salvage regimen.
     - For B-ALL that are refractory or in second or later relapse, treatment with CAR-T cell therapy (tisagenlecleucel) may be considered.
     - Allogeneic hematopoietic stem cell transplant is considered if a morphologic remission is obtained.

SPECIAL CONSIDERATIONS IN ACUTE LEUKEMIAS

1. **What are the medical emergencies in leukemias?**
   - Leukostasis: Leukostasis needs to be treated aggressively with intravenous (IV) hydration, cytoreduction with hydroxyurea (or steroids in cases of lymphoblastic leukemias), and leukapheresis. Avoid red blood cell transfusions until cytoreduction has reduced the risk of leukostasis.
   - *DIC:* DIC needs to be treated aggressively with supportive blood and blood product transfusions and disease control. Suspect APL in patients with DIC and start ATRA before a cytogenetic or molecular diagnosis is established.
   - *APL:* Patients need to start ATRA immediately even before diagnosis is genetically confirmed to limit the risk of DIC even in patients not presenting with overt DIC.
   - *Differentiation syndrome:* This syndrome develops in APL (ATRA and arsenic are risk factors). The signs and symptoms are fever, weight gain, edema, dyspnea, hypoxia, worsening renal function, opacities on chest imaging, pleural/pericardial effusions, and hypotension. Patients need to be treated with dexamethasone 10 mg every 12 hours. If differentiation syndrome is severe, ATRA (and arsenic) needs to be held and resumed only after it resolves. Starting cytotoxic chemotherapy (if not already done) is considered. Consider differentiation syndrome prophylactic therapy with dexamethasone when starting differentiating therapy, especially in those with high-risk APL.
   - *Tumor lysis syndrome:* This syndrome could be spontaneous in aggressive hematologic malignancies or induced by therapy. Patients typically have elevated uric acid, potassium, and phosphorus, low calcium, and worsening renal function. Patients should be treated prophylactically with IV hydration, allopurinol or febuxostat, and monitoring for tumor lysis syndrome through checking creatinine, potassium, phosphorus, uric acid, and calcium two to three times a day during the early days of therapy. Rasburicase can also be considered prophylactically in highly proliferative malignancies if the risk of tumor lysis syndrome is elevated and particularly if the renal function is not normal. Treatment of tumor lysis syndrome includes aggressive IV hydration, aggressive measures to correct electrolyte abnormalities, allopurinol or febuxostat, and rasburicase in select cases. Glucose-6-phosphate dehydrogenase (G6PD) deficiency should be investigated, if suspected, before administration of rasburicase.

Hairy Cell Leukemia

EPIDEMIOLOGY

1. **What is the median age at diagnosis of hairy cell leukemia (HCL)?**
   - 52 years of age

2. **What is the incidence of HCL?**
   - About 600 to 800 new cases per year in the United States (2% of all leukemias)

ETIOLOGY AND RISK FACTORS

1. **Is HCL more common in males or females?**
   - More common in males (with male to female ratio of 4:1)

PATHOLOGY

1. **What genetic mutation is seen in virtually all cases of HCL?**
   - *BRAF* V600E, although this is not known to be a disease-initiating mutation

SIGNS AND SYMPTOMS

1. **What are the typical clinical manifestations of HCL?**
   - Pancytopenia, including monocytopenia
   - Fever and other constitutional symptoms
   - Infections
   - Bleeding
   - Fatigue and other symptoms of anemia
   - Organomegaly (splenomegaly) is common

DIAGNOSIS

1. **What is the common microscopic appearance of HCL?**
   - Hair-like projections from the leukemia cells
   - Fried-egg appearance on bone marrow biopsy
   - Leukemic cells stain brightly with CD20
   - Bone marrow may be hypocellular (need to differentiate from AA and hypoplastic MDS)
   - Bone marrow fibrosis often present

2. **How is the diagnosis established?**
   - Typical clinical manifestations with immunophenotype by flow cytometry
   - HCL immunophenotype: CD11c+, CD25+, CD103+, CD123+, CD20+, CD22+, CD52+, cyclin D1+, annexin A1+, BRAF V600E+
   - Hairy cell variant immunophenotype: CD25–, CD123–, annexin A1–, BRAF V600E–

PROGNOSTIC FACTORS

1. **Does the hairy cell variant respond better or worse to treatment?**
   - The hairy cell variant (immunophenotype CD11c+, CD25–, CD103–, CD123–) tends not to respond as well to purine nucleoside analogue-based therapy. Consideration should be given to treatment with sequential purine nucleoside analogue-based therapy followed by rituximab.

TREATMENT

1. **When do we initiate therapy in HCL?**
   - Watch and wait strategy is recommended unless one of the following criteria for starting therapy is met:
     - Symptomatic disease that interferes with daily activities (e.g., fatigue with no other reason, symptomatic splenomegaly)
     - Anemia (hemoglobin <11 g/dL)
     - Thrombocytopenia (platelet <100,000/microL)
     - Neutropenia (ANC <1,000)

2. **What are the treatment options for HCL?**
   - Cladribine (7-day continuous infusion, or 1- to 2-hour bolus IV daily for 5 days, or subcutaneously daily for 5–7 days, or weekly for 5–6 weeks)
   - Alternative option: pentostatin IV every 2 weeks until maximal response (every 3 weeks if neutrophil count falls far below the baseline)
   - CR achieved in about 70% to 90% of patients, with a relapse rate of approximately 30% to 40% (at 10–15 years)

3. **How are patients followed after therapy?**
   - Improvement in peripheral blood counts may require weeks to months.
   - Bone marrow to document CR should be done at 3 to 4 months.
   - After CR, CBCs are typically obtained every 1 to 3 months until they plateau and then every 3 to 6 months thereafter.

4. **How are patients with relapsed HCL treated?**
   - If initial remission was for more than 2 years, consider repeating therapy with the same agent.
   - If the remission was for less than 2 years, consider the alternative purine nucleoside analogue, combination of a purine nucleoside analogue with rituximab, vemurafenib (although this remains off-label), or moxetumomab (in those who have received at least two prior systemic therapies, including treatment with a purine nucleoside analogue).

5. **How are patients with resistant HCL treated?**
   - Consider an alternative purine nucleoside analogue, the combination of a purine nucleoside analogue with sequential rituximab, vemurafenib (although this remains off-label), or moxetumomab (in those who have received at least two prior systemic therapies, including treatment with a purine nucleoside analogue).

QUESTIONS

1. A 40-year-old man presents to his primary care physician (PCP) with symptoms of fatigue and easy bruising. A complete blood count (CBC) reveals a white blood cell (WBC) count of 85, hemoglobin of 8.8, and platelet count of 31. The WBC differential reveals 83% circulating blasts, with Auer rods present. Bone marrow biopsy is performed and confirms the diagnosis of acute myeloid leukemia (AML). The patient begins induction chemotherapy with anthracycline and cytarabine in a standard 3 + 7 fashion using daunorubicin 90 mg/m² and cytarabine 100 mg/m². Human leukocyte antigen (HLA) typing is sent on admission, and he is found to have a 10/10 HLA matched sibling. With which of the following genetic findings would you more strongly consider consolidation therapy with high-dose cytarabine in first complete remission (CR1)?
   A. Karyotype demonstrating -5,-7,-8.
   B. Normal male karyotype with *TP53* mutation
   C. t(v;11q23.3), that is, KMT2A rearrangement
   D. Normal cytogenetics with *NPM1* mutation without *FLT3-ITD*

2. A 55-year-old woman presents to the ED with complaints of fatigue, dyspnea on exertion, vision changes, and headaches. Routine blood work reveals a white blood cell (WBC) count of 1,160, hemoglobin of 7.5, and platelet count of 60. Review of the peripheral smear shows 80% blasts with Auer rods. Physical exam confirms the presence of retinal hemorrhages bilaterally and she has an SpO_2 of 80% off of supplemental oxygen. What is the next most important step in management?
   A. Order stat CT-PE protocol and call ophthalmology consult.
   B. Transfuse 2 units of packed red blood cells (PRBCs).
   C. Obtain an echocardiogram.
   D. Arrange for urgent leukapheresis, initiate fluids, and begin hydroxyurea.

3. A 45-year-old woman completed multiagent chemotherapy including an anthracycline, cyclophosphamide, and radiation therapy for breast cancer 1.5 years ago. She has been free of disease since but on routine blood work she was noted to have a white blood cell (WBC) count of 0.5, hemoglobin of 8, and platelet count of 53. Prior laboratory testing following completion of chemotherapy revealed a normal complete blood count. Bone marrow biopsy establishes the diagnosis of acute myeloid leukemia (AML). Which cytogenetic abnormality is she most likely to have?
   A. 11q23 abnormality
   B. t(8;21)(q22;q22.1)
   C. t(15;17)(q24;q21)
   D. Normal karyotype, NPM1 mutation

4. A 43-year-old woman is 11 days into therapy with all-trans retinoic acid (ATRA) and arsenic trioxide for a diagnosis of low-risk acute promyelocytic leukemia (APL). She had been doing well, but develops hypoxia, conversational dyspnea, and bilateral lower extremity edema. Chest x-ray reveals bilateral pulmonary infiltrates without features of organization. What is the most appropriate step in management?
   A. Check a procalcitonin level.
   B. Start dexamethasone 10 mg twice daily for presumed differentiation syndrome.
   C. Order a stat CT-PE protocol and initiate a heparin drip as pulmonary embolism is your leading diagnosis.
   D. Perform a stat bedside transthoracic echocardiogram for suspected therapy-induced cardiomyopathy.

5. A 67-year old man is transferred to your center for acute myeloid leukemia. He has no known prior medical history. Initial laboratory assessment demonstrates a uric acid of 16, potassium of 9, calcium of 6.5, and a creatinine elevated to 4 from a normal baseline. His EKG shows peaked T waves. In addition to acute management of hyperkalemia and hypocalcemia corrections, what are the next steps in management?
   A. Initiate aggressive fluid resuscitation and give rasburicase (0.2 mg/kg), with plan to recheck labs in 6 to 8 hours.
   B. Place an emergent trialysis catheter to initiate dialysis.

C. Start low-dose cytarabine for cytoreduction.

D. Start dexamethasone.

6. **A 39-year-old woman is diagnosed with Philadelphia chromosome negative (Ph–) B-cell acute lymphoblastic leukemia (ALL). After undergoing intensive induction with an asparaginase-based multiagent chemotherapy regimen, she achieves a complete remission (CR) but had evidence of minimal residual disease. She then underwent early intensification and interim maintenance therapy. A repeat bone marrow aspiration and biopsy continued to demonstrate a morphologic remission, but also minimal residual disease testing (0.7%). She has a human leukocyte antigen (HLA)-matched related sibling. What is the best strategy for additional therapy?**
   A. Reinduction with an asparaginase-based chemotherapy regimen
   B. Consolidation with maintenance chemotherapy
   C. Consolidation with maintenance chemotherapy followed by an autologous stem cell transplant
   D. Initiation of blinatumomab

7. **A 74-year-old man presents to his primary care physician (PCP) for his annual exam. He is noted to have palpable splenomegaly and describes early satiety. He is otherwise asymptomatic. A complete blood count (CBC) demonstrates a white blood cell (WBC) count of 2.4 with an absolute neutrophil count (ANC) of 0.8, hemoglobin of 8.5, and platelets of 163. Additionally, monocytopenia is noted on differential.** ˙
   Review of peripheral smear demonstrates presence of lymphocytes with villous projections and a diagnosis of hairy cell leukemia is confirmed by flow cytometry. What is the next step in management?
   A. Initiate cladribine intravenously daily for 5 days.
   B. Start *BRAF*-targeted therapy.
   C. Monitor symptoms and blood counts; no treatment at this time.
   D. Refer for bone marrow transplant.

8. **A 65-year-old female presents to the ED after several days of epistaxis. On review of her laboratory studies, you note a hemoglobin of 8.2g/ dL, white blood cells of 17,000/microL, and platelets of 13,000/microL. Peripheral smear review demonstrates atypical-appearing cells which are identified as lymphoblasts by flow cytometry. Fluorescence in situ hybridization (FISH) demonstrates *BCR/ABL*. The patient has no known comorbidities and is completely independent. What is her optimal frontline therapy?**
   A. Dasatinib + hyper-CVAD
   B. Dasatinib + steroids
   C. Pediatric-inspired regimen (i.e., CALGB 10403)
   D. Supportive care only

9. **A 37-year-old woman presents to the ED with heavy menstrual bleeding, now lasting 9 days. This is extremely atypical for her. Her blood counts demonstrate a white blood cell (WBC) count of 4.5, hemoglobin of 8.5, and platelets of 100. Her international normalised ratio (INR) is noted to be 3.4. Her partial thromboplastin time (PTT) is 50. Fibrinogen**

is collected and is 85. Review of her peripheral blood smear is remarkable for large WBCs with abundant Auer rods, a hypergranular cytoplasm, and sliding plate nuclei. What is her most likely diagnosis and what approach should be used for evaluation after managing her coagulopathy?

A. The patient most likely has an underlying infection and blood cultures should be sent.

B. Her presentation is most consistent with a form of von Willebrand disease and evaluation to classify this should be initiated.

C. The patient has acute promyelocytic leukemia (APL) and testing for *PML-RARA* should be sent.

D. The patient has acute lymphoblastic leukemia and peripheral blood flow cytometry should be sent.

10. An 85-year-old man presents to the ED for worsening fatigue. He has a history of coronary artery disease, systolic heart failure, chronic obstructive pulmonary disease (COPD) (on home oxygen), and dementia. He spends most of his day in his chair and ambulates short distances with a walker. Initial evaluation reveals a white blood cell (WBC) count of 35, hemoglobin of 8, and platelets of 45. Peripheral blood smear reveals the presence of circulating blasts confirmed to account for 45% of his WBCs. Subsequent analysis demonstrated a monosomal karyotype and his next generation sequencing (NGS) is remarkable only for a *TET2* mutation. He is admitted to leukemia service and his family emphasizes that his quality of life was quite good before he became visibly unwell over the past 2 weeks. They state that the patient would want antineoplastic therapy. What therapy do you recommend?

A. Cytarabine with daunorubicin administered in a "7+3" fashion.

B. Enasidenib alone

C. Low-dose cytarabine

D. Liposomal cytarabine and daunorubicin

ANSWERS

1. **D. Normal cytogenetics with *NPM1* mutation without *FLT3-ITD*.** The
   National Comprehensive Cancer Network (NCCN) identifies a number of
   adverse risk genetic changes including, but not limited to, the options
   presented in **A, B,** and **C.** The recommendation for standard postremission
   therapy for these higher risk lesions would be an allogeneic hematopoietic
   stem cell transplant. Alternatively, the presence of the *NPM1* mutation
   without *FLT3-ITD* is a well validated favorable-risk group. As such, the
   recommendation for standard postremission therapy is with high-dose
   cytarabine.

2. **D. Arrange for urgent leukapheresis, initiate fluids, and begin
   hydroxyurea.** This patient is suffering from life-threatening leukostasis as
   evidenced by complaints of dyspnea, vision changes, and headaches. She
   needs emergent leukapheresis, fluids, and initiation of a cytoreductive
   agent. Neither an urgent ophthalmologic exam nor an echocardiogram will
   alter your initial recommendations. Despite moderate anemia, transfusion
   of red cells in a patient with active leukostasis would be contraindicated at
   this time due to concerns for exacerbating the stasis.

3. **A. 11q23 abnormality.** The multiagent chemotherapy this patient received
   in treatment for her breast cancer has put her at risk for a treatment-
   related myeloid neoplasm. The short latency of 1.5 years between
   treatment and onset of AML and a lack of prior blood count abnormalities
   favor topoisomerase inhibition (anthracycline) as the mechanism of
   leukemogenesis. Treatment-related myeloid neoplasms caused by
   topoisomerase inhibitors are often associated with translocation 11q23
   KMT2A (previously known as the mixed lineage leukemia gene [MLL]).
   Alkylating agents, on the other hand, would be expected to have a longer
   latency period of 5 to 10 years, tend to be associated with antecedent
   treatment-related myelodysplastic syndrome, and are associated with
   complex cytogenetics as well as monosomy 5 or 7.

4. **B. Start dexamethasone 10 mg twice daily for presumed differentiation
   syndrome.** Differentiation symptom occurs in 2% to 30% of patients
   receiving ATRA or arsenic trioxide. Signs and symptoms include
   leukocytosis, dyspnea, fever, pulmonary edema or infiltrates, effusions,
   weight gain, and bone pain. Classically, it develops 10 to 12 days after
   initiation of therapy. Treatment includes prompt initiation of steroids as
   well as discontinuation of the differentiating agent, depending on the
   severity of symptoms.

5. **A. Initiate aggressive fluid resuscitation and give rasburicase (0.2 mg/kg),
   with plan to recheck labs in 6 to 8 hours.** The patient has evidence of tumor
   lysis syndrome (TLS), which has caused the hyperkalemia, hypocalcemia, and
   a decline in renal function. Given abnormalities in potassium and calcium, the
   former should be lowered and the latter should be corrected. Intravenous
   hydration is a cornerstone of therapy for hyperuricemia and fluids should
   be used liberally in tolerant patients. In this case, since renal function is
   impaired with

a high uric acid, rasburicase should be utilized. If his kidney function does not improve despite appropriate management of tumor lysis, then dialysis can be considered. Given that this is an emergent situation, glucose-6-phosphate dehydrogenase (G6PD) testing need not be completed, but evaluation for hemolysis should be included in laboratory assessment.

6. **D. Initiation of blinatumomab.** Minimal residual disease (MRD) positivity at the time of allogeneic hematopoietic stem cell transplant is associated with an increased risk of relapse. As such, additional therapy is needed with a goal of achieving an MRD-negative state. In this case, blinatumomab, a bispecific T-cell engager (BITE) targeting CD19, has demonstrated activity and has been Food and Drug Administration (FDA)-approved for patients achieving a morphologic remission with minimal residual disease. The FDA approval was based on the MT103-203 (BLAST) trial, which was an open-label, multicenter, single-arm study that included patients with B-cell ALL who were ≥18 years of age, had received at least three chemotherapy blocks of standard ALL therapy (e.g., induction, intensification, and consolidation), were in morphologic CR, and had marrow MRD at a level of ≥0.1% using an assay with a minimum sensitivity of 0.01%. Providing additional cytotoxic chemotherapy in a patient who has already received three cycles of chemotherapy is unlikely to produce a significant response. Likewise, proceeding with a transplant with active disease, while not contraindicated, is likely to be associated with a higher risk of relapse.

7. **A. Initiate cladribine intravenously daily for 5 days.** In this case, the patient has hairy cell leukemia and anemia with a hemoglobin <11. Indications for therapy in hairy cell leukemia include systemic symptoms, splenic discomfort, recurrent infection, anemia (hemoglobin <11), thrombocytopenia (platelet count <100), or neutropenia (ANC <1).

8. **A. Dasatinib + hyper-CVAD.** This patient has Philadelphia chromosome positive B-ALL and thus dasatinib should be incorporated in her treatment plan. CALGB 10403 would be an option if she was under 40 years of age and fit. Steroids + dasatinib would be an option if she were not fit, but she has no known comorbidities. Supportive care should always be discussed with the patient, but would not be recommended in an otherwise healthy patient.

9. **C. The patient has acute promyelocytic leukemia (APL) and testing for *PML-RARA* should be sent.** The patient's heavy menstrual bleeding is most likely the result of coagulopathy that has arisen in the setting of APL. This is a common presentation of APL in young women. After aggressively managing her coagulopathy, molecular testing should be sent to confirm the diagnosis.

10. **C. Low-dose cytarabine.** This is a frail, elderly patient with acute myeloid leukemia (AML) whose family states that his goals of care would include therapy. If this patient is deemed a candidate for therapy, daunorubicin and cytarabine or liposomal daunorubicin and cytarabine would be too toxic to administer in light of age and comorbidities. Furthermore, the

latter is reserved for individuals with therapy-related AML or in those who had antecedent myelodysplastic syndrome. Enasidenib could be considered if he had an *IDH2* mutation, but his NGS was normal. Ultimately, low-dose cytarabine would be an appropriate option for this patient. It is important to explain that this is not a curative intent therapy and is instead aimed at debulking his AML to extend life and hopefully improve his overall quality of life.

Myelodysplastic Syndromes

14

Charles E. Foucar, Rami N. Khoriaty, and Dale Bixby

EPIDEMIOLOGY

1. **What is the median age at diagnosis for myelodysplastic syndrome (MDS)?**
   - 70 to 75 years old

2. **What is the incidence of MDS?**
   - 10,000 to 15,000 new cases per year in the United States (likely an underestimation)

ETIOLOGY AND RISK FACTORS

1. **What is the etiology of MDS?**
   - The exact etiology is uncertain.
   - 90% of MDS cases arise de novo, 5% to 10% cases are therapy-related, and 1% to 2% of cases have an inherited genetic predisposition.

2. **What are the common risk factors for MDS?**
   - Older age (incidence rises exponentially with age)
   - Male sex (55% of cases are in men; 45% are in women)
   - Exposure to chemotherapeutic agents (alkylating agents, anthracyclines, and other topoisomerase II inhibitors)
   - Radiation exposure
   - Exposure to benzene and other organic solvents
   - Congenital disorders: Down syndrome, neurofibromatosis type 1, Fanconi anemia, congenital neutropenic disorders, dyskeratosis congenita, *GATA2* mutations, and others

CLASSIFICATION

1. **What are the subtypes of MDS according to the World Health Organization (WHO) classification?**
   - **NOTE: The 2022 WHO classification system has divided MDS into genetically defined subgroups and morphologically defined subgroups.**

TABLE 14.1

MDS With Defining Genetic Abnormalities	Blasts	Cytogenetics
MDS with low blasts and isolated 5q deletion (MDS-5q)	<5% BM and <2% PB	5q deletion alone, or with one other abnormality other than monosomy 7 or 7q deletion

(continued)

TABLE 14.1 (*continued*)

MDS With Defining Genetic Abnormalities	Blasts	Cytogenetics
MDS with low blasts and *SF3B1* mutation (MDS-*SF3B1*)*	<5% BM and <2% PB	Absence of 5q deletion, monosomy 7, or complex karyotype; *SF3B1* mutation
MDS with biallelic *TP53* inactivation (MDS-bi*TP53*)	<20% BM and PB	Usually complex, two or more *TP53* mutations, or one mutation with evidence of *TP53* copy number loss or cnLOH

MDS, Morphologically Defined	Blasts	Cytogenetics
MDS with low blasts (MDS-LB)	<5% BM and <2% PB	5q deletion alone, or with one other abnormality other than monosomy 7 or 7q deletion
MDS, hypoplastic ** (MDS-h)	<5% BM and <2% PB	Absence of 5q deletion, monosomy 7, or complex karyotype; *SF3B1* mutation
MDS with increased blasts 1 (MDS-IB1)	5%–9% BM or 2%–4% PB	
MDS with increased blasts 2 (MDS-IB2)	10%–19% BM or 5%–19% PB or Auer rods	
MDS with fibrosis (MDS-f)	5%–19% BM; 2%–19% PB	

*Detection of ≥15% ring sideroblasts is a substitute for *SF3B1* mutation.

**≤25% bone marrow cellularity, age-adjusted.

Note: Dysplasia is considered present if it involves at least 10% of a lineage; this is required for a morphologic diagnosis of MDS.

MDS, myelodysplastic syndrome.

2. **What are the subtypes of MDS according to the International Consensus Criteria (ICC)?**

TABLE 14.2

	Dysplastic Lineages	Cytopenia	Cytoses	Blasts	Cytogenetics	Mutations
MDS with mutated *SF3B1* (MDS-SF3B)	≥1	≥1	0	<5% BM and <2% PB	Any, except isolated del(5q), −7/ del(7q), abn 3q26.2, or complex	SF3B1 (≥10% VAF) without multihit TP53 or RUNX1

(*continued*)

TABLE 14.2 (*continued*)

	Dysplastic Lineages	Cytopenia	Cytoses	Blasts	Cytogenetics	Mutations
MDS with del(5q)	≥1	≥1	Thrombocytosis allowed	<5% BM and <2% PB	Del(5q) with up to one additional except −7/del(7q)	Any except multihit TP53
MDS-NOS (without dysplasia)	0	≥1	0	<5% BM and <2% PB	−7/del(7q) or complex	Any, except multihit TP53 or SF3B1 (≥10% VAF)
MDS-NOS (single lineage dysplasia)	1	≥1	0	<5% BM and <2% PB	Any, except not meeting criteria for MDS-del(5q)	Any, except multihit TP53;not meeting criteria for MDS-SF3B1
MDS-NOS (with multi-lineage dysplasia)	≥2	≥1	0	<5% BM and <2% PB	Any, except not meeting criteria for MDS-del(5q)	Any, except multihit TP53; not meeting criteria for MDS-SF3B1
MDS with excess blasts (MDS-EB)	≥1	≥1	0	5%–9% BM, 2%–9% PB	Any	Any, except multihit TP53
MDS/ AML	≥1	≥1	0	10%–19% BM or PB	Any, except AML-defining	Any, except NPM1, Bzip, CEBPA, or TP53
MDS with mutated TP53	Any	Any	N/A	0%–9% BM or PB	Any	Multihit TP53 mutation, or TP53 mutation (VAF >10%) and complex karyotype often with loss of 17p
MDS/ AML with mutated TP53	Any	Any	N/A	10%–19% BM or PB	Any	Any somatic TP53 mutation (VAF > 10%)

AML, acute myeloid leukemia; MDS, myelodysplastic syndrome; N/A, not applicable.

SIGNS AND SYMPTOMS

1. What are the common signs and symptoms of MDS?
- Incidental cytopenias
- Infections (due to neutropenia)
- Bleeding (due to thrombocytopenia)
- Fatigue and other signs/symptoms of anemia

DIAGNOSTIC CRITERIA

1. What are the diagnostic criteria for MDS?
- See the preceding regarding specific WHO/ICC definitions and cutoffs. However, broadly speaking, diagnosis is established with the following criteria:
  - The patient must have one or more persistent cytopenias.
  - Bone marrow examination may show dysplasia in one or more lineages.
  - In the absence of dysplasia, the identification of an elevated blast percentage in the peripheral blood and/or bone marrow aspirate can also establish the diagnosis of MDS.
  - A diagnosis of MDS may also be made in the correct clinical setting if MDS-specific karyotypic abnormalities or molecular mutations (e.g., *TP53* or *SF3B1*) are present.
  - MDS-specific cytogenetic changes include −7/del(7q), −5/del(5q), −13/del(13q), del(11q), and i(17q) or t(17p), among many others.
    NOTE: −Y, del 20q, and +8, while commonly seen in patients with MDS, are not MDS-defining cytogenetic changes.

TABLE 14.3 ■ Chromosomal Changes Diagnostic of Myelodysplastic Syndrome

Unbalanced Changes	Balanced Abnormalities
−7/del(7)q)	t(11;16)(q23;p13.3)
−5/del(5(q)	t(3;21)(q26.2;q22.1)
i(17q) or t(17p)	t(1;3)(p36.3;q21.1)
−13 or del(13q)	t(2;11)(p21;q23)
del (11)(q)	inv(3)(q21q26.2)
del(12p) or t(12p)	t(6;9)(p23;q34)
del (9)(q)	Complex karyotype (three or more chromosomal abnormalities) involving one or more of the preceding abnormalities
idic(X)(q13)	

PROGNOSTIC FACTORS

1. How are patients with MDS stratified into different risk groups?
- The International Prognostic Scoring System (IPSS) stratifies MDS into four risk groups: low risk (IPSS score 0), intermediate-1 risk (IPSS score 0.5–1), intermediate-2 risk (IPSS score 1.5–2), and high risk (IPSS score 2.5–3.5). Patients with low,

intermediate-1, intermediate-2, and high-risk MDS by IPSS have median overall survivals of 5.7, 3.5, 1.2, and 0.4 years, respectively.
- The IPSS scoring system should only be used at diagnosis in non–therapy-related MDS and, if the patient is referred to a tertiary care center, can only be calculated at the time of referral.

TABLE 14.4 ■ IPSS Scores

	0	0.5	1	1.5	2
Percentage of bone marrow blasts	<5	5–10	–	11–20	>20
Karyotype*	Good	Intermediate	Poor	–	–
Number of cytopenias[†]	0–1	2–3		–	–

*Good karyotype risk: normal, –Y, del(5q), del(20q); poor karyotype risk: complex karyotype (≥3 abnormalities), chromosome 7 abnormalities; intermediate karyotype risk: all others.

[†]Neutropenia: absolute neutrophil count <1,800; anemia: hemoglobin <10; thrombocytopenia: platelets <100,000.

IPSS, International Prognostic Scoring System.

- More recently, the IPSS has been updated and revised (IPSS-R) utilizing a larger patient cohort. It has additional risk groups of cytogenetic changes and has added the degree of anemia and thrombocytopenia into the model system. The original IPSS-R applies to only treatment-naïve patients, but several retrospective analyses have suggested but not proven that it may be recalculated prior to therapy as well as after receiving disease-modifying therapy.
- Patients with very low (IPSS-R 2), low (>1.5–3), intermediate (>3–4.5), high (>4.5–6), and very high risk (>6) MDS by IPSS-R have median overall survival of 8.8, 5.3, 3.0, 1.6, and 0.8 years, respectively.

TABLE 14.5 ■ Revised IPSS

	0	0.5	1	1.5	2	3	4
Bone marrow blasts	≤2		>2 to >5		5–10	>10	
Cytogenetics*	Very good		Good		Intermediate	Poor	Very poor
Hemoglobin	≥10		8 to <10	<8			
Platelets	≥100	50–100	<50				
Absolute neutrophil count	≥0.8	<0.8					

*Very good karyotype includes –Y or del(11q); good karyotype includes normal karyotype, del(5q), del(12p), del(20q), or a double abnormality including del(5q); intermediate karyotype includes del(7q), +8, +19, i(17q), and any other single or double independent clones; poor karyotype includes –7, inv(3)/t(3q)/del(3q), double abnormalities including –7/del(7q), or three abnormalities; very poor karyotype includes complex karyotype (≥3 abnormalities).

IPSS, International Prognostic Scoring System.

- A third scoring system for MDS (WHO prognostic scoring system [WPSS]) can be recalculated throughout the disease course. However, it uses diagnostic criteria from the 2008 WHO classification of MDS and is therefore less commonly utilized.
- Lastly, a scoring system incorporating molecular information to prognosticate patients (IPSS-M) was recently published that risk-stratifies patients into six categories (very low, low, medium low, medium high, high, and very high). It uses 31 genes in addition to cytogenetic and hematologic data. It remains to be seen how this will guide therapy in the future.

INDICATIONS FOR TREATMENT

1. **What are the indications for therapy in MDS?**
   - Transfusion dependence or symptoms related to cytopenias
   - Intermediate-2 or high-risk MDS (based on IPSS)

TREATMENT

1. **How is initial therapy chosen for MDS?**
   - Patients should be risk-stratified according to the systems described above. Approach to treatment is dependent on risk score, indication for treatment, and associated cytogenetic changes such as del(5q).

2. **What is the treatment of choice for patients with low- or intermediate-1-risk MDS with symptomatic/transfusion-dependent anemia and del(5q) as the sole cytogenetic abnormality?**
   - Lenalidomide (10 mg/day) is the treatment of choice for these patients. Transfusion-dependent patients with low- or intermediate-1-risk MDS and del(5q) have an approximately 67% chance of becoming transfusion-independent (for median duration of ~2–2.5 years) and approximately 44% chance of achieving complete cytogenetic response with lenalidomide.

3. **Is lenalidomide indicated for patients with low/intermediate-1-risk MDS with symptomatic or transfusion-dependent anemia but lacking del(5q)?**
   - Lenalidomide results in an overall response rate of 26% in patients with low/intermediate-1-risk MDS without del(5q). This response rate is lower than that achieved with erythropoietin-stimulating agents (ESAs) in patients with an appropriate erythropoietin level or with DNA methyltransferase inhibitors. Lenalidomide, as a single agent, is therefore not generally recommended as frontline therapy for MDS patients without del(5q) and is not currently Food and Drug Administration (FDA)-approved for this indication.

4. **What is the treatment of choice for patients with low- or intermediate-1-risk MDS with symptomatic/transfusion-dependent anemia but lacking del(5q)?**
   - The treatment of these patients is based on the erythropoietin level and the number of red blood cell (RBC) transfusions per month.
   - For patients with EPO 500 mU/mL:
     - Guidelines recommend treatment with an ESA in MDS with transfusion-dependent anemia with serum EPO 500 mU/mL.

- The chance of responding to an ESA increases with lower EPO levels and fewer transfusions. For example, patients with an EPO level <100 and <2 transfusions per month have a 74% chance of responding to an ESA, while patients with an EPO of 100 to 500 and more than two transfusions per month have a 23% chance of responding to an ESA. Of note, patients with an EPO >500 have a 7% chance of responding to an ESA, which underlies the recommendation against using ESAs in these patients.
- It must be remembered that these percentages were calculated in patients receiving 10,000 U of erythropoietin 5 days/week. Optimal dosing with less frequent administration of different doses of erythropoietin has not been established, nor has the optimal use of darbepoetin (Aranesp). Neither erythropoietin nor darbepoetin is currently FDA-approved in patients with MDS.
- Most responses to ESAs occur within 8 weeks of treatment, although some patients might respond after 12 weeks of treatment. The median time of response is ~2 years. Dose escalation should be considered if a patient fails to respond to initial therapy.
- Occasionally, the addition of off-label filgrastim or the off-label use of single-agent lenalidomide may lead to erythroid responses in these patients failing an ESA alone.
- Luspatercept-aamt is another option in patients with very low- through intermediate-risk MDS with ringed sideroblasts (MDS-RS) or in patients with MDS/myeloproliferative neoplasm with ring sideroblasts and thrombocytosis (MDS/MPN-RS-T) who either have an elevated baseline erythropoietin level (>200 U/L) or fail ESAs and require two or more RBC transfusions over 8 weeks.
- For patients with EPO ≥500 mU/mL:
  - Luspatercept-aamt can be considered as first-line treatment in patients with MDS-RS or MDS/MPN-RS-T with an EPO level >200.
  - Patients with EPO ≥500 mU/mL without a diagnosis of MDS-RS or MDS/MPN-RS-T could be treated with either DNA methyltransferase inhibitors (azacitidine or decitabine) and/or with RBC transfusions. An oral formulation of decitabine coupled with the cytidine deaminase inhibitor **cedazuridine** (Inqovi) is approved for intermediate or higher risk MDS.

5. When is iron chelation used in MDS?
- Currently, no iron chelation therapy is FDA-approved for patients with myeloid neoplasms, although it is occasionally considered in those who have received curative intent therapy such as an allogeneic stem cell transplant as part of therapy for iron overload due to blood transfusions.

6. What is the treatment of choice for patients with low- or intermediate1-risk MDS with thrombocytopenia and/or neutropenia?
- Patients could be observed, if the thrombocytopenia and/or neutropenia are not severe.
- Azacitidine or decitabine, two FDA-approved DNA methyltransferase inhibitors, if the thrombocytopenia and/or neutropenia are significant. As noted previously, oral decitabine plus cedazuridine (Inqovi) is also approved for intermediate or higher risk MDS.
- Allogeneic stem cell transplant (alloSCT) or a clinical trial can be considered in those who fail to respond or experience disease progression.

7. **When is immunosuppressive therapy (antithymocyte globulin and cyclosporine) considered in MDS?**

   ▪ Antithymocyte globulin and cyclosporine could be considered in a specific subgroup of patients with low/intermediate-1-risk MDS with one or more of the following characteristics: younger age (age <60), hypocellular bone marrow, <5% blasts, presence of a paroxysmal nocturnal hemoglobinuria clone, presence of an HLA-DR15 haplotype, or presence of *STAT3* mutated T-cell clones.

8. **What are the treatment options for patients with intermediate-2/ high-risk MDS?**

   ▪ AlloSCT is the only curative modality in MDS and should be strongly considered in this patient population. Administration of azacitidine or decitabine prior to transplant is not routinely recommended because it has not been shown to add value in patients planning to proceed with alloSCT; however, this could be considered in patients whose alloSCT is expected to be delayed, but patients should be informed that it will not improve their relapse-free survival or overall survival regardless of their response to therapy. Additionally, complications of therapy may delay and prevent transplant in some patients.

   ▪ Patients who are not candidates for or who decline alloSCT should be considered for treatment with azacitidine, decitabine, or oral decitabine/cedazuridine. Azacitidine is the only one of these two drugs that was shown in a randomized control trial to confer a survival benefit compared with best supportive care. However, this is felt to be due to the different designs of the azacitidine and decitabine trials, and both drugs are considered to have equal value in MDS.

9. **For how many cycles of a hypomethylating agent should be given?**

   ▪ Patients receiving azacitidine or decitabine who are not candidates for alloSCT should continue receiving these drugs unless their MDS progresses or they develop side effects prohibiting their use if they are responding to therapy. Patients should receive a minimum of four to six cycles of azacitidine or decitabine before declaring the patient unresponsive to therapy.

SPECIAL CONSIDERATIONS

1. **What is chronic myelomonocytic leukemia (CMML)?**

   ▪ CMML is an overlap syndrome between MDS and myeloproliferative neoplasms and has features of both.

   ▪ MDS features include dysplasia and cytopenias (neutropenia, anemia, and/or thrombocytopenia).

   ▪ Myeloproliferative features include leukocytosis and monocytosis.

2. **How is CMML diagnosed?**

   ▪ CMML is characterized by absolute monocytosis (≥500/microL and ≥10% of the peripheral blood leukocytes), less than 20% blasts in blood and bone marrow, and the presence of clonality (defined as abnormal cytogenetics or at least one myeloid neoplasm-associated mutation with a VAF of at least 10%).

- If no clonality is identified, then monocytosis (≥1,000/microL and ≥10% of the peripheral blood leukocytes) as well as evidence of dysplasia (increased blasts and/or dysplasia in at least 10% of the cells in one lineage) are required for the diagnosis.
- CMML can only be diagnosed after ruling out other myeloid neoplasms (such as chronic myeloid leukemia [CML], polycythemia vera [PV], essential thrombocythemia [ET], or primary myelofibrosis [PMF]) and secondary causes of monocytosis.
- *PDGFRA, PDGFRB, FGFR,* and *PCM1-JAK2* rearrangements should be ruled out, particularly in cases with concomitant eosinophilia.

3. How is CMML classified?

- CMML can be subdivided into CMML-1 (<5% blasts in PB and <10% in BM) and CMML-2 (5%–19% blasts in PB and 10%–19% blasts in the marrow or Auer rods).
- WHO also continues to recognize two clinical behaviors of CMM. A myelodysplastic CMML (MD-CMML), defined as a white blood cell (WBC) count <13 × 10⁹/L, and myeloproliferative CMML (MP-CMML), where the WBC is ≥13 × 10⁹/L.

4. How is CMML treated?

- Asymptomatic patients with no significant anemia or thrombocytosis could be observed. Hydrea could be utilized in these patients if they have a significantly increased leukocyte count or symptomatic splenomegaly.
- The only curative option for CMML is alloSCT. Patients who require therapy should be directed toward alloSCT if clinically appropriate. CMML has its own prognostic scoring systems (CPSS, CPSS-mol, etc.), although the optimal prognostic tool remains unknown.
- Patients who require therapy but are not candidates for alloSCT or in whom alloSCT has to be significantly delayed should be treated with hypomethylating agents, azacitidine, decitabine, or oral decitabine/cedazuridine.

5. What is clonal hematopoiesis of indeterminate potential (CHIP)?

- CHIP is characterized by the acquisition of a gene mutation in a population of hematopoietic stem and progenitor cells that confers a survival advantage in the absence of a detectable hematologic malignancy.
- To diagnose CHIP, a somatic mutation has to be present at >2% allelic frequency (in blood or bone marrow) in the setting of normal blood counts and no clinical or pathologic evidence of hematologic malignancy. Greater than 4% for X-linked gene mutations in males is required.
- CHIP does not include monoclonal B-cell lymphocytosis (MBL) or MGUS, which are precursors to CLL and MM, respectively.
- The incidence of CHIP increases with age and it is present in at least 10% of people >65 years old.
- The most common mutations associated with CHIP occur in *DNMT3A, TET2,* and *ASXL1.*
- Morphologic dysplasia is not present in CHIP.
- CHIP is associated with a small risk of transformation to a hematologic malignancy (MDS or acute myeloid leukemia) estimated at about 1% per year, although risk stratification remains an area of investigation.
- CHIP is associated with increased risk of coronary artery disease and stroke.

6. **What are the definitions of other indolent myeloid disorders on the same spectrum as CHIP?**

TABLE 14.6

	ICUS	IDUS	CHIP	CCUS
Cytopenia*	Yes	No	No	Yes
Dysplasia	No	Yes	No	No
Clonality†	No	No	Yes	Yes

*Cytopenias are formally defined as hemoglobin <13 g/dL in males and <12 g/dL in females, absolute neutrophil count of <1.8 × 10⁹/L for leukopenia, and platelets <150 × 10⁹/L.

†Clonality refers to a population of myeloid cells with an acquired gene mutation.

CCUS, clonal cytopenia of undetermined significance; CHIP, clonal hematopoiesis of indeterminate potential; ICUS, idiopathic cytopenia of undetermined significance; IDUS, idiopathic dysplasia of undetermined significance.

QUESTIONS

1. A 65-year-old woman had a complete blood count (CBC) performed for fatigue, which showed white blood cell (WBC) count 5.0 (absolute neutrophil count [ANC] 2.5), hemoglobin 8.5 g/dL (mean corpuscular volume [MCV] 104), and platelets 505. Iron, vitamin B_{12}, and folic acid levels were normal. The patient had a bone marrow biopsy, which showed a hypercellular marrow, with dysplasia in the erythroid lineage, but normal myeloid and megakaryocytic lineages. There were 1.5% blasts seen in the aspirate smear. Cytogenetics showed del(5q) as the sole abnormality. Which of the following is the best treatment option for the patient at this point?
   A. A hypomethylating agent (azacitidine, decitabine, or oral decitabine/cedazuridine)
   B. Allogeneic bone marrow transplantation
   C. Lenalidomide as single agent
   D. Lenalidomide + a hypomethylating agent
   E. Red blood cell transfusions only

2. A 64-year-old man presents with a transfusion-dependent anemia (2 units of red cells every 6 weeks). Otherwise, he has a normal white blood cell (WBC) count of 6 and absolute neutrophil count (ANC) of 4, as well as a normal platelet count of 250. A bone marrow aspirate and biopsy demonstrated myelodysplastic syndrome (MDS) with dysplasia in the erythroid lineage only. There were 1.8% blasts seen in the aspirate smear and no increased ringed sideroblasts. Cytogenetics showed del 20q. Serum erythropoietin level is 90. Which of the following is the best treatment option for this patient?
   A. Red blood cell (RBC) transfusions only
   B. Allogeneic stem cell transplantation
   C. Lenalidomide as single agent
   D. Erythropoietin-stimulating agent
   E. Hypomethylating agent

3. A 62-year-old man with no other comorbidities and a good performance status was diagnosed with myelodysplastic syndrome (MDS) 2 years ago. He was on observation because he had mild cytopenias initially and he was asymptomatic. Over the recent few months, his counts started to drop, and his most recent complete blood count (CBC) showed white blood cell (WBC) count of 1, absolute neutrophil count (ANC) of 0.5, hemoglobin of 8.5, and platelets of 40. A bone marrow biopsy was repeated and demonstrated a hypercellular marrow with dysplasia in all lineages, 12% blasts on the aspirate smear, and a complex karyotype. Which of the following is the best treatment option for this patient?
   A. Red blood cell transfusions only
   B. Allogeneic stem cell transplant (alloSCT)
   C. Lenalidomide
   D. Erythropoietin-stimulating agent in combination with thrombopoietin-stimulating agent
   E. Hypomethylating agent

4. A 78-year-old man with a history of coronary artery disease, chronic obstructive pulmonary disease (COPD), and hypertension has high-risk myelodysplastic syndrome (MDS) with pancytopenia (white blood cell [WBC] count 0.8, absolute neutrophil count [ANC] 0.3, hemoglobin 8.5, platelets 35). Bone marrow showed 11% blasts and cytogenetics demonstrated a complex karyotype. Which of the following is the best treatment option for this patient?
   A. Red blood cell transfusions only
   B. Allogeneic stem cell transplant (alloSCT)
   C. Lenalidomide
   D. Erythropoietin-stimulating agent in combination with thrombopoietin-stimulating agent
   E. Hypomethylating agent

5. A 59-year-woman has a diagnosis of chronic myelomonocytic leukemia (CMML), with the most recent complete blood count (CBC) showing a white blood cell (WBC) count of 40,000 (absolute neutrophil count [ANC] 25, absolute monocyte count [AMC] 10), hemoglobin of 7.5, and platelets of 200. Her spleen is palpated 6 cm below the left costal margin. A recent bone marrow aspiration and biopsy showed 7% blasts. Cytogenetics demonstrated trisomy 8 in 10 out of 20 metaphases examined (47, XX, +8 [10] / 26, XX[10]). Next-generation sequencing shows mutations in both *ASXL1* and *RUNX1*. She has fatigue and shortness of breath on moderate exertion. The patient has no other comorbidities. She is found to have CPSS-mol score of 6 (high risk). Which of the following is the best treatment option for this patient?
   A. Allogeneic stem cell transplant (alloSCT)
   B. Lenalidomide
   C. Erythropoietin-stimulating agent in combination with thrombopoietin-stimulating agent
   D. Hypomethylating agent

6. A 77-year old man presents for ongoing management of his myelodysplastic syndrome with excess blasts (MDS-EB-2). He was originally diagnosed 3 months ago after presenting to his primary care with fatigue and a complete blood count that demonstrated white blood cell count of 0.1, hemoglobin of 6.4, and platelets of 21. A bone marrow biopsy was performed and showed dysplasia in >10% of erythroid and megakaryocyte lineages, as well as a complex karyotype. 12% blasts were measured on the marrow aspirate. The patient presents after two cycles of decitabine to consider treatment with a third cycle. He continues to receive biweekly transfusions of packed red blood cells and platelets and remains neutropenic. He is not a candidate for allogeneic stem cell transplant and is tolerating treatment well. What is the best treatment approach for this patient?

A. Switch to azacitidine.

B. Continue treatment with decitabine.

C. Treat with luspatercept.

D. Stop treatment and recommend palliative transfusions.

ANSWERS

1. **C. Lenalidomide as single agent.** This patient has low-risk myelodysplastic syndrome (MDS) with symptomatic anemia and del(5q) as the sole cytogenetic abnormality (5q syndrome). Lenalidomide 10 mg/day is the treatment of choice for this patient. Prior studies have shown that 67% of patients with the 5q syndrome treated with lenalidomide no longer needed transfusions and 45% had a complete cytogenetic response.

2. **D. Erythropoietin-stimulating agent.** This patient has low-risk MDS with transfusion-dependent anemia, no del(5q), and no other cytopenias. Because his erythropoietin level is low and he gets less than 2 units of RBC transfusions a month, his chance of responding to erythropoietin-stimulating agents is ~74%. Guidelines recommend trial of erythropoietin-stimulating agents if EPO is <500. It can take 8 to 12 weeks before response is seen.

3. **B. Allogeneic stem cell transplant (alloSCT).** This is a patient with high-risk MDS. AlloSCT is the only curative modality. A retrospective analysis showed that patients with high-risk MDS have better overall survival if they undergo alloSCT. Hypomethylating agents prior to alloSCT are not routinely recommended and have not been shown to add value in patients planning to proceed with alloSCT; therefore, hypomethylating agents should be considered in patients whose alloSCT is expected to be delayed or who are not candidates for alloSCT. This patient has a good performance status and does not have other comorbidities and would be a candidate for alloSCT.

4. **E. Hypomethylating agent.** This is a patient with high-risk MDS. Although alloSCT is the only curative modality, this patient is not a candidate for alloSCT. Hypomethylating agents are the agents of choice. Studies have demonstrated that a hypomethylating agent (azacitidine) given to intermediate-2- or high-risk (International Prognostic Scoring System) MDS patients delayed progression to acute myeloid leukemia (AML) and improved overall survival compared with supportive care alone.

5. **A. Allogeneic stem cell transplant (alloSCT).** The patient has CMML-1 with symptomatic anemia. Using the CMML-mol scoring system, she has high-risk disease. Much like in myelodysplastic syndrome, the only curative option is alloSCT and should be considered in patients with intermediate or higher risk disease. If alloSCT has to be delayed, then a hypomethylating agent should be strongly considered as a bridge to curative intent therapy.

6. **B. Continue treatment with decitabine.** This patient has received two cycles of decitabine and remains cytopenic and transfusion-dependent. However, it can take three to four cycles of therapy to see a hematologic response and therefore this patient should receive more cycles prior to being deemed a treatment failure. There is no evidence to support switching between hypomethylating agents, and luspatercept is only considered to treat anemia refractory to erythropoietin stimulating agents in very-low, low-, or intermediate-risk MDS with ringed sideroblasts (MDS-RS).

Non-Hodgkin Lymphoma— Aggressive B-Cell Lymphoma

15

Radhika Takiar and Yasmin H. Karimi

INTRODUCTION

Aggressive B-cell non-Hodgkin lymphomas (NHLs) comprise a group of mature B-cell neoplasms that are clinically aggressive neoplasms, presenting most often in the fifth and sixth decade of life with acute onset of B symptoms and are usually curable with combination chemotherapy. This heterogeneous group of diseases includes diffuse large B-cell lymphoma (DLBCL), Burkitt lymphoma (BL), mantle cell lymphoma (MCL), primary mediastinal B-cell lymphoma (PMBL), and high-grade B-cell lymphoma (HGBL), among others. The World Health Organization (WHO) classification for B-cell NHL (Figure 15.1) was updated in 2017, changing "B-cell lymphoma, unclassifiable, with features intermediate between DLBCL and Burkitt lymphoma" to "high-grade B-cell lymphoma with MYC and BCL2 and/or BCL6 rearrangements."

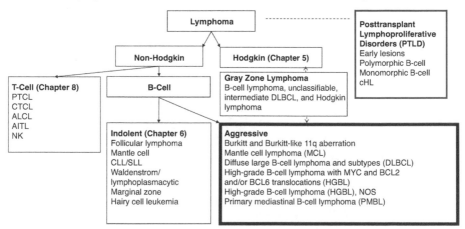

FIGURE 15.1 ■ World Health Organization (WHO) 2017 classification of mature B- and T-cell neoplasms.

AITL, angioimmunoblastic T cell lympoma; ALCL, anaplastic large cell lymphoma; cHL, classic Hodgkin lymphoma; CLL, chronic lymphoma; CTCL, cutaneous T cell lymphoma; NK/T, natural killer/T cell lymphoma; NOS, not otherwise specified; PTCL, peripheral T cell lymphoma; SLL, small lymphocytic lymphoma.

EPIDEMIOLOGY

1. **How common are NHLs and what is the most common subtype of aggressive B-cell NHL?**
   - 80,000 (4% of all new cancer cases) new cases of NHL in 2022 and B-cell lymphomas comprise 85% of all cases of NHL in the United States, stable incidence since 1990
   - DLBCL the most common subtype of NHL, comprising approximately 30% of all NHLs

2. **What are the risk factors associated with aggressive B-cell NHL?**
   - Infection, most commonly HIV, is associated with DLBCL as well as Epstein–Barr virus (EBV) associated with BL in Africa and DLBCL in the older adult.
   - Iatrogenic immunosuppression in organ transplantation leading to dysregulated B-cell proliferation and susceptibility to EBV infection is also a risk factor.

DIAGNOSTIC WORKUP

1. **How do you make a tissue diagnosis of an aggressive B-cell NHL?**
   - Excisional biopsy of FDG avid lymph node as detected on PET-CT is preferred. Core needle biopsy is acceptable for inaccessible lymph nodes. Fine needle aspiration should be avoided since nodal architecture is difficult to fully assess.
     - H&E staining reveals diffuse infiltration by medium or large lymphoid monomorphic cells with high nuclear to cytoplasmic ratio and high mitotic rate.
     - Immunohistochemistry (IHC) stains are usually positive for B-cell markers CD19, CD20, CD22, and CD79a, and variably positive for CD5, CD10, sIg, cyclin D1, BCL2, BCL6, and MUM1 depending on subtype.
       NOTE: TdT, a marker of lymphoid immunoblasts, is negative. If positive, this should prompt consideration of a diagnosis of acute lymphoblastic leukemia/lymphoma (ALL) rather than NHL.
     - Ki-67, a marker of cell proliferation, is usually >90%.
   - Aggressive B-cell NHLs arise from the germinal center of lymph nodes except for MCL (Figure 15.2).
     - Diffuse large B-cell usually originates from germinal center B-cells that express C10+, but can arise from activated B-cells that usually lose CD10+ and can express MUM1.
     - BL and HGBL usually originate from germinal center B-cells.
     - MCL originates from the mantle zone and therefore is usually CD5+.

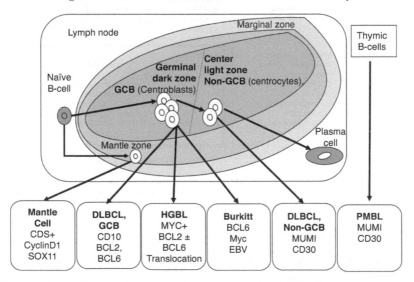

FIGURE 15.2 ■ Immunohistochemistry expression of aggressive B-cell NHL.

B-cell NHL, B-cell non-Hodgkin lymphoma; DLBCL, diffuse large B-cell lymphoma; HGBL, high-grade B-cell lymphoma; PMBL, primary mediastinal B-cell lymphoma.

■ Hints:
- If DLBCL and CD10+, it is germinal center type
- If cyclin D1 positive by IHC and t(11;14) present by fluorescence in situ hybridization (FISH), it is MCL.
- BL expresses CD10, BCL6, and MYC, but rarely expresses BCL2.

2. How is the cell of origin of DLBCL determined and how does the cell of origin impact survival?

■ IHC staining and use of the Hans criteria (among others) as outlined in Figure 15.3

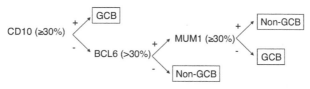

FIGURE 15.3 ■ Hans algorithm to determine DLBCL cell of origin.

DLBCL, diffuse large B-cell lymphoma; GCB, germinal center subtype.

■ DLBCL, GCB Type: better survival due to good response to R-CHOP (rituximab, cyclophosphamide, doxorubicin, vincristine, and prednisone) therapy (5-year overall survival [OS]: 70%–75%)
■ DLBCL, non-GCB type: usually activated B-cell, inferior survival due to poor response to R-CHOP therapy (5-year OS: 50%)
■ Risk of central nervous system (CNS) relapse: tends to be higher among patients with non-GCB type

3. What does dual expresser mean in the context of DLBCL and how does it impact survival?

■ Expression of c-Myc ≥40% and BCL2 ≥50% or BCL6 ≥50% by IHC defines a higher risk subgroup of DLBCL called "double expressor." Dual expression predicts inferior survival when treated with R-CHOP therapy (3-year progression-free survival (PFS) 46% vs. 65% and 3-year OS 46% vs. 75%) and has a higher risk of CNS relapse, but has a better prognosis when compared with HGBL with MYC and BCL2 and/or BCL6 translocations.

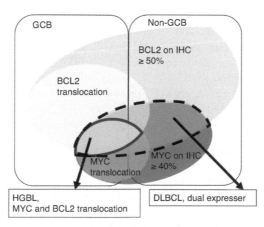

FIGURE 15.4 ■ DLBCL dual expresser versus HGBL MYC and BCL2 translocation.

DLBCL, diffuse large B-cell lymphoma; GCB, germinal center subtype; HGBL, high-grade B-cell lymphoma; IHC, immunohistochemistry.

4. **How is HGBL with MYC and BCL2 and/or BCL6 rearrangements distinguished from a dual-expresser DLBCL?**
   ■ All patients with DLBCL should be tested for MYC rearrangements by FISH to aid in the diagnosis of "double hit" lymphomas. If MYC FISH is positive, FISH for BCL2 and BCL6 should be performed. Double-hit lymphoma (DHL) is defined by MYC rearrangement and either BCL2 or BCL6 rearrangement. This contrasts with double-expressor lymphoma, which is classified based on IHC and protein expression rather than chromosome rearrangements. Triple-hit lymphoma (THL) is defined by MYC rearrangement with both BCL2 and BCL6 rearrangements.

5. **What are the chromosomal translocations as detected by FISH and oncogenes (and function) associated with aggressive B-cell NHL?**

TABLE 15.1 ■ Common Translocations in Aggressive B-Cell NHL

NHL B-Cell Subtype	Cytogenetics	Oncogene	Function
HGBL	t(14;18)	BCL2	Antiapoptosis
c-Myc and BCL2 or	t(3;14)	BCL6	Antiapoptosis
BCL6 translocation	t(2;8), t(8;14), t(8;22)	cMyc	Transcription factor
Mantle cell lymphoma	t(11;14)(q13;q32)	Cyclin D1	Cell cycle regulator
Burkitt lymphoma	t(8;14), most common	cMYC	Transcription factor
	t(2;8), t(8;22)		

HGBL, high-grade B-cell lymphoma; NHL, non-Hodgkin lymphoma.

STAGING AND SPECIAL CONSIDERATIONS

1. **What imaging and testing are required to complete staging prior to treatment of aggressive B-cell lymphomas?**
   ■ PET-CT recommended and adequate to assess bone marrow involvement
   ■ Staging: Ann Arbor Staging system
   ■ Diagnostic lumbar puncture (LP) for all patients with HGBL, BL, and select patients with DLBCL who have clinical suspicion for CNS involvement based on symptoms or exam (see Table 15.3); check cell counts, protein, glucose, cytology, and flow cytometry on cerebrospinal fluid (CSF) examination
   ■ MRI of the brain considered for patients with BL
   ■ Labs: complete blood count (CBC), lactate dehydrogenase (LDH), HIV testing, hepatitis B surface ag/ab, core IgG+IgM
   ■ Fertility counseling recommended
   ■ MUGA/transthoracic echocardiogram (TTE) if treating with anthracycline

2. **How are response to therapy and ongoing remission monitored (role of PET scan)?**
   ■ Repeat PET-CT after two to three cycles of chemotherapy to determine interval response to initial therapy, then after completion of chemotherapy but before planned radiation therapy (RT) if indicated.
      ● Complete response (CR) is considered if FDG uptake on PET-CT is less than or equal to uptake in the liver (Deauville 1, 2, or 3), with no FDG uptake in the bone marrow.

- Partial response (PR) is considered if FDG uptake on PET-CT is greater than that of the liver (Deauville 4 or 5), but reduced compared with pretreatment PET-CT.
- Obtain posttreatment PET-CT 6 to 8 weeks after completion of therapy.
  - If PR to therapy, no response to therapy, or disease progression on interim or posttreatment PET-CT with biopsy-proven persistent disease, proceed to second-line therapy.
  - If CR, proceed to observation with history and physical exam (H&P) and labs every 3 months for years 1 to 2, every 6 months for year 3, and annually thereafter.

NOTE: False positive PET scans are frequent; therefore, biopsy of PET-positive disease should be considered prior to change in treatment.

NOTE: Surveillance imaging has not been shown to have improved survival in retrospective studies.

3. **What are the hallmarks of tumor lysis syndrome (TLS), what are the risk factors, and how should TLS be monitored and prevented?**
   - BL presents the highest risk of spontaneous tumor lysis and TLS with initiation of cytotoxic chemotherapy due to highly proliferative nature.
   - Laboratory hallmarks of TLS include elevated potassium, uric acid, and phosphorous, and low calcium.
   - Risk factors for TLS based on the National Comprehensive Cancer Network (NCCN) include bone marrow involvement, elevated white blood cells, evidence of spontaneous TLS, and decreased renal function at baseline.
   - Prevent by starting high-risk patients on allopurinol and hydration.
   - Monitor uric acid, potassium, phosphorus, creatinine, calcium, and LDH.
   - Treat TLS with allopurinol and hydration with normal saline in cases with evidence of TLS. Consider febuxostat if renal failure and rasburicase when uric acid is >12.

4. **What is the role of hepatitis B prophylaxis in patients infected with hepatitis B who need treatment with rituximab?**
   - Treatment with rituximab may cause hepatitis B reactivation.
     - If there is active hepatitis B virus (HBV) disease with positive polymerase chain reaction (PCR) viral load, treat for HBV.
   - Prophylactic antiviral therapy is recommended for patients who are HBsAg or HBcore IgG- or IgM-positive with negative HBV PCR viral load.
     - Provide prophylaxis with entecavir during and for 12 months after treatment with anti-CD20 antibody while monitoring HBV PCR viral loads during treatment for patients with active infection.

NOTE: Avoid lamivudine due to resistance.

5. **In terms of anti-CD20 antibodies used to treat aggressive B-cell NHL, what is the role of obinutuzumab, subcutaneous injection of rituximab, and rituximab biosimilars?**
   - Rituximab is a murine type I antibody localizing CD20 intracellularly and resulting in CDC (complement-dependent cytotoxicity) but minimal direct cell death (DCD).
     - There are multiple Food and Drug Administration (FDA)-approved rituximab biosimilars that can be substituted for rituximab in all subtypes B-cell NHL.
   - Subcutaneous rituximab hycela hyaluronidase can be substituted for infusional rituximab after first infusional dose of rituximab in R-CHOP regimen to treat DLBCL but not for other types of aggressive B-cell NHL.

- Obinutuzumab is a fully humanized type II anti-CD20 antibody with homotypic adhesion resulting in DCD and more potent ADCC (antibody-dependent cellular cytotoxicity).
  - G (obinutuzumab)-CHOP failed to show PFS, OS, or improved safety benefit compared with R (rituximab)-CHOP in the phase 3 clinical trial GOYA and therefore is currently not used to treat DLBCL.
  - Although FDA-approved for the indication, use of obinutuzumab in the treatment of aggressive B-cell lymphoma is not included in the NCCN guidelines and has not been widely adopted.
  - Per the ORCHARRD trial, there is no role for using obinutuzumab in the salvage setting either.

TREATMENT

The following section outlines the treatment for aggressive B-cell NHL type that includes DLBCL, HGBL with translocations of MYC and BCL2 and/or BCL6 (HGBL DHL/THL), BL, MCL, and PMBL summarized in Table 15.2.

DIFFUSE LARGE B-CELL LYMPHOMA

DLBCL is the most common subtype of NHL and comprises approximately 30% of all NHLs.

1. **What are the risk factors that determine prognosis in patients with DLBCL?**
   See Tables 15.3 and 15.4

2. **What are the risk factors for CNS recurrence?**
   - Use of CNS prophylaxis for DLBCL is an area of constant debate in regard to when it is indicated and how it should be given due to lack of prospective data showing clinical benefit with use.
   - It is also unclear if intra thecal (IT) MTX is sufficient in the prevention of CNS relapse as it does not penetrate the brain parenchyma.
   - The largest retrospective review (2,300 patients) to date has been performed across 21 institutions internationally to evaluate rates of CNS relapse with or without the use of CNS prophylaxis among patients with high-risk disease (DLBCL with CNS-International Prognostic Index [IPI] scores of 4–6, HGBL, or primary breast/testicular DLBCL). At a median follow-up of ~6 years, there was no difference in adjusted 5-year risk of CNS relapse between patients who received CNS prophylaxis compared with those who did not.
   - CNS prophylaxis is no longer standardly included in treatment; however, very-high-risk patients should have a risk/benefit discussion with their treating physician.

3. **What is the first-line treatment for DLBCL by stage?**
   - Treatment at all stages is with curative intent.
   - Stages I to II, nonbulky: three cycles R-CHOP followed by involved field radiation therapy (IFRT), or four cycles R-CHOP
   - Stages II bulky to IV: six cycles of R-CHOP, IFRT to the "bulky" areas considered
     - R-CHOP is standard first-line therapy. R-CHOP should be given in 21-day cycles (R-CHOP-21).

TABLE 15.2 ■ Treatment for Aggressive B-Cell NHL

Subtype (% of NHL)	Staging	First-Line Therapy	CNS PPX	Anti-CD20 Maintenance	Second-Line Therapy	Third-Line Therapy
DLBCL (30%)	■ PET-CT ■ Consider LP if clinical suspicion for CNS involvement	■ I–II nonbulky: 3 × R-CHOP + ISRT or 4 cycles of R-CHOP alone ■ II bulky–IV: 6 × R-CHOP ■ Cardiac issues: 6–8 × R-CEOP No role for consolidative ASCT	Consider in rare circumstances with multiple CNS risk factors	No	■ Primary refractory or relapse <12 months: CAR-T ■ Relapsed: chemo (R-ICE, R-GemOx, R-DHAP); if CR HDT/ASCT or if PR CAR-T ■ Nontransplant: R-GemOx, R-GDP, tafasitamab/ lenalidomide ■ Non-GC: ibrutinib, R2	■ Polatuzumab vedotin + BR ■ Loncastuximab ■ Tafasitamab + lenalidomide ■ Selinexor ■ Clinical trial
HGBL DH/TH NOS (2%–5%)	■ PET-CT ■ Consider LP if suspicion for CNS involvement	■ R-DA-EPOCH ■ R-CODOX-M ■ R-Hyper-CVAD No role for consolidative ASCT	Consider based on patient risk factors	No		
BL (1%–2%)	■ PET-CT ■ LP	■ CODOX-M ■ Hyper-CVAD ■ DA-R-EPOCH No role for consolidative ASCT	Yes	No	■ Transplant: R-DHAP, R-GDP and if CR HDT/ASCT ■ If localized add ISRT	■ Clinical Trial

(continued)

TABLE 15.2 ■ Treatment for Aggressive B-Cell NHL *(continued)*

Subtype (% of NHL)	Staging	First-Line Therapy	CNS PPX	Anti-CD20 Mainte-nance	Second-Line Therapy	Third-Line Therapy
MCL (5%)	■ PET-CT ■ BmBX for cytopenias ■ EGD/colo if clinical suspicion for GI involvement ■ Consider LP if clinical suspicion for CNS involvement	■ Age <65 transplant: AraC-based regimen followed by HDT/ASCT ■ Age ≥65 nontransplant: BR ■ TP53-mutated: clinical trial or BTK inhibitor	No	Yes, after HDT/ASCT every 2 months for 3 years	■ BTK inhibitors ■ Nontransplant: BR, R-CHOP, R2 ■ BTK inhibitors (ibrutinib, zanubrutinib) ■ Ibrutinib plus venetoclax ■ R2 ■ Bortezomib-based regimen	■ CAR-T cell therapy ■ Clinical trial
PMBL (2%–4%)	■ PET-CT	■ 6 × DA-EPOCH-R ■ 6 × R-CHOP + RT	No	No	■ See DLBCL	■ Anti-CD19 CAR-T ■ Pembrolizumab
AIDS-related (1%–2%)	■ PET-CT ■ EBER-ISH ■ HHV-8 ■ LP ■ CD4+/T-cell subset	■ ART ■ HIV BL: same as BL ■ HIV DLBCL: EPOCH-R ■ HIV PBL: Velcade-EPOCH	Yes	No	■ BV-R-ICE, R-ICE, ESHAP, and if candidate HDT/ASCT	

(continued)

TABLE 15.2 ■ Treatment for Aggressive B-Cell NHL (continued)

Subtype (% of NHL)	Staging	First-Line Therapy	CNS PPX	Anti-CD20 Maintenance	Second-Line Therapy	Third-Line Therapy
PTLD	■ PET-CT ■ EBER-ISH	■ Early: RI ■ Polymorphic or monomorphic: RI, and if persistent disease rituximab monotherapy followed by CHOP if not in a CR after single-agent rituximab				

ART, antiretroviral therapy; ASCT, autologous stem cell transplant; BL, Burkitt lymphoma; BR, bendamustine and rituximab; BTK, Bruton tyrosine kinase; CART, can stay as abbreviated; CNS, central nervous system; CR, complete response; DH/TH, double hit/triple hit; DLBCL, diffuse large B-cell lymphoma; EBER-ISH, Epstein-Barr encoding region in situ hybridization; GC, germinal center; GI, gastrointestinal; HDT, high-dose chemotherapy; HGBL, high-grade B-cell lymphoma; HHV8, should stay as abbreviated; ISRT, involved site radiotherapy; LP, lumbar puncture; MCL, mantle cell lymphoma; NHL, non-Hodgkin lymphoma; NOS, not otherwise specified; PBL, plasmablastic lymphoma; PMBL, primary mediastinal B-cell lymphoma; PPX, prophylaxis; PR, partial response; PTLD, posttransplant lymphoproliferative disorder; R2, rituximab and lenalidomide; R-CEOP, rituximab, cyclophosphamide, etoposide, vincristine and prednisone; RI, reduction in immunosuppression; RICE, rituximab, ifosfamide, carboplatin, etoposide; RT, radiation therapy.

TABLE 15.3 ■ Revised-International Prognostic Index (R-IPI) for DLBCL

	Score	R-IPI Risk	5-Year OS
■ Age >60: 1 point	0	Low	94%
■ LDH 1 × ULN: 1 point	1	Low	79%
■ Ann Arbor stage III–IV: 1 point	2	Low intermediate	79%
■ >1 extranodal site: 1 point	3	High intermediate	55%
■ Performance status ≥2: 1 point	4–5	High	55%

DLBCL, diffuse large B-cell lymphoma; LDH, lactate dehydrogenase; OS, overall survival; ULN, upper limit of normal.

TABLE 15.4 ■ CNS IPI Prognostic Model to Assess the Risk of CNS Relapse in DLBCL

Risk Factors	Score	IPI Risk	CNS Prophylaxis Recommended?
■ Age >60: 1 point	0–1	Low	No
■ Performance status ≥2: 1 point	2–3	Intermediate	No
■ LDH > normal: 1 point ■ Ann Arbor stage III–IV: 1 point	4–6	High	Consider in very-high-risk patients*
■ Extranodal ≥2 sites: 1 point			
■ Kidney/adrenal gland involvement: 1 point			
Special Cases: HIV lymphoma, testicular lymphoma, high-grade B-cell lymphoma, primary cutaneous lymphoma, and stage IE DLBCL of the breast			Consider in very-high-risk patients*

*The role of CNS prophylaxis in DLBCL.

CNS, central nervous system; DLBCL, diffuse large B-cell lymphoma; IPI, International Prognostic Index; LDH, lactate dehydrogenase.

- Multiple prior randomized trials have added other agents to R-CHOP without demonstrating superiority to R-CHOP alone. More recently, the POLARIX trial was performed which compared R-CHOP with polatuzumab vedotin (antibody-drug conjugate with anti-CD79b monoclonal antibody conjugated to monomethyl auristatin E) with R-CHP. Although the pola-R-CHP group had an improved 2-year PFS, this has not yet translated to an OS benefit. The standard of care for frontline therapy is still R-CHOP.

  NOTE: Monitor for signs of congestive heart failure (CHF), neuropathy, myelosuppression, and liver or renal dysfunction.

  NOTE: Frontline treatment currently is not dependent on the DLBCL subtype (GCB vs. non-GCB); however, response rate to R-CHOP is inferior in the non-GCB subtype compared with GCB and also inferior in dual expressers (BCL2+ and MYC+ by IHC).

- Add growth factor granulocyte colony stimulating factor (G-CSF) if >65 years of age or neutropenic fever developed.

- CNS prophylaxis: Consider CNS prophylaxis in very-high-risk patients after individualized discussions.
- Parenchymal CNS disease: Incorporate high-dose systemic methotrexate to R-CHOP cycles with growth factor. IT chemotherapy is insufficient to treat CNS parenchymal disease.
- Leptomeningeal disease: Incorporate IT methotrexate or cytarabine twice weekly until CNS is negative for lymphoma concurrent with systemic therapy. Consider high-dose systemic methotrexate in addition to systemic therapy.
- For patients >80 years old, consider a dose-reduced regimen with R-miniCHOP.

NOTE: If anthracycline is contraindicated, consider R-CEOP (rituximab, vincristine, cyclophosphamide, etoposide, and prednisone).

NOTE: There is no definitive role for high-dose chemotherapy/autologous stem cell rescue (HDT/ASCR) in the first-line setting.

NOTE: There is no role for maintenance rituximab.

4. **What are the second- and third-line treatments for relapsed or refractory DLBCL and what are the outcomes?**
   - Prognosis is poor if there is short (<6 months) duration of response or no response to first-line therapy, with OS of 13% at 4 years.
   - Prognosis is better if there is at least 12 months of disease-free survival, with OS of 40% at 4 years.
   - Relapse usually occurs within 2 years. Relapses after 5 years are uncommon.
   - For primary refractory disease or early relapse (within the first 12 months), patients should be referred for evaluation for anti-CD19 chimeric antigen receptor T cell therapy (CAR-T) with axi-cel or liso-cel based on ZUMA-7 and TRANSFORM trials.
   - In patients who have later relapses (>12 months) and are candidates for autologous stem cell transplant (ASCT), salvage chemotherapy regimens that can be used as bridging include the following:
     - R- (rituximab) plus ICE (ifosfamide, carboplatin, etoposide)
     - Gemcitabine-based regimen (R-GDP [gemcitabine, dexamethasone, cisplatin] or R-GemOx [gemcitabine, oxaliplatin])
     - R-DHAP (dexamethasone, high-dose cytarabine, cisplatin)
   - The goal for ASCT-eligible candidates is to achieve CR, then proceed to high-dose chemotherapy with typically R-BEAM (rituximab, carmustine, etoposide, cytarabine, melphalan) and ASCR.
   - Patients who are not transplant candidates or who have progressed after ≥2 prior lines of therapy are eligible for the following therapies:
     - Polatuzumab vedotin with bendamustine and rituximab (pola-BR)
     - Tafasitamab (anti-CD19 Ab) and lenalidomide
     - Loncastuximab tesirine (antibody drug conjugate bound to pyrrolobenzodiazepine (PBD) payload)
     - Selinexor (XPO1 inhibitor)
     - Clinical trials

5. **Special case: What are special features of transformation of follicular lymphoma to DLBCL?**
   - Transformation from follicular lymphoma to DLBCL occurs at a rate of approximately 3% per year and is associated with poor clinical outcomes. Prognosis is better in previously untreated patients with a localized area of transformation.

- Consider transformation if a patient with follicular lymphoma demonstrates disproportionately rapid growth of a lymph node group, elevated LDH, recurrent B symptoms, or an isolated area on a PET with disproportionately higher FDG uptake. Biopsy the more intensely PET-avid lymph node to identify transformed disease.
- If previously untreated, treat initially with R-CHOP, followed by RT if localized.
- If CR, consider 2 years of rituximab maintenance if persistent follicular lymphoma (FL), although this has only demonstrated a PFS benefit and not OS benefit. Additionally, there are both financial and health-related toxicities of long-term treatment with rituximab due to B-cell depletion, which has more implications in the era of Covid-19, and therefore rituximab maintenance is not commonly used.
- If PR to R-CHOP and there is persistent, localized, FDG-avid, biopsy-proven disease, consider ISRT or RIT (yttrium 90-ibritumomab tiuxetan plus rituximab) to achieve CR prior to HDT/ASCR.
- If the patient has previously received R-CHOP, treat with second-line salvage regimens such as R-ICE (rituximab, ifosfamide carboplatin, and etoposide), R-DHAP, and R-GemOx/R-GDP, followed by HDT/ASCT.

BURKITT LYMPHOMA

BL is among the most aggressive lymphomas with three variants: sporadic (1%–2% of all lymphomas in American adults), immunodeficiency-associated (HIV, post-organ transplant, congenital immunodeficiency), and endemic (most common childhood malignancy in equatorial Africa, associated with EBV infection). Histologically, BL has a diffuse growth pattern with medium-sized cells and a high mitotic rate (Ki-67 nearly 100%) with the classic "starry sky appearance" due to presence of necrotic cells on pathology. Another hallmark finding of BL is the presence of cMYC translocation, typically t(8;14) and less commonly, t(2;8) or t(8;22). Approximately 5% of BL cases lack MYC translocation and are classified as Burkitt-like lymphoma with 11q aberration.

1. **What are the risk factors that determine prognosis in patients with BL (per the NCCN guidelines)?**
   - Low risk: normal LDH, stage I, with single extra-abdominal nodal mass <10 cm or completely resected abdominal mass
   - Otherwise considered high risk

2. **What are the frequent clinical features of BL?**
   - Constitutional symptoms
   - Spontaneous TLS
   - Bone marrow involvement in up to 70% of patients at presentation
   - Leptomeningeal involvement in up to 30% to 40% of patients at presentation
   - Bulky abdominal (in adults) adenopathy

3. **What is the preferred initial treatment for BL?**
   - Treatment at all stages is with curative intent and requires intensive multiagent inpatient chemotherapy regimens that include IT chemotherapy for CNS treatment or prophylaxis as well as systemic methotrexate to treat CNS disease. Patients require hospitalization with each cycle of therapy and often require outpatient platelet/blood transfusions and require G-CSF with each cycle of

systemic therapy. There have not been randomized trials comparing the chemotherapy regimens and thus the optimal treatment often depends on institutional preference, CNS involvement, and patient comorbidities/performance status. A retrospective study comparing CODOX-M/IVAC, Hyper-CVAD, and R-EPOCH showed no difference in outcomes.

- R-CHOP is not an adequate therapy.
- CODOX-M (cyclophosphamide, vincristine, doxorubicin, high-dose methotrexate) alternating with IVAC (ifosfamide, etoposide, high-dose cytarabine), with intrathecal methotrexate or AraC. Addition of rituximab may further improve outcomes in these patients.
- R-Hyper-CVAD (rituximab, hyperfractionated cyclophosphamide, vincristine, doxorubicin, dexamethasone, alternating with high-dose methotrexate and cytarabine) with intrathecal methotrexate results in similar outcomes to CODOX-M.
- DA-R-EPOCH (dose-adjusted etoposide, prednisone, vincristine, cyclophosphamide, doxorubicin, and rituximab) is used only if there is not parenchymal CNS involvement.

NOTE: If the patient presents with symptomatic CNS disease, start with the arm of therapy that contains CNS-penetrating agents.

NOTE: All patients with BL should receive CNS prophylaxis with systemic methotrexate and/or IT chemotherapy with methotrexate or cytarabine.

NOTE: Consolidation therapy is provided only in special cases or in the context of clinical trial but is not standard of care.

4. **What is the prognosis and second-line therapy for relapsed or refractory BL?**
   - Prognosis is very poor (<4 months) and there is no definitive second-line therapy. These patients should be considered for clinical trials, if available.
   - If relapse occurs >6 to 18 months after initial therapy, consider DA-R-EPOCH, R-ICE, and R-GDP, followed by HDT/ASCT.
   - If localized, consider palliative ISRT.

5. **HGBL, translocations of MYC and BCL2 and/or BCL6 (double/triple-hit lymphoma), and NOS**
   - HGBL double/triple hit, previously B-cell lymphoma, unclassifiable, with features intermediate between DLBCL and BL, is a new subtype WHO 2017 classification based on a group of lymphomas that are aggressive large B-cell lymphomas, usually of GC type, that have translocation of MYC and BCL2 and rarely BCL6 by FISH, resulting in poor prognosis and inferior response to R-CHOP therapy.
   - HGBL, NOS appears blastoid or intermediate between DLBCL and BL but lack MYC and BCL2 and/or BCL6 translocations. Histologic features are intermediate between DLBCL and BL: presence of "starry sky" pattern, some large cells, and Ki-67 >90%.

6. **What are the risk factors that determine prognosis in patients with translocation MYC + BCL2 ± BCL?**
   - Based on revised IPI score (see Table 15.3)

7. **What are the frequent clinical features of HGBL DHL/THL or NOS?**
   - They present with poor prognosis parameters, including elevated LDH, bone marrow involvement, and CNS involvement (~10%).

8. **What is the first line of therapy for treatment of HGBL, translocation MYC + BCL2 ± BCL, or NOS?**
   - There is no standard of care.
     - R-CHOP results in inferior outcomes and patients are not likely to achieve CR.
     - R-DA-EPOCH results in superior PFS (22 vs. 8 months) compared with R-CHOP, but studies have failed to demonstrate improvement in OS.
     - In fit patients with high IPI scores, consider intensive chemotherapy regimens with R-Hyper-CVAD or CODOX-M, which demonstrate similar PFS as R-DA-EPOCH.
     - Consider consolidative RT for localized disease
     - Consider CNS prophylaxis.
       NOTE: There is no PFS or OS benefit to consolidation therapy with high-dose chemotherapy/ASCT following R-DA-EPOCH but can be considered in certain cases.

9. **What is the second-line treatment for relapsed or refractory HGBL DHL/THL or NOS?**
   - Relapsed/refractory disease is treated in the same manner as DLBCL.

MANTLE CELL LYMPHOMA

MCL is a rare subtype of B-cell lymphoma characterized by t(11;14)(q13;q32) translocation that results in overexpression of cyclin D1 and cell cycle dysregulation. Approximately 85% to 90% of cases are considered conventional nodal MCL (cMCL). About 10% of cMCL present as a blastoid or pleomorphic variant, which tends to be more aggressive. Approximately 10% to 15% of cases are non-nodal disease that behave as indolent lymphomas and possess certain low-risk features including circulating disease, IGHV hypermutation, SOX11 expression, and low Ki-67 <30%.

1. **What are the risk factors that determine prognosis in patients with MCL?**
   - The Mantle Cell Lymphoma International Prognostic Index (MIPI) can be used to predict prognosis as outlined in Table 15.5.
   - Mutations in TP53 predict poor outcomes regardless of MIPI, with a median OS in TP53-mutated patients of 1.8 years versus >7 years in patients with nonmutated TP53.

TABLE 15.5 ■ MIPI Mantle Cell Lymphoma International Prognostic Index

Risk Factors	Score	MIPI Risk	Median OS
■ Age	<5.7	Low	NR; 5-year OS 60%
■ ECOG	5.7–6.2	Intermediate	51 months
■ LDH			
■ WBC	≥6.2	High	29 months

ECOG, Eastern Cooperative Oncology Group; LDH, lactate dehydrogenase; MIPI, Mantle Cell Lymphoma International Prognostic Index; NR, not reached; OS, overall survival; WBC, white blood cell.

2. **What is the typical first-line treatment for MCL by stage?**
   - There is no standard of care for MCL.
   - MCL is incurable with high propensity for relapse, although outcomes have improved with the introduction of novel agents into the treatment paradigm.
     - In indolent cases, a watch and wait approach does not negatively impact OS.
     - Stages I to II, contiguous-nonbulky:
       - RT alone with IFRT
       - Could consider less aggressive chemoimmunotherapy regimens such as BR (bendamustine, rituximab)
     - Stages II bulky to IV (without TP53 mutation):
       - If patient is young (<65 years), fit, and a stem cell transplant candidate, consider an aggressive cytarabine-based regimen. Addition of cytarabine improves PFS to 8 years and the median OS of more than 10 years. Potential regimens are listed below and would be followed by HDT and ASCT with maintenance rituximab posttransplant every 8 weeks for 3 years (as this has demonstrated long-term PFS and OS benefits).
         - NORDIC regimen (rituximab, maxi-CHOP alternating with HD MTX and cytarabine)
         - Alternating R-CHOP/R-DHAP
         - R-Hyper-CVAD
         - BR/AraC
       - If patient is older (≥65 years) or not a transplant candidate, consider less aggressive therapy such as the following:
         - Six cycles of BR (does not require maintenance), which is the preferred regimen over R-CHOP in those unfit for transplant
         - Six cycles of R-CHOP (requires maintenance with rituximab every 8 weeks for 3 years)
         - Six cycles of VR-CAP (bortezomib, rituximab, cyclophosphamide, doxorubicin, prednisone; no evidence for maintenance)
         - Rituximab with lenalidomide (R2)
     - TP53-mutated MCL patients tend to be chemotherapy-refractory with poor prognosis. They should be considered for clinical trials as upfront therapy, and if not a trial candidate then use of novel agents such as Bruton tyrosine kinase (BTK) inhibitors is the preferred approach.

3. **What is the prognosis and subsequent therapy for relapsed or refractory MCL?**
   - If refractory disease or shortened duration of response to initial chemoimmunotherapy (less than the expected PFS), consider second- and third-generation single-agent BTK inhibitors acalabrutinib, zanubrutinib, or the combination first-generation BTK inhibitor ibrutinib with rituximab. Second- and third-generation have higher specificity and fewer off-target effects, specifically lower incidence of atrial fibrillation and bleeding.
   - If the patient is a transplant candidate and there was PR to first-line chemoimmunotherapy, consider treating with a first-line regimen not previously received.
   - If the patient is refractory to or relapses after first-line chemoimmunotherapy and second-line BTK inhibitor, consider lymphodepleting chemotherapy with cytarabine and fludarabine, followed by CD19-directed CAR-T with brexucabtagene autoleucel (Tecartus).

- At any point, a clinical trial is a reasonable approach, especially since novel agents such as bispecific antibodies are showing promising results for relapsed/refractory MCL.
  NOTE: Avoid bendamustine in patients that are candidates for CAR-T cell therapy due to T-cell depletion that hinders collection of T-cells for adoptive therapy.

PRIMARY MEDIASTINAL B-CELL LYMPHOMA

PMBL arises from thymic B-cells in young (30s–40s) females as mediastinal (stage I/II) disease and can present with superior vena cava (SVC) syndrome and pleural or pericardial effusion. Widespread extranodal involvement is uncommon on initial presentation; however, it can be seen at relapse.

1. **What are the risk factors that determine prognosis in patients with PMBL?**
   - IPI is not helpful in predicting outcomes.
   - Risk factors that predict poor prognosis are controversial and may include male sex, advanced stage disease at diagnosis, and elevated LDH.

2. **What is the typical first-line treatment for PMBL by stage?**
   - There is no standard of care and optimal first-line therapy is debated.
   - Treatment at all stages is with curative intent.
   - Regimens that do not require radiation are ideal in the first-line setting to decrease sequela of mediastinal radiation in young women.
     - Six cycles of DA-EPOCH-R: preferred approach to avoid mediastinal radiation
     - Six cycles of R-CHOP followed by RT
       NOTE: Residual masses on PET-CT are common after completion of therapy; biopsy is recommended prior to further therapy as many residual PET-positive masses are ultimately negative.

3. **What is the prognosis and subsequent therapy for relapsed or refractory PMBL?**
   - Treat as DLBCL.
   - Pembrolizumab 200 mg every 3 weeks was approved based on KEYNOTE-170, which demonstrated 3-year PFS of 34% and OS of 45%.
   - Anti-CD19 CAR-T with axicabtagene ciloleucel and lisocabtagene maraleucel are approved after ≥2 prior lines of therapy, although there were a limited number of patients included in these trials with PMBL histology.
   - One could consider axi-cel or liso-cel for second-line therapy per ZUMA-7 or TRANSFORM trials, respectively, although no patients on ZUMA had PMBL and a small proportion on TRANSFORM had PMBL.

4. **AIDS-related B-cell lymphomas**
DLBCL, BL, and primary central nervous system lymphoma (PCNSL) are the most common subtypes of NHL in patients with HIV. Primary effusion (PEL) and multicentric Castleman's are associated with human herpes virus 8 (HHV-8) infection and are less common causes of AIDS-related lymphoma. Plasmablastic lymphoma (PBL) is a rare AIDS-associated lymphoma and is an aggressive subtype involving the jaw and oral cavity. EBER-ISH is recommended for all patients diagnosed with AIDS-associated lymphomas.

5. **What are the risk factors and prognosis of patients with AIDS-related lymphoma?**
   - The 5-year OS in patients with HIV-associated DLBCL, BL, and PCNSL is 50%, 44%, and 23%.
   - Risk factors that portend poor prognosis include older age, lymphoma occurrence while on antiretroviral therapy (ART), CD4+ less than 50/microL at diagnosis, and high HIV RNA viral load.
     - In HIV-infected patients with DLBCL treated with ART and R-CHOP, PFS did not differ from their HIV-negative counterparts.

6. **What is the first-line therapy and special considerations for treating patients with AIDS-related lymphoma?**
   - Treatment is with curative intent.
   - Use G-CSF prophylaxis for all patients.
   - Provide prophylaxis against viral reactivation with acyclovir and pneumocystis jiroveci pneumonia (PJP) prophylaxis with Bactrim.
   - Hold rituximab therapy when CD4+ count is less than 50 to 100/mcL.
   - ART should be administered during chemotherapy. However, zidovudine, cobicistat, and ritonavir should be avoided given their interaction with CYP3A4.
   - CNS prophylaxis is recommended due to high risk of CNS involvement and relapse.
   - For treatment of HIV-associated BL, treat per section.
   - For treatment of HIV-associated DLBCL, HHV-8-associated DLBCL, or PEL, EPOCH-R is the preferred regimen.
   - For treatment of HIV-associated PBL, treat with EPOCH ± bortezomib (preferred), CODOX-M/IVAC, or Hyper-CVAD ± rituximab, and consideration of HDT/ASCT for patients with high-risk features (IPI >2, MYC translocation, TP53 deletion).

7. **What is the prognosis and second- and third-line therapy for relapsed or refractory AIDS-related lymphoma?**
   - Poor prognosis with 1-year OS of 35%
   - Bortezomib-R-ICE, R-ICE, or ESHAP (etoposide, methylprednisolone, cytarabine, cisplatin), followed by HDT/ASCT.

8. **Posttransplant lymphoproliferative disorder (PTLD)**
   - PTLDs are a heterogenous group of lymphomas that occur after solid organ transplant or allogeneic hematopoietic cell transplant resulting from immunosuppression and the EBV. PTLD after solid organ transplant involves the grafted organ and after allogeneic ASCT involves the donor organ.

9. **Which transplants are associated with a higher incidence of PTLD?**
   - PTLD can be seen after solid organ transplants with the highest risk after heart and lung (5%–10%) > liver (1%–6%) > pancreatic (<5%) > kidney (<3%) transplants.
     - PTLD after allogeneic HSCT depends on the degree of human leukocyte antigen (HLA) matching: highest haploidentical (>20%) > unrelated donors (4%–10%) > umbilical cord (4%–5%) > match-related donor (1%–3%).

10. **What are the two main categories of PTLD?**
    - Late onset (~50%): >1 year from transplant, EBV-negative, more likely germinal center type
    - Early onset: occurs within 1 year from transplant, EBV-positive, non-GCB type

11. **What are the WHO classifications and risk factors that determine prognosis in PTLD?**
    - Early-lesion (nondestructive) PTLD: plasmacytic hyperplasia, infectious mononucleosis, follicular hyperplasia; occurs within 1 year and tends to be EBV-positive.
    - Monomorphic PTLD (B-cell, T-cell and NK-cell subtype): most common type of PTLD, with most common subtype being DLBCL
    - Polymorphic PTLD: typically EBV-positive, more common among children
    - Classic Hodgkin lymphoma PTLD: typically EBV-positive, least common subtype

12. **What is the first-line therapy for PTLD?**
    - Treatment depends on the subtype of lymphoma. Treatment with antiviral therapy is debated as 40% of EBV-associated lymphoproliferative disorders in immunocompromised patients have replicating EBV and therefore antivirals can be considered in patients with early or polymorphic PTLD.
    - In majority of cases of PTLD, frontline therapy entails reduction in immunosuppression.
    - Early-lesion (nondestructive) PTLD: Reduce immunosuppression and if CR then, monitor. If there is persistent/progressive disease despite reduction of immunosuppression, treat with rituximab weekly for 4 weeks or radiation for localized disease. Monitor EBV load by PCR.
    - For monomorphic and polymorphic PTLD, the treatment approach is similar and done in a sequential fashion:
      - Reduction in immunosuppression
      - Rituximab monotherapy weekly for 4 treatments
      - Addition of CHOP among those with persistent disease after rituximab monotherapy
    - If Hodgkin lymphoma subtype, treat as Hodgkin lymphoma.

QUESTIONS

1. **A 59-year-old female presents with night sweats, weight loss, and palpable lymphadenopathy. On laboratory studies, she has a white blood cell (WBC) count of 12/mcL, hemoglobin of 12 g/dL, and platelet count of 120/mcL. Lactate dehydrogenase (LDH) is 450 U/L. A PET scan is performed, which demonstrates fluorodeoxyglucose (FDG)-avid lymphadenopathy in cervical, axillary, mesenteric, and inguinal lymph nodes. An excisional lymph node biopsy is performed. Morphology reveals sheets of large, atypical lymphocytes. Flow cytometry is positive for CD20, CD10, and surface immunoglobulin, and negative for CD5 and cyclin D1. Fluorescence in situ hybridization (FISH) is performed, which is negative for BCL6 and MYC but positive for BCL2. What would be the most appropriate treatment for her lymphoma?**

A. R-CHOP with consolidative radiation
B. R-CHOP followed by consolidative high-dose chemotherapy/autologous stem cell transplant (HDT/ACST) in first complete remission (CR1)
C. R-CHOP for six cycles
D. R-CHOP for six cycles followed by maintenance rituximab in CR1

2. **A 30-year-old female presents with shortness of breath and swelling in her neck. A CT of the thorax reveals a large mediastinal mass as well as axillary and cervical lymphadenopathy. PET scan redemonstrates activity in these areas. A lymph node biopsy is performed, which is consistent with a primary B-cell mediastinal lymphoma. Which of the following is the appropriate treatment regimen?**
   A. Treatment with rituximab, cyclophosphamide, and fludarabine
   B. Treatment with R-Hyper-CVAD
   C. Treatment with dose-adjusted EPOCH with rituximab
   D. Radiation therapy first to the mediastinum because of impending superior vena cava syndrome
   E. Treatment with rituximab and bendamustine

3. **A 46-year-old female with history of heart transplantation 5 years ago presents with inguinal lymphadenopathy. She undergoes an excisional lymph node biopsy, which reveals a monomorphic posttransplant lymphoproliferative disorder (PTLD). PET shows scattered fluorodeoxyglucose lymph nodes above and below the diaphragm. She denies any fever, chills, or weight loss. Her labs reveal a white blood cell (WBC) count of 7.7/mcL, hemoglobin of 13 g/dL, and platelet count of 160/mcL. Her comprehensive metabolic panel is unremarkable. Her lactate dehydrogenase (LDH) is 165 U/L. She undergoes a PET scan, which shows low-level uptake only in her right inguinal lymph nodes. Her immunosuppression is reduced, yet she still has persistent disease. What would be the next step in treatment of her PTLD?**
   A. Observe and repeat her PET scan in 3 months.
   B. Treat with rituximab weekly for 4 weeks alone.
   C. Treat with R-CHOP.
   D. Further reduce immunosuppressive therapy.

4. **A 45-year-old male presents with hematochezia for the past month. Fecal occult blood test is positive and he has a colonoscopy with evidence of a 3-cm mass in the ascending colon. Biopsy of this mass is positive for a B-cell lymphoma which is CD5-positive, and CD10- and CD23-negative with t(11;14). Ki-67 is 80% and TP53 is unmutated. PET-CT reveals mediastinal lymphadenopathy in addition to fluorodeoxyglucose (FDG)-avid colonic mass. He is otherwise healthy with Eastern Cooperative Oncology Group (ECOG) performance status of 0. What would be the optimal frontline therapy for his lymphoma?**
   A. Bendamustine-rituximab
   B. Cytarabine-based regimen followed by consolidative high-dose chemotherapy/autologous stem cell transplant (HDT/ACST) and maintenance rituximab
   C. Observation
   D. Acalabrutinib

5. A 60-year-old male presents with night sweats and palpable lymphadenopathy. He is referred to your clinic because he was recently diagnosed with diffuse large B-cell lymphoma (DLBCL). A PET scan reveals fluorodeoxyglucose (FDG)-avid lymph nodes in his cervical, axillary, inguinal, and retroperitoneal lymph nodes. He initiates R-CHOP and interim PET after three cycles shows progressive disease with new FDG-avid adrenal lesions and liver lesions. Biopsy of a liver lesion confirms DLBCL. Which of the following would be the best approach to treatment?
   A. Continuation of R-CHOP for another three cycles and repeat PET
   B. Anti-CD19 CAR-T
   C. Escalation to DA-R-EPOCH
   D. Salvage chemotherapy with R-ICE followed by high-dose chemother-apy/autologous stem cell transplant (HDT/ACST)

6. A 69-year-old male presents with night sweats and weight loss. He is found to have diffuse lymphadenopathy above and below the diaphragm. He undergoes an excisional lymph node biopsy of an axillary node, which is consistent with diffuse large B-cell lymphoma. Which of the following tests are needed before considering initiating rituximab therapy?
   A. Cytomegalovirus (CMV) serologies
   B. Herpes simplex virus (HSV) serologies
   C. Hepatitis B surface antigen, hepatitis B surface antibody
   D. Respiratory virus panel
   E. Epstein–Barr virus (EBV) serologies

ANSWERS

1. **C. R-CHOP for six cycles.** The diagnosis is diffuse large B-cell lymphoma (DLBCL) and frontline therapy entails R-CHOP for six cycles. Given the diffuse lymphadenopathy, there is not a role for consolidative radiation therapy (RT). There is not a role for consolidation with HDT/ASCT or maintenance rituximab.

2. **C. Treatment with dose-adjusted EPOCH with rituximab.** Dose-adjusted EPOCH with rituximab has been shown to have a high cure rate and obviate the need for radiation therapy in patients with primary B-cell mediastinal lymphoma, and currently is a preferred regimen. The other treatment options are not appropriate or indicated in primary B-cell mediastinal lymphoma.

3. **B. Treat with rituximab weekly for 4 weeks alone.** Reduction of immunosuppressives is the most appropriate first step in the management of her PTLD. However, if there is persistent disease despite reduction in immunosuppression, then the next-line therapy is addition of rituximab. Observation is not appropriate in this situation. If after rituximab she still has disease, CHOP can be added.

4. **B. Cytarabine-based regimen followed by consolidative high-dose chemotherapy/autologous stem cell transplant (HDT/ACST) and rituximab maintenance.** The diagnosis is mantle cell lymphoma that is highly aggressive with high Ki-67. Since TP53 is negative, standard frontline treatment would be with chemoimmunotherapy followed by ASCT. After ASCT, rituximab maintenance has been shown to improve overall survival. Observation would not be appropriate since he has gastrointestinal (GI) bleeding from disease that warrants treatment. Acalabrutinib would be considered if TP53-mutated disease was identified since these patients tend to have poor outcomes with chemotherapy. Bendamustine-rituximab is an option, although typically reserved for transplant-ineligible or older patients who could not tolerate cytarabine-based intensive regimens.

5. **B. Anti-CD19 CAR-T.** This patient has progressive disease on standard of care R-CHOP for DLBCL, which suggests primary refractory disease. Based on recent trials (ZUMA-7 and TRANSFORM), the next best approach would be anti-CD19 CAR-T. The continuation of R-CHOP is incorrect since he has progressed on this already. Escalating to DA-R-EPOCH or trying salvage chemotherapy would also be ineffective in primary refractory disease.

6. **C. Hepatitis B surface antigen, hepatitis B surface antibody.** Rituximab has a risk of reactivating hepatitis B and therefore hepatitis B infection needs to be checked prior to therapy.

Non-Hodgkin Lymphoma: Low Grade

16

Shannon A. Carty

EPIDEMIOLOGY

1. **Classify lymphomas into indolent or aggressive categories.**

TABLE 16.1 ■ Subtypes of Indolent and Aggressive Non-Hodgkin Lymphoma

Indolent	Aggressive
■ Follicular lymphoma	■ Diffuse large B-cell lymphoma
■ Marginal zone lymphoma	■ Burkitt lymphoma
■ Small lymphocytic lymphoma/chronic lymphocytic leukemia	■ Lymphoblastic lymphoma
	■ Mantle cell lymphoma*
■ Lymphoplasmacytic lymphoma/ Waldenstrom macroglobulinemia	■ Primary mediastinal large B-cell lymphoma
■ Cutaneous T-cell lymphoma (mycosis fungoides and Sézary syndrome)	■ Anaplastic large cell lymphoma
	■ Angioimmunoblastic T-cell lymphoma
■ Mantle cell lymphoma*	■ Extranodal NK/T-cell lymphoma
	■ Peripheral T-cell lymphoma not otherwise specified

*Can have indolent and aggressive presentations and is discussed in Chapter 15.

ETIOLOGY AND RISK FACTORS

1. **What risk factors are associated with the development of non-Hodgkin lymphoma (NHL)?**
   - ■ Farming (exposure to herbicides and pesticides, such as organochlorine, organophosphate, and phenoxyacid compounds)
     - Infections (see the next question)
     - Immunosuppressive drug use
     - Autoimmune diseases
     - Post-solid organ transplantation

2. **What infections are associated with lymphoma and what is the associated subtype of lymphoma?**
   - ■ HIV: AIDS-associated lymphoma
     - Epstein–Barr virus (EBV): Burkitt lymphoma in Africa, posttransplant lymphoproliferative disorders, NK/T-cell lymphoma, diffuse large B-cell lymphoma (DLBCL) of the older adult

- Human T-cell leukemia virus type 1 (HTLV-1): adult T-cell leukemia/lymphoma
- *Helicobacter pylori:* mucosa-associated lymphoid tissue (MALT) lymphoma
- Human herpesvirus-8: body cavity lymphoma
- Hepatitis C: splenic marginal zone lymphoma
- *Chlamydia psittaci:* orbital adnexal lymphoma
- *Campylobacter jejuni:* intestinal lymphoma
- *Borrelia burgdorferi:* cutaneous MALT lymphoma

STAGING

1. How is NHL staged?
- Ann Arbor staging system

TABLE 16.2 ■ Ann Arbor Staging System

Stage	Location
I	Disease confined to one lymph node region or lymphatic organ (i.e., spleen)
II	Disease localized to one side of the diaphragm but involving two or more regions
III	Disease on both sides of the diaphragm
IV	Diffuse disease involving at least one extra-lymphatic site (such as liver, bone marrow, lungs)
Additional designations:	
A	No "B" symptoms
B	Fevers, night sweats, >10% unintentional weight loss
E	Extranodal involvement by direct extension
X	Bulky disease: >10 cm or involving >one-third of the mediastinum

SIGNS AND SYMPTOMS

1. What are the common presenting signs and symptoms of NHLs?
- Lymphadenopathy
  - B symptoms
    - Fever (temperature >38°C)
    - Drenching night sweats
    - Unintentional weight loss (>10% loss within a 6-month period of time)
    - Anorexia
    - Fatigue
  - Splenomegaly

DIAGNOSTIC FEATURES

1. **What are the immunophenotypic markers of the indolent NHLs?**

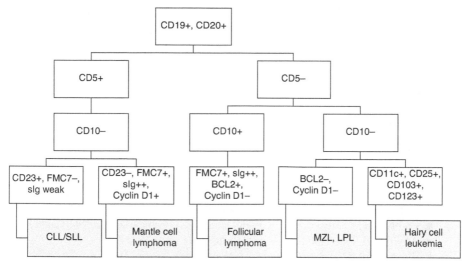

FIGURE 16.1 ■ Immunophenotypic markers for indolent non-Hodgkin B-cell lymphomas.

CLL, chronic lymphocytic leukemia; LPL, lymphoplasmacytic lymphoma; MZL, marginal zone lymphoma; sIg, surface immunoglobulin; SLL, small lymphocytic lymphoma.

2. **What are the chromosomal translocations and their oncogene (and function) associated with indolent NHLs?**

TABLE 16.3 ■ Chromosomal Translocations in Non-Hodgkin Lymphomas

Non-Hodgkin Lymphoma Subtype	Cytogenetics	Oncogene	Function
Follicular lymphoma	t(14;18)(q32;q21)	BCL2	Antiapoptosis
Mantle cell lymphoma	t(11;14)(q13;q32)	Cyclin D1	Cell cycle regulator
Marginal zone lymphoma/ extranodal marginal zone lymphoma	t(11;18)(q21;q21) Others: t(14;18), t(1;14), t(3;14)	API2-MALT	Resistance to *Helicobacter pylori* treatment
Lymphoplasmacytic lymphoma	t(9;14)(p13;q32) Rare, nonspecific	PAX-5	Deregulation of PAX-5 gene

Follicular Lymphoma

GRADE AND PROGNOSTIC FACTORS

1. **How do we determine the grade of follicular lymphoma (FL)?**
   - Grade 1 to 2 is defined by ≤15 centroblasts per high-power field.
   - Grade 3 is defined by >15 centroblasts per high-power field.
   - Grade 3b is defined by sheets of centroblasts.

2. What are the poor prognostic factors associated with FL?

- Follicular Lymphoma International Prognostic Index (FLIPI) at the time of diagnosis can help predict outcomes.

TABLE 16.4 ■ FLIPI Score and Risk Groups

Criteria*	Risk Group
Age >60	Low (0–1 points)
Number of nodal sites >4	Intermediate (2 points)
Elevated LDH	High (3–5 points)
Hemoglobin level <12 g/dL	
Ann Arbor stage III or IV	

*One point for each.

LDH, lactate dehydrogenase.

- According to the Groupe d'Etude des Lymphomes Folliculaires (GELF) criteria, the following are the poor prognostic factors:
  - Involvement of three or more nodal sites, each with a diameter of at least 3 cm
  - Any nodal/extranodal mass with a diameter of at least 7 cm
  - Presence of B symptoms
  - Splenomegaly
  - Pleural effusion or ascites
  - Cytopenia(s)
  - Circulating tumor cells (>5,000 malignant cells/mm³)

TREATMENT

1. What are treatment options for limited-stage (I–II) grade 1 to 2 FL <7 cm?

- Involved site radiation therapy (ISRT) for stage I or contiguous stage II
  - Some may add anti-CD20 monoclonal antibody ± chemotherapy in certain circumstances.
- Anti-CD20 monoclonal antibody ± chemotherapy for noncontiguous stage II
  - Some may add palliative ISRT.
- Observation if toxicity outweighs benefit

2. What are the indications for treatment of advanced-stage FL?

- According to the GELF criteria, the following factors can help guide initiation of treatment:
  - Involvement of three or more nodal sites, each with a diameter of at least 3 cm
  - Any nodal/extranodal mass with a diameter of at least 7 cm
  - Presence of B symptoms
  - Splenomegaly
  - Pleural effusion or ascites
  - Cytopenia(s) due to disease
  - Circulating tumor cells (>5,000 malignant cells/mm³)

3. When treatment is indicated, what are first-line treatment regimens for stage III/IV grade 1/2 FL?

- Fit patients
  - Bendamustine + rituximab or obinutuzumab

- CHOP (cyclophosphamide, doxorubicin, vincristine, and prednisone) + rituximab or obinutuzumab
- CVP (cyclophosphamide, vincristine, and prednisone) + rituximab or obinutuzumab
- Lenalidomide + rituximab
- Rituximab monotherapy (low tumor burden)
- For older adults or for those who are expected to poorly tolerate the preceding regimens
  - Rituximab monotherapy
  - Chlorambucil + rituximab
  - Cyclophosphamide + rituximab

4. How do you treat grade 3 FL or an aggressive presentation of FL?

- Grade 3a FL management is controversial and should be individualized.
- Grade 3b FL is treated like DLBCL.

5. What is the role of maintenance rituximab or obinutuzumab?

- Maintenance therapy is optional.
- After single-agent rituximab, retreatment with rituximab at recurrence provides comparable disease control to maintenance rituximab.
- In the PRIMA trial, rituximab (every 8 weeks for up to 2 years) after R-CVP (rituximab, cyclophosphamide, vincristine, and prednisone) or R-CHOP (rituximab, cyclophosphamide, doxorubicin, vincristine, and prednisone) improved progression-free survival (PFS), but not overall survival (OS).
- In the GALLIUM trial, obinutuzumab maintenance after obinutuzumab-based chemoimmunotherapy resulted in improved PFS, but no difference in OS, compared with rituximab maintenance after rituximab-based chemoimmunotherapy.
- In the FIT trial, ibritumomab tiuxetan (Y-90) after response to rituximab-containing regimens improved PFS, but not OS.

6. What are subsequent treatment regimens for relapsed/refractory grade 1 to 2 FL?

- Chemoimmunotherapy
  - First-line regimen that has not been previously used (see above)
  - Lenalidomide with rituximab or obinutuzumab
  - Obinutuzumab monotherapy
- Radioactive monoclonal antibody (radioimmunotherapy)
  - Ibritumomab tiuxetan (Y-90)
    - Requires bone marrow cellularity >15%, bone marrow lymphoma involvement <25%, and platelet count >100,000
- Anti-CD19 chimeric antigen receptor-T (CAR-T) cell therapy (axicabtagene ciloleucel or tisagenlecleucel; after two prior therapies)
- EZH2 inhibitor tazemetostat (after two prior therapies in EZH2 mutation-positive or EZH2 wild-type with no satisfactory alternative options)
- Copanlisib, phosphoinositide 3-kinase (PI3K) inhibitor (after two prior therapies) NOTE: Other PI3K inhibitors have been withdrawn from the market or under approval consideration due to safety concerns in 2021 to 2022.
- CD20 × CD3 bispecific antibodies

7. **How should we treat histologic transformation of FL to aggressive lymphoma (such as DLBCL)?**
   - Transformed FL should be treated the same way as a DLBCL (see details in Chapter 14).

Marginal Zone Lymphoma

SIGNS AND SYMPTOMS

1. **What is the clinical presentation of extranodal marginal zone (MALT) lymphoma?**
   - Signs and symptoms from involvement of the gastrointestinal (GI) tract, respiratory tract, salivary gland, kidney, prostate, lung, eye (conjunctiva), and other involved organs.
     - It is associated with autoimmune diseases, such as Sjögren syndrome or Hashimoto thyroiditis.

2. **What is the clinical presentation of splenic marginal zone lymphoma?**
   - Presenting symptoms include splenomegaly, circulating lymphocytosis, and cytopenias.
     - Peripheral circulating malignant lymphocytes may display villous cytoplasmic projections.

TREATMENT

1. **What is the initial treatment for stage I or II gastric *H. pylori*-positive MALT lymphoma?**
   - *H. pylori* is treated with antibiotics.
   - If t(11;18) is present, then ISRT is also added (or rituximab if radiation is contraindicated).

2. **What are the initial treatment options for stage I or II gastric *H. pylori*-negative MALT lymphoma?**
   - ISRT
     - Single-agent rituximab (if radiation is contraindicated)

3. **What is the follow-up and subsequent management of stage I/II gastric MALT lymphoma?**
   - Repeat endoscopy and biopsy.
     - After 3 months if antibiotic treatment alone
       - If *H. pylori* remains positive, then treat with second-line antibiotics.
       - If lymphoma remains and the patient has symptoms, then ISRT.
     - After 3 to 6 months when ISRT or rituximab given
       - If *H. pylori* remains positive, consider additional antibiotic treatment.
       - If lymphoma remains, then use first-line chemoimmunotherapy.
   - After remission has been achieved, then endoscopy is repeated every 3 to 6 months for 5 years, then annually.
     - Recurrences can be treated with ISRT if not previously given or with observation until indications for chemoimmunotherapy arise (symptoms, GI bleeding, bulky disease, rapid progression, or threatened end-organ function).
     - Chemoimmunotherapy options are similar to those used in FL.

4. **What is the treatment of stage III/IV MALT lymphoma that involves the stomach?**
   - Observation until a clinical indication for treatment arises
   - First-line chemoimmunotherapy or palliative radiation
   - Endoscopy follow-up the same as localized disease

5. **What is the treatment for nongastric, noncutaneous MALT lymphoma?**
   - Localized disease (stage I/II) is managed with ISRT, surgery in select locations, rituximab, or observation.
   - Advanced disease is treated with palliative ISRT or observation until an indication for chemoimmunotherapy arises.

6. **What is the treatment for nodal marginal zone lymphoma?**
   - Nodal marginal zone lymphoma is managed similar to grade 1 to 2 FL.

7. **What is the initial treatment for symptomatic, splenic marginal zone lymphoma without hepatitis C infection?**
   - Single-agent rituximab (preferred) or splenectomy

8. **What is the treatment for symptomatic, splenic marginal zone lymphoma with hepatitis C infection?**
   - Treat hepatitis C infection first.
   - If resolution of the lymphoma does not occur, then treat similar to splenic marginal zone without hepatitis C.

9. **What is the treatment for asymptomatic, splenic marginal zone lymphoma?**
   - Observation
   - Treatment of hepatitis C

Lymphoplasmacytic Lymphoma/Waldenstrom Macroglobulinemia

DIAGNOSIS

1. **What are some additional tests needed during workup for lymphoplasmacytic lymphoma (LPL)?**
   - Bone marrow biopsy: typically requires demonstration of infiltration by a lymphoplasmacytic cell population for diagnosis
   - Quantitative immunoglobulins, serum protein electrophoresis with immunofixation, and serum free light chains to detect monoclonal gammopathy
   - Labs and imaging to rule out multiple myeloma
   - *MYD88* mutation testing (present in ~90% of cases) on bone marrow
   - *CXCR4* gene mutation testing if considering ibrutinibx

SIGNS AND SYMPTOMS

1. **What is the clinical presentation of LPL?**
   - Monoclonal gammopathy, hyperviscosity syndrome (30%), neuropathy, amyloidosis, cryoglobulinemia, and cold agglutinin disease

TREATMENT

1. **What are the indications for treatment of LPL?**
   - Hyperviscosity syndrome
     - Organomegaly
     - Cryoglobulinemia
     - Cold agglutinin disease
     - Cytopenia
     - Other disease-related symptoms

2. **What are some treatment regimens for LPL?**
   - Chemoimmunotherapy
     - Bendamustine + rituximab
     - Rituximab + cyclophosphamide + dexamethasone/prednisone
     - Others (R-CHOP, fludarabine ± rituximab, FCR [fludarabine, cyclophospha-mide, rituximab], cladribine ± rituximab)
   - Ibrutinib ± rituximab
   - Zanubrutinib
   - Proteasome inhibitor-based regimens
     - Bortezomib/rituximab
     - Bortezomib/dexamethasone (VD)
     - Bortezomib/dexamethasone/rituximab (RVD)
     - Carfilzomib/rituximab/dexamethasone (CRD)
   - Single-agent rituximab to be avoided in patients with a markedly elevated serum immunoglobulin M (IgM)/serum viscosity without prior plasmapheresis due to concern for IgM flare, which can temporarily cause marked elevation in IgM and subsequent hyperviscosity

3. **What is the treatment for hyperviscosity syndrome related to Waldenstrom macroglobulinemia?**
   - Plasmapheresis in emergent situations, then proceed with definitive therapy

Small Lymphocytic Lymphoma

For details about small lymphocytic lymphoma, see Chapter 17.

QUESTIONS

1. A 53-year-old male presents with several months of abdominal bloating, early satiety, fatigue, and 15-lb weight loss. Complete blood count is notable for a white blood cell count of 13.2 (75% lymphocytes), hemoglobin 8.9, and platelet count of 95,000. Peripheral blood smear shows frequent, atypical, small lymphoid-appearing cells with surface villous projections. CT imaging of the abdomen shows a spleen 24 cm in maximum dimension. He undergoes a bone marrow biopsy which shows intrasinusoidal lymphocytic infiltrates staining positive for CD20; negative for CD3, CD5, CD10, cyclin D1, BCL2, CD25, and CD103; and showing immunoglobulin (Ig) light chain restriction. Peripheral blood

flow cytometry shows the same phenotype. Which of the following infections is most likely to be detected in this patient?
A. Epstein–Barr virus
B. Human T-cell leukemia virus type 1 (HTLV-1)
C. *Chlamydia psittaci*
D. Hepatitis C virus
E. Human herpesvirus-8

2. A 57-year-old male presents with 1 year of slowly enlarging lymph nodes in the neck and inguinal regions. He denies pain in the lymph nodes, fever, drenching sweats, weight loss, or fatigue. Complete blood count is normal. He undergoes an excisional lymph node biopsy. Immunohistochemical staining on neoplastic cells show they are CD20+, CD5−, CD10+, BCL2+, BCL6+, and cyclin D1−. Surface immunoglobulin (sIg) is bright. Centroblasts are observed at <15 per high powered field. Ki-67 is <20%. Which of the following is the most likely to be detected on fluorescence in situ hybridization?
A. t(9;14)(p13;q32)
B. t(11;18)(q21;q21)
C. t(11;14)(q13;q32)
D. t(14;18)(q32;q21)

3. A 45-year-old female presents with enlarged lymph nodes in her axillary and inguinal regions. An excisional lymph node biopsy is performed and consistent with follicular lymphoma, grade 2. She has no symptoms, continues to work full time, and has an Eastern Cooperative Oncology Group (ECOG) performance score of 0. A complete blood count is normal. A PET scan reveals uptake in her cervical, axillary, and inguinal lymph nodes, and all nodes are less than 3 cm. She does not demonstrate any splenomegaly. Her bone marrow biopsy is negative for involvement of her follicular lymphoma. What is the appropriate initial step in management?
A. Treatment with rituximab and bendamustine
B. Treatment with rituximab, cyclophosphamide, doxorubicin, vincristine, and prednisone (R-CHOP)
C. Observation
D. Treatment with rituximab monotherapy for four doses

4. The same patient described in Question 3 returns to the clinic in 3 months. She has developed nightly drenching sweats and 15-lb weight loss. A repeat PET-CT shows interval slight enlargement in several of her lymph nodes, which all have similar levels of fluorodeoxyglucose F18 (FDG)-avidity as her initial PET-CT. She undergoes treatment with rituximab, cyclophosphamide, doxorubicin, vincristine, and prednisone (R-CHOP) for symptomatic follicular lymphoma. Her posttreatment PET scan reveals complete remission. She has come to your clinic today and asks about the role of maintenance rituximab after chemotherapy. Which of the following best describes the role of maintenance rituximab when compared with surveillance?

A. Rituximab can prolong her time to progression and prolong her overall survival.

B. Rituximab can prolong her time to progression but overall survival is not changed.

C. Rituximab does not change her time to progression but can improve overall survival.

D. Rituximab decreases her risk of lymphoma transformation.

5. **A 68-year-old female returns to the clinic for biopsy-confirmed, relapsed, low-grade follicular lymphoma. She was previously treated with R-CHOP and obtained a complete remission for 1 year before relapsing with symptomatic disease, at which point she was treated with rituximab and lenalidomide. She obtained partial response before developing symptomatic progression. She has an Eastern Cooperative Oncology Group (ECOG) performance status of 1 and is interested in more therapy. No EZH2 mutation was detected. Her medical history includes hypertension for which she takes two antihypertensive medications and insulin-dependent type 2 diabetes mellitus. She would prefer to be on a fixed-duration therapy. Which of the following treatments would be the most reasonable in her case?**
   A. Copanlisib
   B. Tazemetostat
   C. Ibrutinib
   D. Axicabtagene ciloleucel
   E. Venetoclax

6. **A 56-year-old male presents with progressive abdominal pain and weight loss. He was first evaluated by a gastroenterologist and underwent an upper endoscopy which revealed a gastric ulcer and mild mucosal erythema of the gastric wall. Biopsy of the ulcer is consistent with gastric mucosa-associated lymphoid tissue (MALT) lymphoma.** *Helicobacter pylori* **testing on the biopsy specimen is positive. Complete blood counts and comprehensive metabolic panel are within normal range. CT scan of the abdomen and pelvis does not identify any abnormalities. He is considered to have stage II disease. He begins antibiotic treatment for the** *H. pylori.* **Identification of which of the following abnormalities is most predictive of lack of response to antibiotics?**
   A. t(3;14)
   B. t(11;14)
   C. t(11;18)
   D. t(14;18)

7. **The patient in Question 6 is identified to have the translocation predicting poor response to antibiotics alone. He is managed with antibiotic therapy and involved site radiation therapy. He had significant side effects from the radiation therapy, but gradually recovered completely. Three months after completion of therapy, repeat endoscopy and biopsy do not detect any lymphoma, and** *H. pylori* **testing is negative. He continues to undergo surveillance endoscopy**

every 3 to 6 months. Three years later, surveillance endoscopy shows mucosal erythema; biopsy is consistent with recurrent gastric mucosa-associated lymphoid tissue (MALT) lymphoma; *H. pylori* testing is negative. He has no symptoms. He has not observed any melena or bright red blood in his stool. Complete blood count and comprehensive metabolic panel tests are normal. Repeat CT scans do not identify any bulky disease. He enjoys his current job, which involves frequent, long trips overseas, and prefers to avoid interruptions in his work at this time. Which of the following is the best management choice?

A. Observation and repeat endoscopy in several months
B. Treatment with antibiotics alone
C. R-CHOP
D. Repeat involved site radiation therapy
E. Surgical resection

8. A 70-year-old male presents for evaluation of an incidentally discovered elevated immunoglobulin M (IgM) level. Serum protein electrophoresis and immunofixation were previously obtained and detected a monoclonal protein (IgM) at 2.5 g/dL. Serum free light chains are normal. Complete blood count is normal. Serum creatinine is 1.1 and serum calcium is 9.8. Bone marrow biopsy is obtained and is significant for a 20% infiltrate consisting of small lymphocytes, plasmacytoid lymphocytes, and plasma cells. The infiltrate has expression of CD19, CD20, CD22, and IgM, while negative for CD5, CD10, and CD103. PET-CT did not identify bone lesions or splenomegaly, but was notable for mildly enlarged intra-abdominal and inguinal lymph nodes. Vital signs are normal and he is asymptomatic. Which of the following tests would be most useful to support the likely diagnosis?

A. *BCL2* rearrangement
B. Fluorescence in situ hybridization for deletion of 17p
C. *MYD88* mutation testing
D. *BRAF V600E* mutation testing
E. *IRF4/MUM1* rearrangement

ANSWERS

1. **D. Hepatitis C virus.** His clinical picture, peripheral blood smear, immunophenotype on flow cytometry, and bone marrow are suggestive of a marginal zone lymphoma. The massive splenomegaly and bone marrow pattern (intrasinusoidal lymphoid infiltrate) are most strongly suggestive of a splenic marginal zone lymphoma. The negative CD25 and CD103 argue against hairy cell leukemia, which can also present with splenomegaly and cytopenias. Splenic marginal zone lymphomas have been shown to be associated with chronic hepatitis C infection and can regress after treatment of the hepatitis C. Epstein–Barr virus infections can be seen in Burkitt lymphoma in Africa, posttransplant lymphoproliferative disorders, NK/T-cell lymphoma, and diffuse large B-cell lymphoma (DLBCL) of the older adult. The morphology and immunophenotype of the neoplastic cells in this patient do not fit any of these disorders. HTLV infections are associated with T-cell lymphomas, but the immunophenotype here is consistent with a B-cell disorder. *Chlamydia psittaci* has been associated with orbital adnexal lymphoma, not splenic marginal zone lymphoma (MZL). Human herpesvirus-8 is associated with body cavity lymphoma (also known as primary effusion lymphoma), usually in immunocompromised patients.

2. **D. t(14;18)(q32;q21).** The pattern observed on immunohistochemical stains is most consistent with follicular lymphoma. The most common translocation observed in follicular lymphoma is the t(14;18)(q32;q21), which involves the *IGH* gene on chromosome 14q32 and the *BCL2* gene on chromosome 18q21.

3. **C. Observation.** She has asymptomatic grade 2 follicular lymphoma; observation is appropriate at this time.

4. **B. Rituximab can prolong her time to progression but overall survival is not changed.** The PRIMA trial was a phase 3 trial that randomized patients with follicular lymphoma to observation or maintenance rituximab given every 8 weeks for 2 years in those who responded to first-line chemoimmunotherapy (R-CHOP, R-CVP, or R-FCM). At 10 years, the progression-free survival was 51% in the maintenance rituximab arm versus 35% in the observation arm, a finding that was statistically significant. The overall survival was 80% in both arms. There was no difference in the risk of transformation or quality of life measures. There was an increased risk of infection in the maintenance rituximab arm.

5. **D. Axicabtagene ciloleucel.** Copanlisib and anti-CD19 CAR-T therapy (axicabtagene ciloleucel, tisagenlecleucel) are both options after two prior therapies in patients with follicular lymphoma. The phosphoinositol 3-kinase (PI3K) inhibitor copanlisib is given intravenously and can cause or worsen hypertension or hyperglycemia; since this patient already has poorly managed hypertension and diabetes and prefers a fixed-duration therapy, copanlisib would not be the best choice. Axicabtagene ciloleucel is an anti-CD19 chimeric antigen receptor T-cell therapy and provides

the option to avoid continuous therapy. Tazemetostat is approved in EZH2-mutated follicular lymphoma after two prior lines of therapy, but only recommended in patients without EZH2 mutations with no other alternative options. Single-agent ibrutinib or venetoclax are not currently approved for treatment of follicular lymphoma.

6. **C. t(11;18).** This translocation is predictive of lack of response to antibiotics in *H. pylori*-positive gastric MALT lymphoma. Such cases often require the addition of involved site radiation therapy or rituximab in localized MALT lymphoma. t(1;14), t(3;14), and t(14;18) can also be found in gastric MALT lymphomas, but are not known to predict response to antibiotics.

7. **A. Observation and repeat endoscopy.** This patient had a complete response to antibiotics and involved site radiation therapy for localized gastric MALT lymphoma, then developed recurrence detected by surveillance endoscopy several years later. Patients with advanced stage or recurrent gastric MALT lymphoma can be observed if there are no indications for treatment (gastrointestinal bleeding, bulky disease, threatened end-organ damage, rapid progression). In this case, the patient does not have any indications for treatment and appears to prefer avoiding treatment at this time if able, so observation and repeat endoscopy would be most appropriate. If treatment is indicated, then chemoimmunotherapy would be appropriate at that time.

8. **C. *MYD88* mutation testing.** The patient in this scenario most likely has lymphoplasmacytic lymphoma (LPL). The lack of CRAB features (hypercalcemia, renal insufficiency, anemia, bone lesions), presence of lymphadenopathy, and lymphoplasmacytic features in the bone marrow point toward LPL rather than multiple myeloma. *MYD88* mutations are found in approximately 90% of patients with LPL. *BCL2* rearrangements can be found in B-cell lymphomas, but would not add diagnostic value in this setting. Deletion of 17p can be helpful in making treatment decisions in some B-cell neoplasms, but not in the diagnosis. *BRAF V600E* mutations can be seen in classic hairy cell leukemia (HCL); in this case, HCL appears unlikely based on the negative CD103 and lack of other suggestive features. *IRF4/MUM1* rearrangements can be seen in large B-cell lymphoma with IRF4 rearrangement or in some cases of grade 3b follicular lymphoma.

Chronic Lymphocytic Leukemia

17

Dahlia Sano

EPIDEMIOLOGY

1. **What is the incidence of chronic lymphocytic leukemia (CLL)?**
   - It is estimated that about 20,160 new patients will be diagnosed with CLL in the United States in 2022 (1.1% of all cancer diagnosis), with an estimated death of about 4,410 patients in 2022.
   - The median age at diagnosis is 70 years. It is infrequently seen in people under age 40 and is extremely rare under the age of 20.

2. **What is the median overall survival (OS)?**
   - The 5-year relative survival of CLL is about 88%.

3. **What are the common risk factors for CLL?**
   - Positive family history for CLL or other lymphoid malignancies: first-degree relative of CLL patients with more than double the risk
   - Older age
   - Male sex (male to female ratio of 2:1)
   - More common in North America and Europe than in Asia
   - Chemical exposure: Agent Orange, herbicide, and possibly pesticide exposure

STAGING

1. **How can we stage CLL?**

TABLE 17.1 ■ More Commonly Used in the United States

Rai Stage	Modified Rai Stage	Definition
0	Low risk	Lymphocytosis only (more than 5,000/mm^3 monoclonal lymphocytosis) or >40% of lymphocytes in the bone marrow
I	Intermediate risk	Lymphocytosis and lymphadenopathy (CLL/SLL)
II	Intermediate risk	Stage I with splenomegaly and/or hepatomegaly
III	High risk	Stage 0–II with anemia (hemoglobin <11 g/dL); no other causes of anemia
IV	High risk	Stage 0–III with thrombocytopenia (platelets <100,000/mm^3)

CLL, chronic lymphocytic leukemia; SLL, small lymphocytic lymphoma.

TABLE 17.2 ■ More Commonly Used in Europe

Binet Stage	Definition
A	Less than three nodal sites*
B	Three or more nodal sites*
C	Anemia (hemoglobin <10 g/dL) and/or thrombocytopenia (platelets <100,000/mm³)

*The five nodal sites for Binet staging are cervical (including Waldeyer ring), axillary, inguinal, spleen, and liver.

- CT scans are not needed to stage CLL. Serial CT scans are not indicated in CLL. CT scans should only be obtained to follow and monitor disease progression in patients with new symptoms when peripheral adenopathy is not present. PET scans are usually needed when transformation is suspected.

NOTE: Small lymphocytic lymphoma (SLL) without CLL should be staged based on the Ann Arbor staging system like other lymphomas.

SIGNS AND SYMPTOMS

1. **What is the most common presentation of CLL?**
   - Incidental lymphocytosis during routine labs
   - Asymptomatic lymphadenopathy

2. **What are the common signs and symptoms of CLL?**
   - Fatigue and malaise associated with anemia; can also present as hemolytic anemia
   - Early satiety or abdominal discomfort secondary to splenomegaly
   - B symptoms: fevers, night sweats, and weight loss
   - Recurrent infections due to neutropenia and/or hypogammaglobulinemia
   - Patients with CLL at 7 times higher risk of squamous skin cancer and more than 14 times higher risk of basal skin cancer
   - Patients with CLL at higher risk of developing autoimmune diseases

3. **What are the characteristic peripheral blood smear findings of CLL?**
   - Typical CLL smear: increased number of small mature lymphocytes with clumped chromatin and a narrow rim of cytoplasm; may see anemia, thrombocytopenia, or evidence of hemolytic anemia (increased reticulocytes and nucleated red blood cells)
   - Smudge cells

DIAGNOSTIC CRITERIA

1. **How do you diagnose CLL?**
   - Peripheral blood monoclonal B lymphocyte count ≥5,000/mm³
   - Characteristic peripheral blood lymphocyte flow cytometric immunophenotype: CD5+/CD23+/CD20 (dim)
   - Percentage of prolymphocytes <55% of the lymphocytes
   - Bone marrow biopsy not needed to make the diagnosis of CLL

- Differential diagnosis of increased peripheral blood lymphocytosis: CLL, peripheralized marginal zone lymphoma, and mantle cell lymphoma (MCL); less commonly: follicular lymphoma, Burkitt lymphoma, and diffuse large B-cell lymphoma

2. Define monoclonal B-cell lymphocytosis (MBL).

- If the monoclonal B lymphocyte count is <5,000/mm³ in the setting of a characteristic flow cytometry pattern and absence of lymphadenopathy or hepatosplenomegaly, then the patient's diagnosis is an MBL. MBL has a 1% to 2% per year risk of transforming to CLL. Yearly monitoring is advised.

3. What is prolymphocytic leukemia?

- If monoclonal B lymphocyte count is ≥5,000/mcL and the percentage of prolymphocytes is ≥55% of the lymphocytes, then the patient's diagnosis is prolymphocytic leukemia.

4. What is small lymphocytic lymphoma (SLL)?

- If the clonal B-cells seen within an enlarged lymph node (LN), liver, or spleen have a CLL immunophenotype (CD5+, CD20[dim], CD23+), but the patient does not have a peripheral monoclonal B-lymphocyte count ≥5,000/mcL, then the patient has a diagnosis of SLL.

5. What do you see in flow cytometry in CLL?

- Flow cytometry shows restriction in either kappa or lambda immunoglobulin light chains (monoclonal disease).
- CD5+, CD19+, CD23+, monoclonal B-cell population also typically expresses CD20 dim, CD79b dim, and surface immunoglobulins (sIg) dim.
- It differs from MCL, which is CD5+, CD19+, CD23−. In MCL, cytogenetics (or fluorescence in situ hybridization [FISH]) demonstrates t(11;14) and cyclin D1 is positive immunohistochemically.
- CD23 can be negative in CLL (atypical CLL). Cyclin D1 differentiates atypical CLL from MCL.
- SOX11 is typically positive in MCL but not in CLL.

INDICATIONS FOR TREATMENT

1. How do you treat asymptomatic CLL?

- Careful monitoring without therapy, typically with follow-up visits every 3 to 6 months without surveillance imaging unless indicated for symptoms; average time to first therapy 4 to 5 years from diagnosis

2. What are the indications for therapy?

- New or worsening anemia (Rai stage III disease) not caused by autoimmune hemolytic anemia (AIHA) *or* hemolytic anemia refractory to standard therapy (steroids and rituximab)
- New or worsening thrombocytopenia (Rai stage IV disease) not due to immune thrombocytopenic purpura [ITP]
- Threatened end-organ function due to adenopathy
- Progressive bulky disease (spleen >6 cm below the left costal margin, or LN >10 cm in longest diameter)
- B symptoms: fevers (>100.5°F or >38.0°C for more than 2 weeks with no evidence of infection), night sweats (for >1 month with no evidence of infection), and unintentional weight loss (≥10% in the last 6 months)

■ Severe fatigue resulting in an Eastern Cooperative Oncology Group (ECOG) performance status of ≥2 (rule out other causes of fatigue)

3. **When is therapy for CLL not indicated?**
   ■ Do not treat CLL in the absence of the criteria listed above even if the patient has the following:
     ● Significantly elevated white blood cell (WBC) count
     ● Hypogammaglobulinemia
     ● Paraproteinemia
     ● Presence of autoimmune diseases or other primary malignancy
     ● High-risk cytogenetic features without indications to treat (current trials are evaluating the role of early intervention in asymptomatic CLL with *TP53* mutation)

PROGNOSTIC FACTORS

1. **What are the important FISH testing abnormalities in CLL?**
   ■ 80% of patients with CLL have FISH abnormalities, including the following:
     ● Deletion 13q (~50%)
     ● Trisomy 12 (~20%)
     ● Deletion 11q (~15%)
     ● Deletion 17p (~7%–10%)

2. **What are poor risk features on FISH testing?**
   ■ Deletion 17p
   ■ Deletion 11q

3. **What are the intermediate prognosis risk factors on FISH testing?**
   ■ Trisomy 12
   ■ Normal karyotype on FISH

4. **What generates a favorable prognosis on FISH testing?**
   ■ Deletion 13q with no other abnormality (median OS ~11 years)

5. **What are other prognostic factors in CLL?**
   ■ Mutated *IGHV* (>2% mutation) portends an excellent OS (~22.8 years; exception: patients expressing the *VH3–21* gene have poor survival). Patients with unmutated *IGHV*(≤2% mutation) have shorter OS (~6.6 years).
   ■ *TP53* mutation by DNA sequence determines prognosis. If mutated, then patient has unfavorable prognosis.
   ■ Positive ZAP-70 expression (≥20%), measured by flow cytometry in CD19+/CD5+ cells, predicts short time to treatment (TTT)—2.9 years for those who are ZAP-70-positive versus 9.2 years for those who are ZAP-70-negative (rarely used in clinical practice).
   ■ Positive CD38 (≥30%) predicts for short TTT.
   ■ Complex karyotype (CK; ≥3 chromosome abnormalities in more than one cell on conventional cytogenetics) also determines prognosis.
   ■ Elevated beta-2 microglobulin level is also a prognostic factor.

6. **What are the prognostic models used for CLL?**
   ■ Several prognostic models have been developed for risk stratification and predication of time to first treatment. For example:

- The International Prognostic Index for chronic lymphocytic leukemia (CLL-IPI) stratifies based on TP53 and IGHV mutation status, serum B2M level, clinical stage, and age. The 5-year OS rates were significantly different between these risk groups (93% for low risk, 79% for intermediate, 63% for high risk, and 23% for very high risk).
- The international prognostic score for asymptomatic early-stage chronic lymphocytic leukemia (IPS-E) score stratifies patients with early-stage CLL to calculate time to first treatment. The cumulative risk for the need of treatment after 1 and 5 years of observation was 14% and 61%, respectively, for IPS-E high-risk patients compared with 2% and 28% for intermediate-risk patients and <0.1% and 8% for low-risk patients.
- Progression of disease (POD) within 2 years of first-line therapy has been identified as a prognostic factor for CLL. The overall response rate (ORR) was 53% for those with early POD compared with 80% and 84%, respectively, for those with late POD and no POD. Early POD was also associated with inferior survival.

MANAGEMENT

1. What do you order for newly diagnosed CLL?
- For prognostication: CLL FISH and cytogenetics, TP53 sequencing, CpG-stimulated metaphase karyotype for CK, and molecular analysis for IGHV mutation
- Lactate dehydrogenase (LDH), B2M, uric acid level, and calcium level
- Hepatitis panel and HIV screening
- Haptoglobin, reticulocytes counts, and Coombs test if hemolytic anemia is suspected
- Bone marrow biopsy if unsure about the cause of cytopenia (immune-mediated vs. disease involvement)
- PET scan if transformation is suspected
- Quantitative immunoglobulin level if recurrent infection

2. What are the current available options for therapy?
- Continuous treatment (Bruton's tyrosine kinase inhibitor [BTKi] ± anti-CD20 monoclonal antibody)
- Fixed-duration therapy (venetoclax + anti-CD20 monoclonal antibody) and chemoimmunotherapy (CIT); CIT not recommended in patients with TP53 mutations/17p deletion as they have a short duration of response to chemotherapy

3. What are the currently available BTK inhibitors?
- Acalabrutinib
- Zanubrutinib
- Ibrutinib

NOTE: All BTK inhibitors lead to initial increase in lymphocyte counts that will gradually improve over several weeks after starting therapy.

4. What are the side effects of BTK inhibitors?
- Increased risk of bleeding/bruises due to antiplatelet effect and thrombocytopenia
- Cardiovascular side effects: hypertension and atrial fibrillation (more common with ibrutinib [16% vs. 9% with acalabrutinib]).
- Diarrhea and skin rash (more common with ibrutinib)
- Joint pain and muscle aches
- Headache with acalabrutinib: improves with caffeine
- Cytopenia (more common with zanubrutinib)

5. How long do you hold BTK prior to surgery?

- 3 to 7 days prior to and after surgery depending on if minor or major surgery
- Avoid chemoimmunotherapy (CIT) in patients with TP53 mutation as they are usually refractory to CIT.

6. What are common mutations leading to BTK resistance?

- BTK C481S can lead to resistance to covalent BTK inhibitors (ibrutinib, acalabrutinib, and zanubrutinib). It can be overcome by starting a noncovalent BTK inhibitor (pirtobrutinib, nemtabrutinib).
- BTK V416L, A428D, and M437R,T4741 are resistant to covalent and noncovalent BTK inhibitors.

7. Why should you avoid abrupt discontinuation of BTK inhibitor early in the treatment course?

- Abrupt discontinuation may lead to fast disease progression with severe symptoms.
- If there is disease progression on BTK inhibitor, try to continue therapy until the next agent is available.

8. What are the specific preferred regimens for first-line treatment of CLL?

- Acalabrutinib (A) ± obinutuzumab (O; ELEVATE-TN trial: patients ≥65 years or 18–65 years with comorbidities, 5-year progression-free survival [PFS] 84% in A+O, 72% in A, and 21% in chlorambucil + O; 14% of patients had del(17)(p13.1) and/or mutated TP53; 4-year PFS for this group was 75%)
- Venetoclax + obinutuzumab (5-year PFS 74 % vs. 35% in chlorambucil + obinutuzumab; 13.8% of the patients had TP53 deletion, mutation, or both)
- Zanubrutinib (SEQUOIA trial: 24-month PFS 85% vs. 69% in bendamustine + rituximab; deletion 17 were excluded)
- Ibrutinib (RESONATE-2 Burger et al. NEJM 2015. phase 3 study of ibrutinib compared with chlorambucil: patients (≥65 years) with previously untreated CLL, without del(17p); with up to 8 years of follow-up (range, 0.1–96.6 months; median, 82.7 months), significant PFS benefit was sustained for ibrutinib vs. chlorambucil [hazard ratio {HR}, 0.154; 95% confidence interval {CI}, 0.108–0.220]; at 7 years, PFS was 59% for ibrutinib vs. 9% for chlorambucil; specific to patients with 17p deletion/TP53 mutation, phase 2 studies indicate that ibrutinib results in long-term remissions, despite the lack of deep remissions, with an estimated 5-year PFS of 66%).

9. What other agents can be used in relapse?

- Clinical trials
- May reuse venetoclax + anti-CD20 if relapsed after initial remission
- BTK inhibitors ± anti-CD20 monoclonal antibody
- PI3K inhibitors: duvelisib, idelalisib ± rituximab
- CIT: bendamustine + rituximab, FCR (fludarabine, cyclophosphamide, and rituximab)
- Obinutuzumab
- Lenalidomide ± rituximab
- Allogeneic stem cell transplant

SPECIAL CONSIDERATIONS

1. **What are the causes of anemia in patients with CLL?**
   - The differential diagnosis includes progressive marrow failure from CLL due to direct involvement by disease, splenomegaly, AIHA, and pure red cell aplasia in cases of isolated anemia.
   - Cytopenia(s) from marrow failure secondary to CLL should be documented by a bone marrow biopsy.
   - **Pure red cell aplasia** (diagnosis suspected by lack of reticulocyte response and confirmed by absence of erythroid precursors in the bone marrow): Rule out viral infections including Epstein–Barr virus, cytomegalovirus (CMV), and parvovirus.
   - **AIHA** diagnosis is based on exclusion of other causes of anemia and the presence of elevated LDH, high unconjugated bilirubin, elevated reticulocyte count, low haptoglobin, and positive direct antiglobulin test (DAT).

2. **How is AIHA in patients with CLL treated?**
   - If indication for CLL therapy exists independent of the anemia: Treat the underlying CLL. (Purine analogues may potentially worsen AIHA. Therefore, it is prudent to avoid fludarabine in patients with active AIHA and in patients with a history of AIHA, particularly if purine analogue-induced).
   - If no independent indication for CLL therapy: Treat with prednisone 1 mg/kg/day for 4 weeks + folic acid, followed by a *slow* steroid taper (fast tapers can result in relapse). If no response or if relapse after steroid withdrawal, options include rituximab, intravenous immunoglobulins (IVIG), cyclosporine A, mycophenolate mofetil, azathioprine, daily low-dose oral cyclophosphamide, rituximab, or alemtuzumab. A trial of rituximab and at least one immunosuppressive agent is generally recommended prior to consideration of splenectomy.
   - Treatment-refractory AIHA: Treat CLL with BTK inhibitor.

3. **What is the treatment of patients with CLL and recurrent sinopulmonary infections?**
   - Check serum immunoglobulin G (IgG) levels. If <500 mg/dL, administer monthly IVIG. Adjust dose/interval to maintain nadir IgG of approximately 500 mg/dL.

4. **What anti-infective prophylaxis is indicated in patients receiving purine analogue or alemtuzumab?**
   - Purine analogue
     - Herpes prophylaxis with acyclovir
     - PCP prophylaxis with sulfamethoxazole/trimethoprim or equivalent
   - Alemtuzumab
     - Herpes prophylaxis with acyclovir
     - PCP prophylaxis with sulfamethoxazole/trimethoprim or equivalent
     - Monitor for CMV viremia by polymerase chain reaction every 2 to 3 weeks while on therapy. If present or if viral load is rising, use ganciclovir and consult with infectious disease.

5. **When is Richter's transformation suspected in CLL, what is the risk of transformation, and how is it treated?**
   - Richter's transformation is transformation to diffuse large B-cell lymphoma (DLBCL) or Hodgkin lymphoma.

- RS occurs in approximately 2% to 10% of CLL patients during their disease, with a transformation rate of 0.5% to 1% per year.
- It is suspected in the following:
  - Patients with prominent B symptoms (fevers, night sweats, weight loss)
  - Rapidly enlarging LNs
  - Significantly elevated LDH (in the absence of hemolysis)
  - Pancytopenia common
  - Hypercalcemia ± lytic bone lesions can be seen
- DLBCL transformation can be clonally related to original CLL (more common and worse prognosis [median survival of 1 year] or clonally unrelated [same prognosis as in de novo DLBCL]).
- Patients with del17p13.1, del11q23.1, CDKN2A loss, TP53 disruption, C-MYC activation, and NOTCH1 mutations are at a higher risk of transformation.
- Hodgkin lymphoma transformation typically has a good prognosis.
- Always refer to clinical trial when available.
- Patients with DLBCL transformation should be treated with regimens developed for DLBCL (R-CHOP [rituximab, cyclophosphamide, doxorubicin, vincristine, and prednisone]). Patients should be considered for allogeneic stem cell transplant (autoSCT) after complete response or partial response to initial therapy.
- Patients with Hodgkin lymphoma transformation should be treated with a standard regimen used to treat Hodgkin lymphoma.

QUESTIONS

1. A 57-year-old woman presents with an elevated white blood cell (WBC) count of 55,000/mcL, hemoglobin of 13.5 g/dL, and platelet count of 160,000/mcL. A peripheral flow cytometry is sent and reveals a monoclonal population of cells expressing CD5, CD20 (dim), CD19, and CD23. The cells were negative immunohistochemically for cyclin D1. Which of the following is not associated with a poorer prognosis in this diagnosis?
   A. Deletion 17p
   B. Deletion 11q
   C. ZAP-70 expression greater than 20%
   D. Mutated *IGHV* status
   E. CD38 expression

2. A 55-year-old gentleman with chronic lymphocytic leukemia (CLL) presents with fever, severe fatigue, weight loss, and increased lymphadenopathy. His complete blood counts are significant for a white blood cell (WBC) count of 80,000/mcL, absolute lymphocyte count (ALC) of 70,000/mcL, hemoglobin of 10 g/dL, and platelet count of 102,000/mcL. His CLL fluorescence in situ hybridization (FISH) reveals a del(17p). He is initiated on ibrutinib 420 mg PO daily and has mild diarrhea but otherwise tolerates therapy in his first week. On his subsequent labs in 2 weeks, his WBC has increased to 180,000/mcL, ALC 160,000/mcL, while hemoglobin and platelet counts were stable. In 1 month, his WBC has increased to 225,000/mcL, ALC 200,000/mcL, while hemoglobin and platelet counts remained stable. His palpable lymphadenopathy has resolved. What is the next appropriate step in the management of his CLL?

A. Perform CT of the chest/abdomen/pelvis to evaluate for bulky disease in areas that are not palpable by exam.
B. Switch therapy to idelalisib.
C. Continue ibrutinib 420 mg PO daily.
D. Increase ibrutinib to 560 mg PO daily.
E. Refer him for a reduced intensity allogeneic bone marrow transplantation.

3. A 45-year-old gentleman presents to the clinic for the first time with a new diagnosis of chronic lymphocytic leukemia (CLL). He feels well and denies any fever, chills, night sweats, or weight loss. He was noted to have an elevated white blood cell (WBC) count of 40,000/mcL and absolute lymphocyte count (ALC) of 35,000/mcL on routine bloodwork. Hemoglobin level and platelet counts were within normal. Fluorescence in situ hybridization (FISH) analysis was positive for 17p deletion. How do you mange?
A. Monitor every 3 to 6 months.
B. Start treatment with Bruton tyrosine kinase inhibitor (BTKi).
C. Start treatment with acalabrutinib +obinutuzumab.
D. Refer for stem cell transplant.
E. Perform PET scan.

4. A patient with chronic lymphocytic leukemia (CLL) who has been followed up for 2 years presented to the ED with severe headache. CT of the head showed epidural hematoma. His complete blood count showed elevated white blood cell count at 150,000/mcl with absolute lymphocyte count of 132,000/mcl, hemoglobin level of 7 g/dL, and platelet count of 7,000/mcL. Coombs test was negative and fluorescence in situ hybridization was positive for 11q deletion. The patient received platelet transfusion and his hematoma stabilized. Bone marrow biopsy showed 90% involvement by CLL. How do you treat this patient?
A. Ibrutinib
B. Acalabrutinib
C. Venetoclax with obinutuzumab
D. Chlorambucil

5. A 47-year-old woman with known chronic lymphocytic leukemia (CLL) presents to the clinic with worsening lymphadenopathy, night sweats, and shortness of breath. Her white blood cell (WBC) count is 102,000/mcL, hemoglobin 8 g/dL, and platelet count 90,000/mcL. Calcium is elevated at 12 mg/dL. Her CLL fluorescence in situ hybridization (FISH) demonstrates a deletion 17p. PET scan shows high uptake in the left axillary lymph nodes (SUV of 24). Ultrasound-guided core biopsy shows diffuse large B-cell lymphoma. Which of the following would be the most appropriate frontline therapy option?
A. Fludarabine, cyclophosphamide, and rituximab (FCR)
B. Rituximab, cyclophosphamide, doxorubicin, vincristine, and prednisone (R-CHOP)
C. Ibrutinib
D. Bendamustine and rituximab (BR)
E. Venetoclax with obinutuzumab

ANSWERS

1. **D. Mutated *IGHV* status.** This is associated with a better prognosis in chronic lymphocytic leukemia (CLL) than unmutated *IGVH* status, which is associated with unfavorable prognosis. Options A, B, C, and E have all been associated with unfavorable prognosis in CLL.

2. **C. Continue ibrutinib 420 mg PO daily.** Increased peripheral lymphocytosis after initiating treatment with ibrutinib therapy is common and may last for several months. The development of peripheral lymphocytosis secondary to ibrutinib has not been shown to be detrimental to long-term clinical outcomes.

3. **A. Monitor every 3 to 6 months.** The patient is asymptomatic with normal counts and is at high risk of needing therapy soon given the 17p deletion. Consider enrolling in clinical trial if available.

4. **C. Venetoclax with obinutuzumab.** Bruton tyrosine kinase inhibitor can increase risk of bleeding and worsening thrombocytopenia. Try to avoid in situations where there is major bleeding or severe thrombocytopenia.

5. **B. Rituximab, cyclophosphamide, doxorubicin, vincristine, and prednisone (R-CHOP).** Always refer patients with Richter's transformation to clinical trial if available. If no available trial, the standard of care is treatment with R-CHOP.

Multiple Myeloma and Other Plasma Cell Neoplasms

18

Jason Chen and Erica Campagnaro

EPIDEMIOLOGY

1. **What are plasma cell neoplasms?**
   - According to the 2022 update of the World Health Organization (WHO) Classification of Haematolymphoid Tumours, plasma cell neoplasms fall under the category of B-cell lymphoid proliferations and lymphomas and include those listed in Box 18.1:

BOX 18.1 ■ Plasma Cell and Monoclonal Gammopathy-Related Disorders

---

Monoclonal gammopathies
   - Monoclonal gammopathy of undetermined significance (MGUS)
     - IgM
     - Non-IgM
   - Monoclonal gammopathy of renal significance (MGRS)
   - Cold agglutinin disease

Plasma cell neoplasms
   - Plasmacytoma (solitary plasmacytoma of bone and extramedullary plasmacytoma)
   - Plasma cell myeloma (also called myeloma, multiple myeloma, or MM)
   - Plasma cell neoplasms associated with paraneoplastic syndrome
     - POEMS: polyneuropathy, organomegaly, endocrinopathy, monoclonal protein, skin changes
     - TEMPI: telangiectasias, elevated erythropoietin and erythrocytosis, monoclonal gammopathy, perinephric fluid collections, intrapulmonary shunting
     - AESOP: adenopathy and extensive skin patch overlying a plasmacytoma

Diseases with monoclonal immunoglobulin deposition
   - Monoclonal immunoglobulin deposition disease (LCDD and HCDD)
   - Immunoglobulin-related amyloidosis (AL, AH, AHL)

Heavy chain diseases
   - Alpha heavy chain disease
   - Gamma heavy chain disease
   - Mu heavy chain disease

AH, heavy chain; AHL, heavy and light chain; AL, light chain; HCDD, heavy chain deposition disease; IgM, immunoglobulin M; LCDD, light chain deposition disease.

- Among the plasma cell neoplasms, monoclonal gammopathy of undetermined significance (MGUS) and multiple myeloma (MM) are the most common.

2. How common is myeloma?

- MM is the second most common hematologic malignancy, after non-Hodgkin lymphoma.

3. What is the significance of myeloma?

- MM is still considered incurable, accounts for 20% of hematologic malignancy deaths and 2% of all cancer deaths.

ETIOLOGY AND RISK FACTORS

1. What is the etiology of myeloma?

- MM is a cancer of plasma cells (B-cells) usually originating in the bone marrow, caused by clonal somatic genetic mutations leading to abnormal proliferation and protein secretion (monoclonal protein, M-protein).

2. What are the risk factors for myeloma?

- Older age, male gender, African American race, obesity, family history of myeloma, personal history of MGUS, and certain environmental exposures, including herbicides (Agent Orange), radiation, and benzene, are associated with increased risk of myeloma.

SCREENING AND DIAGNOSTIC CRITERIA

1. Who should be evaluated for a potential plasma cell neoplasm?

- Myeloma should be considered when a patient has otherwise unexplained hypercalcemia, renal failure, anemia, bone pain, or lytic bone lesions on imaging.
- Other potential reasons to consider the diagnosis of myeloma include high or low serum total protein, hyperviscosity, neuropathy, frequent infections, and generalized symptoms of advanced malignancy such as weight loss.
- In addition to the above, more rare signs and symptoms of myeloma and other plasma cell neoplasms can include, and are not limited to, coagulation disorder, cardiac or liver failure, lymph node and/or liver/spleen enlargement, and dermatologic abnormalities.

2. What tests are important for assessing plasma cell neoplasms, including myeloma?

- Complete blood count with differential and peripheral blood smear
- Comprehensive metabolic panel to check calcium, albumin, renal, and liver function
- Serum beta-2 microglobulin (B2M) and lactate dehydrogenase (LDH)
- Serum protein electrophoresis (SPEP) with IFIX
- 24-hour urine protein electrophoresis (UPEP) with IFIX
- Serum quantitative immunoglobulins, IgG, IgA, and IgM (IgD and IgE only if suspected)
- Serum kappa and lambda free light chain (FLC) quantification
- Serum viscosity if monoclonal immunoglobulin level is >5 g/dL or symptoms suggestive of hyperviscosity

- Imaging standards for screening for myeloma bone disease , which are evolving
  - Whole-body low-dose CT is preferred to x-ray skeletal survey (more sensitive and specific). When not available, skeletal survey is reasonable.
  - In smoldering myeloma (SMM) and solitary plasmacytoma, whole-body imaging that is more sensitive than bone survey is mandatory. Options include whole-body low-dose CT, whole-body MRI, or PET/CT. If these options are not available, MRI of the spine and pelvis plus a skeletal survey is reasonable. NOTE: Bone lesions in POEMS (polyneuropathy, organomegaly, endocrinopathy, monoclonal gammopathy, skin changes) are typically sclerotic, not lytic. NOTE: Technetium-99m bone scans that are commonly used in other solid organ malignancies (e.g., to detect skeletal metastases from prostate cancer) are NOT helpful in the evaluation of MM and have a false negative rate up to 50%.
- Bone marrow biopsy with flow cytometry, conventional cytogenetics (karyotype), and fluorescence in situ hybridization (FISH) for commonly acquired genetic mutations (MM FISH panel)
- If AL amyloid is suspected, confirmation with Congo red staining ("apple-green birefringence under polarized light") and amyloid protein identification by immunohistochemistry, immunofluorescence (IF), and/or mass spectrometry (gold standard) on the affected tissue

3. What are the diagnostic criteria for active myeloma (requiring treatment)?

- Biopsy-proven plasmacytoma *or* ≥10% clonal bone marrow plasma cells, *and* at least one of the following (**SLiM CRAB** mnemonic):
  - **S** ("sixty"): clonal plasma cells ≥60% of bone marrow cellularity
  - **Li** ("light chain ratio"): involved to uninvolved FLC ratio of ≥100 (the involved FLC must be least ≥100 mg/L)
  - **M**: MRI with >1 focal lesion in the bone or bone marrow (size ≥5 mm)
  - Any plasma cell dyscrasia-related end-organ damage (CRAB criteria)
    - **C**: elevated serum calcium level (calcium >11 mg/dL)
    - **R**: renal insufficiency (creatinine >2 mg/dL or creatinine clearance <40 mL/min)
    - **A**: anemia (hemoglobin <10 g/dL or >2 g/dL below lower normal limit)
    - **B**: lytic bone lesions (one or more) on skeletal survey, CT, MRI, or PET/CT

4. What are the diagnostic criteria for the myeloma precursor conditions?

- MGUS
  - Serum M-protein <3 g/dL
  - Clonal bone marrow plasma cells <10%
  - Absence of end-organ damage attributed to the plasma cell neoplasm
- SMM
  - Serum M-protein ≥3 g/dL and/or urinary monoclonal protein ≥500 mg/24 hours and/or 10% to 59% clonal bone marrow plasma cells
  - Absence of end-organ damage attributed to the plasma cell neoplasm
- Solitary plasmacytoma
  - Solid clonal plasma cell tumor without bone marrow involvement or evidence of end-organ damage attributable to monoclonal plasma cells
  - Patients with a solitary plasmacytoma *and* <10% clonal plasma cells in bone marrow considered to have a solitary plasmacytoma with minimal marrow involvement; treated the same as solitary plasmacytoma, but with higher risk of recurrence or progression to active myeloma.

- POEMS
  - Among the plasma cell neoplasms with an associated paraneoplastic syndrome, POEMS is the most common.
    - Polyneuropathy: required major criteria for diagnosis
    - Organomegaly
    - Endocrinopathy
    - Monoclonal gammopathy: required major criteria for diagnosis
    - Skin changes
  - Also known as osteosclerotic myeloma due to sclerotic bone lesions
  - Associated with increased serum vascular endothelial growth factor (VEGF) and Castleman disease
- AL amyloidosis
  - Primary (AL) amyloidosis is characterized by deposition of amyloid protein composed of monoclonal immunoglobulin light chains (rarely, clonal heavy chains—AH amyloid, or both—AHL amyloid, have been described as well).
  - Amyloid protein deposition damages the affected organ(s), resulting in problems such as nephrotic syndrome, congestive heart failure, malabsorption or bowel motility disorders, neuropathy, pulmonary infiltrates, and so on.
- Monoclonal gammopathies of renal significance (MGRS)
  - MGRS occurs when an abnormal B-cell clone and secreted monoclonal immunoglobulin or fragment is associated with renal injury, despite not meeting criteria for active myeloma.
  - Amyloidosis (AL, AH, AHL) and light chain deposition disease (LCDD) are the most common.
  - Diagnosing MGRS usually requires kidney biopsy with IF and electron microscopic (EM) studies to identify deposit composition and organizational pattern.

PATHOLOGY

1. **What is the cell of origin for the malignant plasma cells of myeloma?**
   - Myeloma cells are postgerminal center plasma cells (a type of differentiated B-cell) identifiable by somatic mutations in the variable region of the immunoglobulin heavy chain gene.

SIGNS AND SYMPTOMS

1. **What are the most common symptoms of active myeloma?**
   - Anemia (73%)
   - Bone pain due to lytic lesions (58%)
   - Increased creatinine (48%)
   - Fatigue (32%)
   - Hypercalcemia (28%)
   - Weight loss (24%)

2. **What are uncommon but important signs and symptoms?**
   - Plasmacytoma (7%)
   - Paresthesia (5%)
   - Spinal cord compression (5%—due to plasmacytoma or vertebral body fracture)

RISK STRATIFICATION

1. **How do we determine prognosis and risk stratification in MM?**
   - Labs: B2M, LDH, albumin, peripheral plasma cell count
   - Mutational testing (marrow): MM FISH panel, karyotype

2. **Which features are associated with high-risk disease and worse prognosis?**
   - Revised International Staging System (R-ISS) stage III disease (see staging criteria that follows)
   - Cytogenetic testing (FISH, karyotype) showing t(4;14), t(14;16), t(14;20), del(1p), gain(1q), del(17p), or hypodiploidy
   - LDH > upper limit of normal (ULN), B2M ≥5.5mg/L
   - Primary plasma cell leukemia (≥5% circulating plasma cells on manual differential)
   - About 15% of people with myeloma with high-risk disease, with a median survival of 2 to 3 years despite standard therapy, and often relapse <12 months after prior therapy

3. **Which features are associated with standard-risk disease and better prognosis?**
   - R-ISS stage I disease (see staging criteria below)
   - Lack of high-risk cytogenetic abnormalities mentioned above; normal LDH and albumin, B2M <3.5mg
   - Median survival 8 to 10 years

4. **Which features are associated with intermediate-risk disease?**
   - R-ISS stage II disease (not meeting the criteria for stage I or III disease)

STAGING

1. **Which staging system is preferred for active myeloma?**
   - The R-ISS

2. **How is active myeloma staged according to the R-ISS?**
   - The R-ISS uses serum B2M, serum albumin, LDH, cytogenetics, and FISH for common mutations. Online calculators are widely available and useful in practice.
     - Stage I: B2M <3.5 mg/L, albumin ≥3.5 g/dL, normal LDH, no del(17p), t(4;14), or t(14;16; 5-year progression-free survival [PFS] and overall survival [OS] 55% and 82%, respectively)
     - Stage II: neither stage I nor stage III (5-year PFS and OS 36% and 62%, respectively)
     - Stage III: B2M ≥5.5 mg/L and LDH greater than ULN or del(17p), t(4;14), or t(14;16) by FISH (5-year PFS and OS 24% and 40%, respectively)

TREATMENT

GENERAL TREATMENT PRINCIPLES

1. **Which plasma cell neoplasms should be treated?**
   - In general, treatment is indicated when a plasma cell clone, its secreted monoclonal immunoglobulin, or fragment of monoclonal immunoglobulin, is causing

clinically significant symptoms or organ damage, or if symptoms or organ damage are expected to occur within the next 2 years without intervention.

■ There is no known benefit from treating MGUS or low-risk SMM; observation is the standard of care. High-risk SMM patients may benefit from treatment with lenalidomide and dexamethasone. The definition of high-risk SMM varies, but the most commonly used model is the "2/20/20" criteria: monoclonal protein >2 g/dL, bone marrow plasma cells >20%, and abnormal involved serum FLC ratio >20.

■ Patients with active myeloma should be treated since, by definition, end-organ damage is present or imminent.

■ Patients with other plasma cell disorders with systemic involvement such as AL amyloidosis also warrant treatment to prevent further organ damage.

■ Patients with a solitary plasmacytoma without meeting the criteria for MM can be treated with local radiation therapy with curative intent.

2. **What are the main factors in determining best frontline therapy for patients with newly diagnosed active myeloma?**
   ■ Disease risk (R-ISS staging)
   ■ Eligibility for high-dose chemotherapy followed by autologous hematopoietic stem cell transplantation (SCT)

3. **How do we define the criteria for disease response to therapy?**
   ■ The International Myeloma Working Group (IMWG) has established response criteria:
     ● Stringent complete response (sCR): no M-protein on IFIX, normal FLC ratio and no clonal plasma cells in the marrow, no residual plasmacytoma
     ● Complete response (CR): no M-protein on IFIX, <5% plasma cells in marrow, no residual plasmacytoma
     ● Very good partial response (VGPR): ≥90% reduction in M-protein, although still detectable
     ● Partial response (PR): ≥50% reduction in serum M-protein plus ≥90% reduction in urine light chains and total 24-hour urine light chains <200 mg; if no measurable serum or urine M-protein at baseline, then ≥50% reduction in serum FLC ratio (involved/uninvolved light chain), and if present ≥50% reduction in plasmacytoma size
     ● Minimal response (MR): ≥25% to 49% reduction in the M-protein or plasmacytoma size
     ● Stable disease (SD): not meeting the preceding criteria
     ● Progressive disease (PD): ≥25% increase in serum or urine M-protein, FLC ratio, bone marrow plasma cell %, new bone lesions or plasmacytomas, new hypercalcemia related to plasma cell disorder
   ■ There are also response guidelines based on minimal residual disease (MRD) testing, either by specialized flow cytometry or next-generation sequencing testing. Results of MRD testing are not yet being used outside of clinical trials for treatment decision-making.

4. **How is newly diagnosed myeloma treated?**
   ■ Most patients receive initial therapy with a triplet (three-drug) regimen, most commonly including a proteasome inhibitor and immunomodulatory agent, along with corticosteroids.

- The most common initial triplet regimens used are VRD (bortezomib, lenalidomide, dex: dexamethasone), CyBorD (cyclophosphamide, bortezomib, dex), DaraRd (daratumumab, lenalidomide, dex).
- VRD is generally preferred for transplant-eligible people based on the phase 3 SWOG S0777 trial.
- For patients who are frail or have contraindications to triplet therapy, consider DaraRd or doublet (two-drug) combinations such as Vd (bortezomib, dex) or Rd (lenalidomide, dex).
- Initial treatment with four-drug combinations, especially DaraVRD (daratumumab, bortezomib, lenalidomide, dex), is becoming more popular due to the randomized phase 2 GRIFFIN study.
  - Food and Drug Administration (FDA)-approved quadruplet treatments for previously untreated myeloma include DaraVMP (daratumumab, bortezomib, melphalan, dex) and DaraVTD (daratumumab, bortezomib, thalidomide, dex)

5. How do you decide what induction therapy to use?

- Disease risk stratification, patient factors (performance status, comorbidities, psychosocial support, patient goals), institutional resources (e.g., infusion and clinical trial availability), eligibility for autologous SCT

6. What happens after induction therapy?

- Consolidation: Patients who achieve an optimal response to induction therapy can receive consolidation with high-dose chemotherapy (melphalan 140 or 200 mg/m^2) followed by autologous SCT if eligible for transplant.
- Maintenance: After autologous SCT or after a longer course of induction therapy (if transplant-ineligible), patients are transitioned to maintenance therapy. Lenalidomide is the only FDA-approved agent at this time, based on several phase 3 trials, including IFM2005-02 and CALGB 100104.

7. What are the key agents used in first-line active myeloma treatment and what are their common toxicities?

- Proteasome inhibitors
  - Bortezomib (Velcade®)
    - Administration: IV or SQ (preferred)
    - Dosing interval: weekly (preferred) or twice weekly
    - Side effects: peripheral (sensory) neuropathy, thrombocytopenia, gastrointestinal (GI) (nausea, diarrhea), herpes zoster reactivation
    - Hepatic metabolism: dose adjustment required with liver dysfunction
    - No renal dose adjustment needed, useful in renal failure or chronic kidney disease (CKD) patients
    - Viral prophylaxis with acyclovir or valacyclovir required to prevent zoster reactivation
- Immunomodulators
  - Lenalidomide (Revlimid®)
    - Administration: oral
    - Dosing interval: daily, usually with week off
    - Side effects: myelosuppression, venous thromboembolism, fatigue
    - Renal metabolism: dose adjustment required with significant renal dysfunction
    - Venous thrombotic event (VTE) prophylaxis: low-dose aspirin (e.g., 81 mg daily), prophylactic low-molecular-weight heparin (LMWH), or prophylactic direct oral anticoagulants (DOAC)

- Teratogen: prescription and administration requiring participation in a REMS (Risk Evaluation and Mitigation Strategy) program
- Corticosteroids
  - Dexamethasone (Decadron®)
    - Administration: oral or IV
    - Dosing interval: weekly or twice weekly
    - Side effects: mental status changes, hyperglycemia, weight gain
    - No renal dose adjustments needed
    - VTE prophylaxis considered when used as higher doses (>160 mg/cycle)
- Monoclonal antibodies
  - Daratumumab (Darzalex®)
    - Mechanism: monoclonal antibody against CD38
    - Dosing interval: depending on trial, usually weekly for cycles 1 to 2, biweekly for cycles 3 to 6, then monthly for cycles 7 onward
    - Administration: IV or SQ
    - Side effects: infusion reactions, increased infection risk
    - Interference with routine blood type and screen testing due to presence of CD38 on red blood cell (RBC) surface; need to let blood bank know ahead of time and check type and screen prior to starting treatment

8. **What is the role of bone-modifying agents (BMA) in myeloma?**
   - BMA decreases the risk of skeletal-related events (SREs), which are pathologic fracture, spinal cord compression, needing radiation, or surgery for bone
   - BMA is recommended for patients with active myeloma, regardless of presence of lytic lesions.
   - Approved BMA for myeloma includes bisphosphonates, pamidronate and zole-dronic acid, and the RANK-L inhibitor denosumab.
   - Optimal duration of treatment with BMA is unknown, but current recommendation for bisphosphonates is every 1 to 3 months for 2 years, after which the decision to continue can be reassessed, depending on remission status. The current recommendation for denosumab is monthly, indefinitely. If denosumab is stopped, administration of a bisphosphonate should be considered to lower risk of rebound fracture.
   - Important side effects of all BMAs include hypocalcemia, osteonecrosis of the jaw, and fragility fractures. Bisphosphonates may cause renal failure and/or mild cytokine release syndrome (CRS; generally described as flu-like symptoms for 1–2 days after administration). Renal function should be routinely monitored on bisphosphonate treatment. Close monitoring and calcium supplementation are recommended with all BMAs, especially in severe renal failure (serum creatinine >3 mg/dL or creatinine clearance (CrCl) <30 mL/min), as there is higher risk of severe, prolonged hypocalcemia.

PRINCIPLES OF AUTOLOGOUS STEM CELL TRANSPLANTATION (SCT) IN MYELOMA

1. **What is the role of autologous SCT in myeloma therapy?**
   - Autologous SCT generally results in higher response rates and prolonged PFS compared with standard therapies; data from phase 3 studies describing its impact on OS are mixed.
   - Autologous SCT should be considered in all MM patients who are eligible, particularly those with high-risk disease.

2. **Who is eligible for an autologous SCT?**
   - The eligibility criteria for autologous SCT are not standardized; the decision for SCT is often individualized rather than based on standard eligibility criteria.
   - Age >75 years, Eastern Cooperative Oncology Group (ECOG) performance status ≥3, and other significant comorbidities (e.g., heart failure, significant pulmonary disease) increase the risk of this treatment and are generally exclusions to autologous SCT.

3. **When are autologous hematopoietic stem cells collected for myeloma patients?**
   - Usually after 2 to 4 months of therapy and/or after cytoreduction of myeloma by ≥50% (at least PR)

4. **When is the best time to complete an autologous SCT?**
   - Autologous hematopoietic cell transplantation (HCT) can be completed to consolidate response "early" (preferred, after first treatment) or "late" (at the time of first relapse, after second treatment).

5. **Can a patient undergo a second autologous SCT?**
   - Yes. Usually, enough hematopoietic stem cells are collected to perform two autologous HCTs.
   - Because of increasing treatment options for relapsed myeloma, use of second autologous HCT is becoming more uncommon. It is generally reserved for consolidation of induction beyond first line of treatment if the response to the first autologous HCT was prolonged, beyond 3 years with maintenance therapy.

PRINCIPLES OF FIRST-LINE THERAPY

1. **What are the initial treatment options for myeloma patients who are autologous SCT candidates (transplant-eligible)?**
   - Key point: Avoid prolonged treatment with alkylating agents (cyclophosphamide or melphalan), or lenalidomide, which can interfere with stem cell collection.
   - The most common induction regimen is the three-drug combination VRD, followed by SCT.
   - After SCT, patients should be started on maintenance therapy to maintain or improve disease response.
   - Standard-risk MM:
     - Induction therapy can be followed by upfront or delayed autologous SCT.
     - Posttransplant maintenance therapy is recommended with lenalidomide.
   - High-risk MM:
     - Use three-drug or four-drug combinations for induction or consider clinical trial.
     - Induction therapy should be followed by early autologous SCT in most patients.
     - Posttransplant maintenance therapy with bortezomib-based regimens (e.g., dose-reduced VRD) or daratumumab-based regimens (e.g., daratumumab with lenalidomide) is recommended by expert opinion; definitive studies are lacking. For patients with t(4;14), maintenance with bortezomib every other week is recommended. Additional agents are sometimes added depending on individual risk and physician discretion.

2. **What are the initial treatment options for myeloma patients who are not autologous SCT candidates (transplant-ineligible)?**
   - Induction therapy regimens similar to transplant-eligible patients

■ Adjustment of treatment doses and schedules as needed for age, performance status, and comorbidity (guidelines available from the European Myeloma Network)

RELAPSED OR REFRACTORY DISEASE

1. What is the definition of PD after initial treatment?

■ PD: ≥25% increase in serum or urine M-protein, FLC ratio, bone marrow plasma cell %, new bone lesions or plasmacytomas, new hypercalcemia related to plasma cell disorder

■ Relapse: development of CRAB criteria (new hypercalcemia, anemia, renal failure, bone lesions)

2. What treatment strategies are available for relapsed disease?

■ If it has been ≥1 year since initial therapy without maintenance, repeating the initial therapy is reasonable.

■ Combination therapy using agents from a different class than those used in prior treatment is preferred. Additional strategies include choosing different agents from already used drug classes and using new combinations of previously used agents.

■ Second autologous SCT can be considered in fit patients who had prolonged response after their first transplant.

■ Allogeneic SCT is generally not recommended due to high treatment-related morbidity and mortality but can be considered in the context of a clinical trial.

■ Generally, the duration and depth of response decline with lines of therapy.

■ B-cell maturation antigen (BCMA)-directed genetically modified autologous T-cell immunotherapy or bispecific BCMA-directed CD3 T-cell engager therapies can be considered after exhausting other standard options. Studies are ongoing to evaluate the role of these newer agents earlier in treatment.

■ In special circumstances, combination chemotherapy is sometimes used for ultra-high-risk myeloma, such as plasma cell leukemia, and for myeloma refractory to several lines of therapy in patients who need urgent cytoreduction due to symptoms related to myeloma. Common combinations include VDT-PACE (bortezomib, dexamethasone, thalidomide, cisplatin, doxorubicin, cyclophosphamide, etoposide) and DCEP (dexamethasone, cyclophosphamide, etoposide, cisplatin).

3. What additional drugs are available for relapsed/refractory disease?

■ Agents for relapsed/refractory disease often given in two-, three- or four-drug combinations depending on the nature of relapse (indolent vs. aggressive), the patient's comorbidities, and the response and tolerance to prior treatment

■ Immunomodulators
  ● Pomalidomide (Pomalyst®): oral, similar side effect profile to lenalidomide including cytopenia and thrombosis risk; also requires REMS program enrollment.

■ Proteasome inhibitors
  ● Carfilzomib (Kyprolis®): IV only, less peripheral neuropathy than bortezomib, possible cardiac toxicity so requires baseline cardiac assessment
  ● Ixazomib (Ninlaro®): oral drug, causes less peripheral neuropathy, but more GI toxicity (e.g., nausea and diarrhea) than bortezomib

■ Monoclonal antibodies
  ● Daratumumab (Darzalex®): IV or SC, anti-CD38 antibody; see the "Principles of First-Line Therapy" section for more information?

- Isatuximab (Sarclisa®): IV anti-CD38 antibody, similar side effect profile to daratumumab
- Elotuzumab (Empliciti®): IV anti-SLAMF7 antibody (glycoprotein expressed on natural killer and myeloma cells), side effects mainly infusion reactions and increased infection risk
- Belantamab mafodotin (Blenrep®): IV antibody-drug conjugate targeting BCMA, major side effect is significant corneal toxicity requiring frequent ophthalmology exams before starting and during treatment
- Teclistamab (Tecvayli®): SC bispecific BCMA-directed CD3 T-cell engager; registration in REMS program and admission to the hospital for monitoring while starting treatment required due to CRS and neurologic toxicity, including immune effector cell-associated neurotoxicity (ICANS)
  - Other cellular therapies
    - Idecabtagene vicleucel (Abecma®): a BCMA-directed genetically modified autologous T-cell immunotherapy; requires autologous T-cell collection and preparation, pretreatment with lymphodepleting chemotherapy, and hospital admission to manage complications such as CRS and ICANS
    - Ciltacabtagene autoleucel (Carvykti®): a BCMA-directed genetically modified autologous T-cell immunotherapy; requires autologous T-cell collection and preparation, pretreatment with lymphodepleting chemotherapy, and hospital admission to manage complications such as CRS and ICANS
  - Other agents
    - Selinexor (Xpovio®): oral selective inhibitor of nuclear export, associated with significant GI toxicity and cytopenia

QUESTIONS

1. **A 55-year-old woman was referred to you after workup of anemia revealed a monoclonal protein (M-protein) of 4.2 g/dL with several lytic lesions on skeletal survey. Immunofixation demonstrates immunoglobulin G (IgG) kappa M-protein. Bone marrow biopsy showed 25% clonal plasma cells, with normal karyotype and fluorescence in situ hybridization (FISH) testing. She is working full time as a registered nurse and runs about 15 miles per week. She wants aggressive therapy to improve her chances of survival if possible. What is your treatment recommendation?**
   A. Bortezomib, lenalidomide, and dexamethasone (VRD), stem cell collection after four cycles, autologous stem cell transplantation (SCT), lenalidomide maintenance
   B. VRD for four cycles, lenalidomide maintenance
   C. VRD, stem cell collection after four cycles, autologous SCT, no maintenance therapy
   D. Lenalidomide and dexamethasone (RD), stem cell collection after four cycles, autologous SCT, lenalidomide maintenance

2. **A 55-year-old woman was recently diagnosed with multiple myeloma and is planning to start treatment with weekly bortezomib, lenalidomide, and dexamethasone. She has no history of bleeding or prior thrombosis. What is the best way to reduce her risk of venous thrombotic events (VTE)?**

A. Warfarin, 1 to 2 mg daily
B. Aspirin 81 mg daily
C. Enoxaparin 1 mg/kg daily
D. Compression stockings
E. None needed

3. **Bisphosphonates in multiple myeloma patients do which of the following?**
   A. Reduce risk of need for future radiation therapy or surgery
   B. Increase risk of fragility fractures
   C. Reduce risk of myeloma-related renal dysfunction
   D. Increase risk of venous thromboembolism
   E. A and B

4. **A 67-year-old man presents with chronic right hip pain and was found to have a 2.4-cm pelvic bone mass on an MRI scan done during workup by primary care provider. PET/CT was done and showed FDG = [^{18}F] Fluorodeoxyglucose uptake in the right pelvis mass, with no other areas of suspicious uptake. Pelvic mass biopsy confirmed a lambda-restricted plasma cell population. Bone marrow biopsy showed 5% lambda-restricted plasma cells. Blood tests were negative for anemia, hypercalcemia, or renal dysfunction, although showed a monoclonal immunoglobulin G lambda protein level of 1.2 g/dL. How would you treat this patient?**
   A. ≥40 Gy radiation to the pelvic plasmacytoma followed by observation
   B. ≥40 Gy radiation to the pelvic plasmacytoma followed by VRD and consideration for autologous stem cell transplantation (SCT)
   C. Surgical resection followed by observation
   D. Surgical resection followed by lenalidomide maintenance therapy

5. **Which of the following characterizes high-risk multiple myeloma (MM)?**
   A. del(5q)
   B. t(11;14)
   C. Trisomy 15
   D. del(17p)

6. **A 61-year-old woman was referred to you after her primary care physician found a monoclonal protein (M-protein) of 3.6 g/dL during a workup for elevated total protein levels. Immunofixation reveals an immunoglobulin A (IgA) kappa M-protein. She has normal hemoglobin, normal serum calcium, normal creatinine, and negative urine Bence Jones protein. Her serum kappa/lambda light chain ratio is 3.6. An x-ray skeletal survey was negative for lytic lesions. Bone marrow biopsy shows 35% monoclonal plasma cells. What is your next step in management?**
   A. Obtain next-generation sequencing (NGS) from bone marrow aspirate to risk-stratify and determine therapy.
   B. Start VRD and refer to bone marrow transplant center in preparation for autologous stem cell transplantation (SCT).
   C. Observation and recheck appropriate labs in 6 to 8 weeks.
   D. Obtain an MRI of the spine and pelvis or PET/CT.

7. **Which of the following is not a component of POEMS syndrome?**
   A. Polyarthralgia
   B. Organomegaly
   C. Endocrinopathy
   D. Monoclonal gammopathy
   E. Skin changes

8. **All the following features are associated with high-risk disease and worse prognosis except:**
   A. Lactate dehydrogenase (LDH) more than the upper limit of normal
   B. Beta-2 microglobulin of 3 mg/L
   C. Presence of 6% circulating plasma cells
   D. Del(1p)
   E. Gain(1q)

9. **All the following combinations of therapeutics for myeloma and mode of action are correct except:**
   A. Daratumumab: anti-CD38 antibody
   B. Elotuzumab: anti-SLAMF7 antibody
   C. Belantamab mafodotin: antibody-drug conjugate targeting CD38
   D. Ixazomib: proteasome inhibitor
   E. Teclistamab: T-cell redirecting bispecific antibody that targets both CD3 and B-cell maturation antigen (BCMA)

ANSWERS

1. **A. Bortezomib, lenalidomide, and dexamethasone (VRD), stem cell collection after four cycles, autologous stem cell transplantation (SCT), lenalidomide maintenance.** This patient has standard-risk active myeloma and should receive triplet combination induction therapy with VRD. A doublet induction therapy (RD) would be considered in a frail patient with comorbid conditions, not for this relatively healthy patient. This patient has a good performance status and should be considered for an autologous HCT after induction, and therefore her stem cells should be collected after approximately the fourth cycle of induction therapy. Not offering upfront autologous SCT would not be standard of care for this patient unless she was deemed transplant-ineligible. All patients who undergo SCT should receive posttransplant maintenance therapy. If the patient were to opt against SCT, then more than four cycles of induction should be used.

2. **B. Aspirin 81 mg daily.** Low-dose aspirin daily is effective in lowering thrombosis risk in people at standard risk for VTE on lenalidomide therapy. Patients at higher risk for thrombosis (e.g., prior thrombosis, high-dose dexamethasone use) may require prophylactic or therapeutic anticoagulants. Low-dose warfarin is inferior to VTE prophylaxis in older adults with myeloma regardless of risk. Prophylactic dosing of enoxaparin (e.g., 40 mg daily) would be another option.

3. **E. A and B.** Bisphosphonates have been shown in several studies to reduce the risk of new skeletal events and reduce myeloma-related bone pain but can increase the risk of fragility fractures, especially with long-term use. Bisphosphonates may cause renal toxicity, so renal function must be monitored and doses adjusted as needed with treatment. Bisphosphonates are not known to increase venous thrombotic events (VTE) risk in myeloma patients.

4. **A. ≥40 Gy radiation to the pelvic plasmacytoma followed by observation.** This patient has a solitary plasmacytoma of bone (SPB) with minimal (<10%) bone marrow involvement that does not meet the criteria for multiple myeloma (MM). Radiation with curative intent (total dose ≥40 Gy) is the standard of care for SPB, and after completing this he would undergo surveillance for his underlying IgG lambda monoclonal gammopathy of undetermined significance (MGUS). PET/CT is important to rule out other bone lesions prior to a diagnosis of SPB with minimal marrow involvement. Surgical intervention for SPB can be considered in certain cases, such as impending fracture or cord compression, which is not the case for this patient.

5. **D. del(17p).** Mutations such as t(14;20), t(14;16), t(4;14), gain(1q), del(1p), and del(17p) are cytogenetic markers of high-risk myeloma, along with elevated lactate dehydrogenase (LDH) or evidence of plasma cell leukemia. Trisomies, del(5q), and t(11;14) are considered standard-risk mutations in myeloma.

6. **D. Obtain an MRI of the spine and pelvis or PET/CT.** This patient likely has smoldering multiple myeloma based on her monoclonal serum protein of ≥3 g/dL and ≥10% clonal plasma cells in her bone marrow, without evidence of end-organ damage. Prior to diagnosing her with smoldering myeloma, however, she needs to be assessed for bone lesions that may have been missed by skeletal survey. This can be completed with whole-body MRI, MRI total spine and pelvis (if whole-body MRI is not available), or PET/CT. Up to 50% of patients without lytic lesions on skeletal survey demonstrate tumor-related lesions using more sensitive imaging methods. NGS testing of bone marrow in myeloma patients is not standard of care, although is often used in the context of clinical trials or minimal residual disease monitoring.

7. **A. Polyarthralgia.** Polyneuropathy, organomegaly, endocrinopathy, monoclonal gammopathy, and skin changes are components of POEMS syndrome.

8. **B. Beta-2 microglobulin of 3 mg/L.** Beta-2 microglobulin ≥5.5mg/L is associated with high-risk disease.

9. **C. Belantamab mafodotin: antibody-drug conjugate targeting CD38.** Belantamab mafodotin is an antibody-drug conjugate targeting bispecific BCMA.

Immunodeficiency-Associated Lymphoproliferative Disorders

19

Darren King and Shannon Ann Carty

DEFINITION

Immunodeficiency-associated lymphoproliferative disorders are a group of lymphoid neoplasms associated with an immunosuppressed state, that is, with primary immune disorders, after solid organ or allogeneic hematopoietic stem cell transplant (HCT), on immunosuppressive medications for autoimmune or rheumatologic disorders, or with HIV infection/AIDS.

Posttransplant Lymphoproliferative Disorders

EPIDEMIOLOGY

1. **What is the incidence of posttransplant lymphoproliferative disorders (PTLDs)?**
   - PTLD is the most common malignancy seen after solid organ transplant (up to 20%) and uncommon after allogeneic HCT.
   - Incidence varies by type of transplant but estimated to be 1% at 10 years.
   - 80% of cases occur within the first year posttransplant, the time of most intense immunosuppression.

ETIOLOGY AND RISK FACTORS

1. **What is the etiology of PTLD?**
   - In the majority of patients (≥70%), it is related to B-cell expansion induced by infection with Epstein–Barr virus (EBV) in the setting of chronic immunosuppression and decreased T-cell surveillance. EBV+ PTLD is most common in the first year post transplant.
   - EBV is a common pathogen and 90% to 95% of U.S. adults are seropositive.
   - EBV-infected B-cells can originate from either the host or the donor.
   - Host-derived PTLD is most common following solid organ transplantation.
   - Donor-derived PTLD is more common following allogeneic HCT.

2. **What are the main risk factors for developing PTLD?**
   - Degree of T-cell immunosuppression (most common immunosuppressive treatments (ISTs) are calcineurin inhibitors [tacrolimus, cyclosporine])
   - Highest in those with multiorgan transplant > lung transplant > liver, stem cell, and heart > renal transplant (least common)
   - Increased risk for PTLD in EBV-seronegative recipients of EBV-positive donor organs

CLASSIFICATION

1. **What are the types of PTLD: World Health Organization classification?**
   - Early (nondestructive) lesions: polyclonal B-cells without signs of transformation to lymphoma, including the following:
     - Plasmacytic hyperplasia
     - Infectious mononucleosis-like lesions
     - Florid follicular hyperplasia
   - Polymorphic PTLD: polyclonal or monoclonal B-cells with malignant transformation but does not meet the criteria for B-cell or NK/T-cell lymphoma
   - Monomorphic PTLD: monoclonal malignant cells that meet the criteria for B-cell or NK/T-cell lymphoma
     - B-cell neoplasms
       - Diffuse large B-cell lymphoma (DLBCL)
       - Burkitt lymphoma
       - Plasma cell myeloma
       - Plasmacytoma-like lesion
       - Other
     - T-cell neoplasms
       - Peripheral T-cell lymphoma
       - Hepatosplenic (gamma-delta) T-cell lymphoma
       - Other
     - Classic Hodgkin lymphoma-type PTLD

SIGNS AND SYMPTOMS

1. **What are the signs and symptoms of PTLD?**
   - B symptoms such as fevers, weight loss, night sweats, failure to thrive, and fatigue
   - Lymphadenopathy
   - 50% of cases presenting with extranodal masses, which may involve the gastrointestinal (GI) tract, lung, liver, and the allografted organ itself

DIAGNOSIS

1. **How is this diagnosed?**
   - Tissue biopsy and histologic evaluation followed by staging with PET/CT

TREATMENT

1. **How is PTLD treated?**
   - Options include reduction in immunosuppression (RI), rituximab, chemoimmunotherapy, radiation, or a combination of therapies. Initial management is dependent on the type of PTLD and RI must be performed in close consultation with the patient's transplant team.
   - Patients receiving chemotherapy-based regimens for PTLD (e.g., R-CHOP [rituximab, cyclophosphamide, doxorubicin, vincristine, and prednisone]) must receive G-CSF support with each cycle, with strong consideration for *Pneumocystis jirovecii* prophylaxis.
   - Based on outcomes data from the PTLD-1 trial, frontline therapy for polymorphic and monomorphic (B-cell type) PTLD may be administered in a sequential, risk-adapted approach.

- Initial therapy with rituximab given weekly for four doses, followed by restaging PET/CT
- In those patients achieving complete remission (CR; approximately 25% of cases), consolidation given as rituximab every 3 weeks for four cycles.
- In cases which fail to achieve CR or progress, chemoimmunotherapy with R-CHOP given every 21 days for four cycles
- An alternative to the sequential risk-adapted approach is to treat upfront with chemoimmunotherapy (e.g., R-CHOP).
- Early lesions: Consider RI alone. If CR achieved, monitor EBV by peripheral blood polymerase chain reaction and graft organ function in the setting of RI. If partial response or persistent/progressive disease despite RI, then treat with rituximab.
- Classic Hodgkin lymphoma-like PTLD: Use similar protocols as those used to treat classic Hodgkin lymphoma, that is, ABVD ± radiation therapy.
- For T-cell-type PTLD, there is no established therapy guideline and standard peripheral T-cell lymphoma therapies are used, including brentuximab vedotin for CD30+ disease.

2. **Is antiviral therapy effective for treatment of PTLD?**
   - There is no established, effective antiviral prophylaxis for EBV-associated PTLD. Patients with EBV-driven PTLD who are refractory to the above therapies may be candidates for EBV-specific cytotoxic T lymphocyte (CTL) therapy, currently undergoing clinical trials.

3. **Is there a role for radiation therapy or surgery in PTLD?**
   - Localized polymorphic PTLD may be treated with involved site radiation therapy (ISRT) or surgical excision alone or in combination with rituximab.

Acquired Immunodeficiency Syndrome-Related Lymphoma

DEFINITION

AIDS-related lymphoma includes non-Hodgkin lymphoma (NHL), Hodgkin lymphoma (HL), primary effusion lymphoma (PEL, human herpesvirus-8 (HHV-8) associated), and central nervous system (CNS) lymphoma.

EPIDEMIOLOGY

1. **What is the incidence of lymphoma in HIV-positive patients?**
   - The incidence of NHL is 1.2% per year.
   - There is a 25% to 40% risk of malignancy in HIV patients, with 10% of those being NHL.
   - AIDS-related lymphoma is more common in males than in females.
   - NHL is an AIDS-defining malignancy.
   - HL is not an AIDS-defining malignancy.
   - There is a 15- to 30-fold increase in HL found in the HIV-positive population.

2. **What is the incidence of PEL?**
   - Primary effusion lymphoma is the least common NHLs, accounting for 1% to 4% of all AIDS-related lymphomas.

3. **What is the incidence of CNS lymphoma?**
   - CNS lymphoma accounts for 15% of NHLs in HIV-positive patients.
   - The incidence is 2% to 6% in HIV-positive patients.

ETIOLOGY AND RISK FACTORS

1. **What are the risk factors for NHL in HIV-positive patients?**
   - Low CD4 count
   - High HIV viral load
   - Decreased incidence of NHL and primary CNS lymphoma with combination antiretroviral therapy

CLASSIFICATION

1. **What are the subtypes of AIDS-related lymphoma?**
   - Systemic NHL
     - DLBCL (75%)
     - Burkitt lymphoma (25%)
     - Plasmablastic lymphoma (<5%)
     - T-cell lymphoma (1%–3%)
     - Indolent B-cell lymphoma (<10%)
   - PEL
   - Primary CNS lymphoma
   - HL

SIGNS AND SYMPTOMS

1. **What are the signs and symptoms of AIDS-related lymphomas?**
   - Systemic NHL and classic HL can present with B symptoms (fever, weight loss, night sweats), lymphadenopathy, and extranodal disease. Also consider cytopenias, hypercalcemia, and labs consistent with tumor lysis syndrome as a presentation.
   - Most commonly involved extranodal sites are the GI tract, bone marrow, liver, lung, and CNS.
   - PEL involves the pleura and pericardium or presents as ascites. Patients can have dyspnea or chest pain.
   - CNS lymphoma presents with headaches, confusion, seizures, visual changes, or focal neurologic deficits.

STAGING

1. **How are patients with AIDS-related lymphoma staged?**
   - The same staging system used for NHL/HL in the HIV-negative population is used.

DIAGNOSIS

1. **How do you diagnose a patient with AIDS-related lymphoma?**
   - Must have HIV infection
   - Biopsy of tissue and histologic confirmation

- PEL: effusion containing malignant cells with HHV-8 virus in the nuclei of these cells
- CNS lymphoma: either by biopsy of brain mass or cerebral spinal fluid evaluation

TREATMENT

1. What are the treatments for AIDS-related lymphomas?

- All patients should be started on antiretroviral therapy if not already on treatment. CR rates for lymphoma are higher in patients who receive concurrent antiretroviral therapy. Choice of antiretroviral therapy must be made in consultation with an infectious disease specialist, with particular attention paid to anticipated time to response as well as potential interactions with chemotherapy drug classes.
- Patients receiving chemotherapy for AIDS-related lymphomas must receive granulocyte colony stimulating factor (G-CSF) support in addition to appropriate antimicrobial prophylaxis (e.g., *P. jirovecii*).
- Frontline recommended therapy for AIDS-related DLBCL and PEL is dose-adjusted (DA) R-EPOCH (rituximab, etoposide, prednisone, vincristine, cyclophosphamide, doxorubicin). In addition to standard dose adjustments per cycle based on cytopenia nadirs, cyclophosphamide dose is also adjusted per baseline CD4+ count. An alternative frontline regimen is R-CHOP. Rituximab is typically omitted from PEL treatment as the disease is usually CD20-negative.
- Burkitt lymphoma is treated with modified R-CODOX-M/IVAC (rituximab, cyclophosphamide, vincristine, doxorubicin, high-dose methotrexate alternating with ifosfamide, etoposide, and high-dose cytarabine). Alternative regimens are DA-R-EPOCH or rituximab, hyperfractionated cyclophoshamide, vincristine, doxorubicin, dexamethasone (R-Hyper-CVAD).
- There is no established therapy guideline for plasmablastic lymphoma; however, emerging regimens typically combine lymphoma-like regimens (e.g., DA-EPOCH) with proteosome inhibitors used in multiple myeloma (e.g., bortezomib). There is no role for rituximab in the treatment of plasmablastic lymphoma as the disease is CD20-negative.
- CNS prophylaxis is recommended for all AIDS-associated NHL except for PEL.
- HL is treated with doxorubicine/adriamycin, bleomycin, vinblastine, dacarbazine (ABVD).
- Primary CNS lymphoma is treated with high-dose intravenous methotrexate. Radiation therapy may play a role in palliation of symptoms.

Iatrogenic Immunodeficiency Lymphoproliferative Disorders in Nontransplant Settings

DEFINITION

Iatrogenic immunodeficiency lymphoproliferative disorders are a group of lymphoid neoplasms associated with an immunocompromised state, such as patients with autoimmune/rheumatic disorders or in the posttransplant period being treated with immunosuppression (see preceding text for PTLDs).

ETIOLOGY

1. **What types of IST are related to iatrogenic lymphoproliferative disorders?**
   - Methotrexate, infliximab (tumor necrosis factor [TNF] alpha-blocker), and mycophenolate mofetil are agents used in autoimmune/rheumatic disorders which are commonly associated with iatrogenic lymphoproliferative disorders.

EPIDEMIOLOGY AND RISK FACTORS

1. **What are the risk factors for developing iatrogenic immunodeficiency lymphoproliferative disorders?**
   - Risk factors include underlying autoimmune disorders, such as rheumatoid arthritis, psoriasis, and inflammatory bowel disease requiring treatment with immunosuppressive therapy.
   - There is a known association between hepatosplenic (gamma-delta) T-cell lymphoma and patients receiving anti-TNF alpha therapy (e.g., infliximab) for inflammatory bowel disease.

PATHOLOGY

   - IST, such as methotrexate (MTX), can impair T-cell-mediated immune surveillance and allow expansion of clonal B-cell population.
     - 40% of MTX-related lymphoproliferative disorders are EBV-positive.
     - It can develop into NHL or HL.

TREATMENT

1. **What are the treatments for IST-related lymphoproliferative disorders?**
   - Stop or reduce underlying IST if possible.
   - Discontinuing MTX in MTX-associated lymphoproliferative disorder can lead to regression in one out of three cases.
   - Regression is rare in cases related to infliximab.
   - Treatment is similar to that in PTLD—use chemoimmunotherapy appropriate to the lymphoma subtype.

QUESTIONS

1. **A 60-year old Caucasian male with untreated AIDS is referred to an oncologist for a newly diagnosed stage IV diffuse large B-cell lymphoma (DLBCL) with bone marrow involvement. He has not started antiretroviral therapy yet. He denies headache, confusion, vision changes, or other focal neurologic changes. His Eastern Cooperative Oncology Group (ECOG) performance status score is 2. What is the optimal treatment regimen?**
   A. Patient with very advanced disease so best supportive care with hospice should be considered
   B. Antiretroviral therapy, chemoimmunotherapy, and prophylactic intrathecal chemotherapy
   C. Chemotherapy alone
   D. Antiretroviral therapy alone

2. **Which of the following is not considered an AIDS-defining malignancy?**
   A. Hodgkin lymphoma
   B. Diffuse large B-cell lymphoma (DLBCL)
   C. Cervical cancer
   D. Burkitt lymphoma

3. **A 52-year-old female presents to the clinic on day 72 following lung transplant. She is taking tacrolimus and prednisone to prevent graft rejection. She reports 1 week of drenching night sweats and general malaise. On physical exam, a 2-cm cervical lymph node is palpated. She undergoes excisional biopsy of the node and pathology shows histologic features of a monomorphic CD20-positive diffuse large B-cell lymphoma (DLBCL), with immunostaining positive for Epstein–Barr virus (EBV). Peripheral blood EBV quantitative polymerase chain reaction (PCR) is markedly elevated at 2,000,000 IU/mL. PET/CT is performed and shows multiple areas of nodal involvement above and below the diaphragm. The patient's tacrolimus is tapered. What is the next step in management?**
   A. Close monitoring of weekly EBV PCR level
   B. Weekly rituximab for four doses followed by PET/CT
   C. Chemoimmunotherapy with R-CHOP for six cycles
   D. Stop tacrolimus entirely

4. **A 65-year-old female who underwent a living donor renal transplant 1 year ago has been diagnosed with a monomorphic B-cell posttransplant lymphoproliferative disorder (diffuse large B-cell lymphoma). Her immunosuppression has been tapered and she has completed 4 weekly doses of rituximab for Epstein–Barr virus (EBV)-positive disease. A restaging PET/CT shows a complete metabolic response. At this time, what is the most appropriate next step in management?**
   A. Close monitoring of weekly EBV polymerase chain reaction level
   B. Consolidation chemoimmunotherapy with R-CHOP for four cycles
   C. Consolidation with rituximab every 3 weeks for four cycles
   D. Consolidation with autologous stem cell transplant

5. **A 56-year-old Caucasian male with a 10-year history of Crohn's disease presents with abdominal pain, bloating, nausea, and vomiting. He has had loss of appetite over the past 3 months and has lost 15 pounds. During your interview, you are told by the patient that his Crohn's disease has been treated with mesalamine, steroids, and methotrexate for many years. He has been off all treatments for the past 2 months due to progressive cytopenias. What is your next step in management?**
   A. Resume treatment with methotrexate.
   B. Obtain a CT scan of the abdomen and pelvis.
   C. Perform an esophagogastroduodenoscopy (EGD).
   D. Check lactate dehydrogenase (LDH).

6. **A 45-year-old woman with AIDS presents with shortness of breath and cough. She had not been taking her antiretroviral therapy and her CD4 count is <100. A chest x-ray (CXR) reveals a large right-sided effusion. She undergoes thoracentesis and the fluid is positive for malignant cells consistent with B-cell non-Hodgkin lymphoma (NHL). Polymerase chain**

reaction (PCR) is positive for human herpesvirus-8 (HHV-8). Her Eastern Cooperative Oncology Group (ECOG) performance status score is 2. What is the preferred treatment?

A. Antiretroviral therapy
B. Best supportive care and hospice
C. Cyclophosphamide, doxorubicin, vincristine, etoposide, and prednisone (dose-adjusted EPOCH) plus rituximab with granulocyte colony stimu-lating factor (G-CSF) support plus antiretroviral therapy
D. Cyclophosphamide, doxorubicin, vincristine, etoposide, and prednisone (dose-adjusted EPOCH) with G-CSF support plus antiretroviral therapy

ANSWERS

1. **B. Antiretroviral therapy, chemoimmunotherapy, and prophylactic intrathecal chemotherapy.** This patient has an AIDS-defining lymphoma. Most non-Hodgkin lymphomas in HIV-infected individuals are of B-cell origin and are frequently associated with Epstein–Barr virus (EBV) infection. Current treatment recommendations for AIDS-associated DLBCL include the following: (a) antiretroviral therapy; (b) chemoimmunotherapy with DA-R-EPOCH (preferred) or R-CHOP (alternative regimen) with G-CSF support; and (c) patients with AIDS-related NHL are at increased risk of central nervous system involvement and therefore administration of prophylactic intrathecal chemotherapy is reasonable.

2. **A. Hodgkin lymphoma.** The three cancers considered as AIDS-defining cancers or malignancies are Kaposi sarcoma, aggressive B-cell non-Hodgkin lymphoma, and cervical cancer.

3. **B. Weekly rituximab for four doses followed by PET/CT.** This patient has posttransplant lymphoproliferative disorder (PTLD). Most cases of PTLD in the setting of allogeneic hematopoietic cell transplantation are due to donor EBV-infected B-cells passed to the host (recipient). Owing to suppressed T-cell activity from tacrolimus, these EBV-infected B-cells may proliferate at a high rate and lead to a lymphoproliferative disorder. Patients can present with constitutional symptoms. Given the presence of a high-grade lymphoma, this patient must begin therapy in addition to having appropriately started to taper tacrolimus. Based on outcomes data from the PTLD-1 trial, an appropriate initial regimen is 4 weekly doses of rituximab followed by restaging PET/CT.

4. **C. Consolidation with rituximab every 3 weeks for four cycles.** This patient with monomorphic B-cell PTLD (DLBCL) has had an excellent response to initial frontline therapy with rituximab, having achieved complete response (CR) per PET/CT. Given outcomes data from the PTLD-1 trial, it is appropriate to proceed with consolidation with single-agent rituximab every 3 weeks for four cycles. Approximately 25% of patients with PTLD will achieve CR with frontline single-agent rituximab.

5. **B. Obtain a CT scan of the abdomen and pelvis.** The patient's symptoms are concerning for an iatrogenic lymphoproliferative disorder due to immunosuppressive therapy (IST) for his Crohn's disease. The most common ISTs associated with iatrogenic lymphoproliferative disorders are methotrexate, infliximab, calcineurin inhibitors, and mycophenolate mofetil. Patients often present with B symptoms (fever, night sweats, anorexia, weight loss). This patient requires imaging tests to evaluate for the presence of lymphadenopathy or extranodal masses. If present, an excisional biopsy should be performed for histologic evaluation. If positive for lymphoma, the next step in management includes withdrawal/tapering of IST ± immunotherapy, chemotherapy, radiation, or a combination of the above.

6. **D. Cyclophosphamide, doxorubicin, vincristine, etoposide and prednisone (dose-adjusted EPOCH) plus antiretroviral therapy.** This patient has a primary effusion lymphoma (PEL). PEL is a rare and aggressive B-cell non-Hodgkin and is an AIDS-defining cancer. It is a lymphoma that usually presents with malignant effusions without tumor masses. HHV-8 virus is strongly associated with PEL. More than 70% of cases occur with concurrent Epstein–Barr virus (EBV) infection. It is associated with a poor prognosis. Although PEL is a B-cell NHL, in most cases these cells do not express CD20. In appropriate patients, optimal treatment consists of combination antiretroviral therapy and chemotherapy (dose-adjusted EPOCH) without rituximab since CD20-negative. G-CSF support is recommended for all patients.

T-Cell and NK-Cell Neoplasms

20

Jonathan Weiss and Ryan Wilcox

INTRODUCTION

Mature T-cell leukemias/lymphomas are a heterogeneous group of cutaneous and systemic diseases with the most common subtype being peripheral T-cell lymphomas (PTCL) and including breast implant-associated anaplastic large cell lymphoma (BIA-ALCL), T-cell large granular lymphocytic leukemia (TGL), adult T-cell leukemia/lymphoma (ATLL), T-cell prolymphocytic leukemia (TPLL), hepatosplenic T-cell (HSTCL), and extranodal NK/T-cell lymphomas, nasal type (ENKL).

Cutaneous T-cell lymphomas (CTCL) include mycosis fungoides and Sézary syndrome, as well as primary cutaneous CD30+ T-Cell lymphoproliferative disorder.

RISK FACTORS

1. **What are the risk factors and associations for various types of T-cell leukemias/lymphomas?**
   - Variable depending on the subtype
     - HSTCL: chronic immunosuppression
     - ATLL: human T-cell leukemia virus type 1 (HTLV-1) infection, most common in the Caribbean islands, southern Japan, and central Africa
     - Enteropathy-associated T-cell lymphoma (EATL): celiac disease
     - ENKL: Epstein–Barr virus (EBV) infection, most common in Asia
     - BIA-ALCL breast implants: lymphoma involving the fibrous capsule around the implant without invasion of the underlying breast tissue

Peripheral T-Cell Lymphoma

The following section outlines the diagnosis, pathology, prognosis, and treatment of the subtypes of PTCL.

1. **What are the subtypes of PTCL and how common are they?**
   - PTCLs are a heterogeneous group of diseases that account for <15% of all non-Hodgkin lymphomas (NHLs) in Western countries.
   - There are many PTCL subtypes and the following are the most common subtypes of nodal PTCL:
     - PTCL, not otherwise specified (NOS)
     - Nodal T-follicular helper cell lymphoma, angioimmunoblastic-type (nTFHL-AI)
     - Anaplastic large cell lymphoma (ALCL), ALK (±)
       - ALK(+) median age of onset 34 years
       - ALK(−) median age of onset 58 years
     - EATL (<5%)

2. **What are the signs and symptoms of patients with various subtypes of PTCL?**
   - Lymphadenopathy (LAD), cytopenias, elevated lactate dehydrogenase (LDH), and advanced-stage disease at presentation, with the following unique features:
     - PTCL-NOS: 50% with concurrent extranodal disease (liver, bone marrow, skin, and gastrointestinal [GI] tract)
     - nTFHL-AI: acute-onset LAD, B symptoms, organomegaly, also associated with eosinophilia, pruritic rash, autoimmune events (rheumatoid arthritis, thyroid disease, vasculitis), polyarthritis, effusions/ascites, polyclonal hypergammaglobulinemia, elevated erythrocyte sedimentation rate (ESR), hypoalbuminemia, and positive Coombs test

3. **How is PTCL staged?**
   - Most subtypes of PTCL are staged according to the Ann Arbor lymphoma staging system.

PATHOLOGY

1. **Are there common genetic mutations seen in nodal PTCL?**
   - ALK(−) ALCL: *DUSP22* (prevalence 30%, possibly favorable prognosis) and *TP63* (prevalence 8%, unfavorable prognosis) rearrangements have been described
   - ALK(+) ALCL: t(2;5), *ALK* rearranged with *NPM*
   - nTFHL-AI: *TET2*, *DNMT3A*, *RHOA*, and *IDH2*

2. **What are the lymph node histopathologic features of nodal PTCL?**
   - PTCL-NOS
     - Effacement of lymph nodes with cells of variable size; sheets of atypical lymphocytes in a paracortical or diffuse pattern; mixture of plasma cells and eosinophils; high mitotic rate; morphologically diverse
   - ALCL
     - Immunophenotypic markers: CD30+
     - Sinusoidal growth pattern (and may mimic metastatic carcinoma)
     - Classic variant: large blastic cells with prominent nucleoli and abundant cytoplasm
       - Hallmark cells: eccentric nuclei, eosinophilic paranuclear hof (Figure 20.1)
   - nTFHL-AI:
     - Partial or complete effacement of lymph nodes; neovascularization or arborizing endothelial venules; nTFHL-AI derived from follicular helper T-cells (explaining the B-cell and follicular dendritic cell expansion observed); typified by a mixture of plasma cells, B-cell immunoblasts, small lymphocytes, eosinophils, follicular dendritic cells, and medium-sized malignant cells with abundant cytoplasm
       - Usually requires excision lymph node biopsy to visualize the neovascularization in order to make the diagnosis

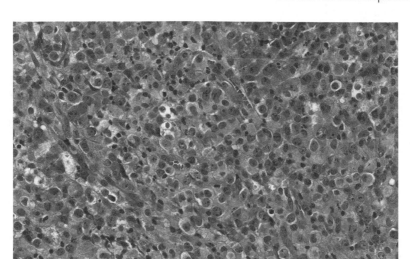

FIGURE 20.1 ■ Hallmark cells with eccentric nuclei and eosinophilic paranuclear hof as seen in anaplastic large cell lymphoma.

Source: Courtesy of Nathaneal Bailey, University of Pittsburgh Department of Pathology.

PROGNOSTIC FACTORS

1. How are patients with PTCL risk-stratified?
■ In general, the International Prognostic Index (IPI) is applicable to PTCL.
■ A similar Prognostic Index for T-Cell lymphoma (PIT) can also be used.

TABLE 20.1

IPI Prognostic Factors	PIT Prognostic Factors
Age >60	Age >60
LDH > ULN	LDH > ULN
ECOG PS ≥2	ECOG PS ≥2
Ann Arbor stage ≥3	Bone marrow involvement
Number of extranodal sites >2	

Note: The number of IPI factors determines the prognostic group: low = 0–1; low–intermediate = 2; high–intermediate = 3; high = 4–5.

ECOG PS, Eastern Cooperative Oncology Group performance status; IPI, International Prognostic Index; LDH, lactate dehydrogenase; PIT, Prognostic Index for T-Cell Lymphoma; ULN, upper limit of normal.

2. How does the prognosis of PTCL compare with aggressive B-cell NHL?
■ Stage-for-stage outcomes are inferior for patients with PTCL compared with those with aggressive B-cell NHL.

3. What is an additional important prognostic factor for ALCL?
■ The presence or absence of an ALK fusion protein significantly affects ALCL prognosis.
■ ALK(+) ALCL has a 5-year overall survival (OS) rate of 70%, while ALK(−) ALCL has a 5-year OS rate of 49%.

TREATMENT

Overall, the survival of patients with untreated PTCL is measured in months and treatment should be initiated once diagnosis is established. Goal is for cure but recognizing that 5-year OS for all comers with PTCL is 10% to 20% with progression-free survival (PFS) at 5 years of approximately 30%, with only a small subset of patients maintaining a durable remission. Treatment for the most common subtypes of PTCL including PTCL-NOS, nTFHL-AI, and ALCL ALK(±) are listed in the following:

1. **What is the first-line therapy for PTCL subtypes?**
   - ALCL
     - Multiagent, anthracycline-based therapy (brentuximab vedotin + Cyclophosphamide, Doxorubicin, Prednisone [CHP]) ± radiation therapy (RT); stage I to II disease: consider three to four cycles of chemotherapy followed by RT
   - PTCL-NOS, nTFHL-AI
     - Consider clinical trial participation
     - Multiagent chemotherapy (Cyclophosphamide, doxorubicin, vincristine, prednisone [CHOP] or Cyclophosphamide, doxorubicin, vincristine, etoposide, prednisone [CHOEP]) for six cycles; stage I to II disease: consider three to four cycles of chemotherapy followed by RT
     - If CD30+, brentuximab vedotin + CHP

2. **What is the role of consolidative autologous stem cell transplant (ASCT) after complete response with first-line therapy?**
   - Patients with ALK(+) ALCL do not typically receive consolidative treatment in first remission due to favorable 5-year OS with chemotherapy.
   - In contrast to DLBCL, most transplant-eligible patients with PTCL-NOS, ALK(−) ALCL, and nTFHL-AI achieving a complete remission with induction first-line therapy (CHOP or CHOEP) undergo consolidation with high-dose therapy and ASCT as this approach appears to be associated with improved PFS/OS.

3. **What is the second-line therapy for PTCL subtypes?**
   - No standard second-line treatment and clinical trials should be considered. Overall response rates in relapsed/refractory PTCL are ~20% to 50%; however, responses are not typically durable.
     - Single-agent regimens: brentuximab (overall response rate [ORR] ~85% in ALCL), belinostat, pralatrexate (limited activity in nTFHL-AI)
   - Consider stem cell transplantation.
     - High dose therapy (HDT)/ASCT can be considered for patients who did not undergo transplant in first complete remission.
     - Allogeneic stem cell transplantation can lead to durable responses in up to 60% of relapsed/refractory cases, but is associated with up to 30% rate of treatment-related mortality.
   - For older adult patients with nTFHL-AI unable to tolerate chemotherapy, consider corticosteroids or immunosuppressive therapy with cyclosporine.

Rare T-Cell Leukemias/Lymphomas

The following section describes the subtype, prognosis, diagnosis, symptoms, and treatment for the rare subtypes of T-cell leukemias/lymphomas plus primary CTCL.

TABLE 20.2 ■ T-Cell Leukemias/Lymphomas

Type/Prognosis	Diagnosis/Pathology	Symptoms	Treatment
T-cell prolymphocytic leukemia ■ Median age 65 years ■ Aggressive ■ Poor prognosis usually <1 year	Usually diagnosed from peripheral blood: ■ Small/medium prolymphocytes (mature postthymic T-cells) ■ IHC panel: TCL1	■ Generalized LAD, hepatosplenomegaly, serous effusion, and skin involvement ■ Lymphocyte count usually >100 ■ Anemia/thrombocytopenia ■ HTLV-1-negative	■ Alemtuzumab IV (anti-CD52) ■ Alemtuzumab + pentostatin ■ FMC* followed by alemtuzumab ■ If CR, alloSCT†
T-cell large granular lymphocytic leukemia ■ Age 45–75 years ■ Indolent ■ Median OS 10 years ■ STAT3 mutations with longer OS	Usually diagnosed from peripheral blood: ■ Mature cytotoxic lymphocytes T-cells ■ >6 months of LGL >2,000 ■ TCR oligo/monoclonal ■ TCRαβ/TIA/granzyme B+ ■ 30% STAT3 mutations SH2 domain (longer OS)	■ Involves peripheral blood, bone marrow, and spleen ■ Concurrent with autoimmune/rheum syndrome (Crohn's, Sjogren's, psoriatic arthritis, rheumatoid arthritis) ■ Indications to treat: ANC <0.5, Hgb <10, Plt <50, symptomatic splenomegaly/B symptoms	■ Low-dose MTX ± prednisone ■ Cyclophosphamide ± prednisone ■ Cyclosporine
Adult T-cell leukemia/lymphoma ■ Median age 58 years ■ Endemic in Japan, Caribbean, and Central Africa ■ Prognosis: smoldering-median overall survival (OS) 2.9 years. Chronic-median OS 5.3 years ■ Acute: OS <2 years acute, lymphoma <2 years	Diagnosis requires HTLV-1 antibodies ■ HTLV-1 P40 transcriptional activate gene within infected lymphocytes ■ Acute: leukemic phase with flower cell ■ CD2/CD3/CD5+ but CD7– ■ CD25+, CD30+/– Alk– ■ TCR receptor rearranged	■ Acute: leukemic phase, elevated WBC with eosinophilia, hyperCa++ ■ Lymphoma: generalized LAD, B symptoms, elevated LDH ■ Chronic/smoldering: exfoliating skin rash, normal WBC, no hyperCa++	■ Acute/lymphoma: Hyper-CVAD‡ DA-EPOCH§, BV+CHP (CD30+ only)‖ followed by alloSCT†, zidovudine + interferon (acute only) ■ Chronic/smoldering: observe, skin-directed therapy or zidovudine + interferon

* FMC (fludarabine, mitoxantrone, and cyclophosphamide).

† AlloSCT (allogeneic stem cell transplant).

‡ Hyper-CVAD (hyperfractionated cyclophosphamide, vincristine, doxorubicin, dexamethasone alternating with high-dose cytarabine and systemic methotrexate).

§ DA-EPOCH (dose-adjusted etoposide, vincristine, cyclophosphamide, doxorubicin, and prednisone).

‖ BV+CHP (brentuximab vedotin plus cyclophosphamide, doxorubicin, and prednisone).

ANC, absolute neutrophil count; CR, complete response; Hgb, hemoglobin; HTLV-1, human T-cell leukemia virus type 1; IV, intravenous; LAD, lymphadenopathy; LDH, lactate dehydrogenase; LGL, large granular lymphocytic leukemia; MTX, methotrexate; OS, overall survival; Plt, platelet; TCR, T-cell receptor; TIA, T-cell restricted intracellular antigen; WBC, white blood cell.

TABLE 20.3 ■ Rare Subtypes of T-Cell Lymphomas

Type/Prognosis	Diagnosis/Pathology	Symptoms	Treatment
Extranodal NK/T-Cell, Nasal Type ■ Poor prognosis 5-year OS 42%	Biopsy of mass: ■ Angiodestructive, CD3ε+ ■ Always EBER-ISH+ ■ 30% TCR rearranged	■ Mass of the paranasal sinus, nasopharynx, and GI involvement, skin ■ Nasal obstruction/epistaxis	■ Radiation + asparaginase cornerstone of therapy ■ Stage I/II nasal disease only: RT alone (if unfit for chemo), RT + cisplatin or RT + DeVIC‡ ■ Stage I–IV extranasal fit: mSMILE* + RT or "sandwich chemoradiation" (2 cycles P-GemOx†, followed by RT, followed by 2–4 cycles P-GemOx) ■ Consolidation autoSCT if extranasal/stage IV
Breast Implant-Associated ALCL ■ Women <50 years ■ Good prognosis: 3-year OS 94%	Diagnosed FNA of effusion or mass: ■ CD30+, Alk− ■ Somatic/germline mutation JAK1/STAT3	■ History of breast implants with ultrasound with effusion or mass	■ Total capsulectomy and excision by surgical oncology plus radiation for incomplete resection
Hepatosplenic T-cell Lymphoma ■ Aggressive median survival <2 years ■ 20% chronic immunosuppression	■ Medium lymphoid cells with sinusoidal infiltration ■ T-cell receptor γδ type ■ Isochrome 7q ■ Trisomy 8	■ Splenomegaly, hepatomegaly, bone marrow; lymph nodes NOT involved ■ Chronic immunosuppression: azathioprine or infliximab	■ ICE followed by alloSCT

*mSMILE. modified etoposide, asparaginase, ifosfamide, methotrexate, and dexamethasone

†P-GemOx (pegaspargase, gemcitabine, oxaliplatin).

‡RT + DeVIC (radiation therapy + dexamethasone, etoposide, ifosfamide, and carboplatin).

ALCL, anaplastic large cell lymphoma; alloSCT, allogeneic stem cell transplant; autoSCT, autologous stem cell transplant; EBER-ISH, Epstein-Barr virus in situ hybridization; FNA, fine needle aspiration; GI, gastrointestinal; ICE, ifosfamide, carobplatin, etoposide; mSMILE, modified smile; OS, overall survival; RT, radiation therapy; TCR, T-cell receptor.

TABLE 20.4 ■ Primary Cutaneous T-Cell Lymphoma

Type/Prognosis	Diagnosis/Pathology	Treatment
Mycosis fungoides ■ Indolent course ■ Can progress/ transform ■ Usually limited to skin **Sézary syndrome** ■ Erythroderma ■ Lymphadenopathy ■ Leukemic involvement (greater than 1,000 Sézary cells/mm³) ■ Mogamulizumab ■ Combination therapy: phototherapy + ECP	■ Pruritic patch/plaque with skin biopsy with aberrant T-cells in the upper dermis/ epidermis or Pautrier microabscesses ■ Peripheral blood smear with cerebriform (Sézary) cell 	**MF (limited to skin):** ■ Topical: corticosteroids, mechlorethamine, retinoids, imiquimod ■ Radiation: radiation to single lesion or total skin ■ Phototherapy UVB ■ ECP **Advanced-staged MF (tumors, nodules, or visceral involvement):** ■ Systemic: brentuximab (anti-CD30) ■ Bexarotene (systemic retinoid) ■ Vorinostat/ romidepsin (HDAC inhibitor) ■ Mogamulizumab (anti-CCR4). ■ Consider allotransplant
Primary cutaneous CD30+ T-Cell lymphoproliferative disorders	■ Punch biopsy of skin lesion with CD30+ T-cells	■ ISRT ■ Systemic: brentuximab

Note: Cutaneous T-cell lymphomas (CTCL) primarily present and can progress to involve lymph nodes, blood and visceral organs. CTCLs are treatable but not curable. Staging is based on percentage of body surface area (BSA) with T1 <10% and T4 >80%.

ECP, extracorporeal photopheresis; HDAC, histone deacetylase; ISRT, involved site radiation; MF, mycosis fungoides.

Source: Image courtesy of Nathaneal Bailey, University of Michigan Department of Pathology.

QUESTIONS

1. Which of the following peripheral T-cell lymphoma (PTCL) subtypes has the best prognosis?
   A. Nodal T-follicular helper cell lymphoma, angioimmunoblastic-type (nTFHL-AI)
   B. ALCL, ALK(+)
   C. Extranodal NK/T-cell lymphoma
   D. ALCL, ALK(−)

2. A 47-year-old Jamaican man presents with an elevated lymphocyte count and his peripheral blood shows some cells with hyperlobated nuclei appearing like clovers. Which pathogen is typically associated with this peripheral T-cell lymphoma (PTCL) subtype?
   A. *Helicobacter pylori*
   B. Epstein–Barr virus (EBV)
   C. HTLV-1
   D. Cytomegalovirus (CMV)

3. A 60-year-old man presents with years of pruritus with large, scattered pink/erythematous patches on his chest, back, upper arms, and thighs. Past biopsies have shown eczema and folliculitis and topical treatments have not resulted in improvement. Repeat biopsy shows mononu-clear cells with cerebriform nuclei in the upper dermis and epidermal keratinocytes with intraepidermal aggregates forming microabscess-like structures. What is the most likely diagnosis?
   A. Sézary syndrome
   B. Atopic dermatitis
   C. Psoriasis
   D. Mycosis fungoides
   E. Infection

4. A 68-year-old man develops joint pain and swelling, fatigue, short-ness of breath, night sweats, lower extremity erythematous rash, and enlarged neck lymph nodes. Labs show a white blood cell count of 10 K/mcL with an absolute lymphocyte count of 0.5 K/mcL, hemoglobin of 6.5 g/dL, platelet count of 130 K/mcL, total bilirubin of 4.5 mg/dL, and lactate dehydrogenase (LDH) >2 × the upper limit of normal. Chest x-ray shows bilateral pleural effusions. What is the most likely diagnosis?
   A. Nodal T-follicular helper cell lymphoma, angioimmunoblastic-type (nTFHL-AI)
   B. Mycosis fungoides
   C. Peripheral T-cell lymphoma, not otherwise specified (PTCL-NOS)
   D. Follicular lymphoma

5. A woman without a significant past medical history and only surgical history of bilateral breast implants presents with right-sided breast full-ness. In addition to a primary breast carcinoma, which of the following is in the differential diagnosis?

A. Nodal T-follicular helper cell lymphoma, angioimmunoblastic-type
B. Peripheral T-cell lymphoma, not otherwise specified (PTCL-NOS)
C. Metastatic disease
D. ALCL, ALK(–)

6. A 67-year-old male with no significant past medical history presents with worsening pruritus and new skin lesions. On exam, he has pink/erythematous patches on his left arm. Biopsy is consistent with mononuclear cells with cerebriform nuclei in the upper dermis and epidermal keratinocytes with intraepidermal aggregates forming microabscess-like structures. What is the best first-line treatment?
A. Brentuximab
B. Mogamulizumab
C. Topical corticosteroids or radiation
D. Vorinostat

7. A 62-year-old male with no significant past medical history presents with night sweats, weight loss, and diffuse lymphadenopathy. Axillary lymph node biopsy shows effaced architecture with solid, cohesive sheets of neoplastic cells with eccentric, horseshoe-shaped nuclei, CD30+, CD2+, CD3+, CD4+, CD43+, CD45+, ALK(–). What is the best first-line treatment?
A. Cyclophosphamide, doxorubicin, vincristine, prednisone (CHOP)
B. Mogamulizumab
C. Brentuximab vedotin + cyclophosphamide, doxorubicin, and prednisone (BV + CHP)
D. Vorinostat

8. A 55-year-old male presents with pruritus, skin lesions, and diffuse erythroderma. Peripheral blood evaluation shows greater than 1,000 Sézary cells/mm^3. He is started on mogamulizumab. Shortly after starting mogamulizumab, he appears to have new, erythematous skin lesions. What is the next best step?
A. Stop mogamulizumab due to disease progression.
B. Biopsy new skin lesion.
C. Continue mogamulizumab.
D. Apply topical corticosteroids and continue mogamulizumab.

9. A 65-year-old male with no significant past medical history presents with night sweats, weight loss, and diffuse lymphadenopathy. Axillary lymph node biopsy shows effaced architecture with solid, cohesive sheets of neoplastic cells with eccentric, horseshoe-shaped nuclei, CD30+, CD2+, CD3+, CD4+, CD43+, CD45+, ALK(–). Decision is made to start the patient on brentuximab vedotin + cyclophosphamide, doxorubicin, and prednisone (BV + CHP). What side effect is most common with brentuximab vedotin?
A. Drug eruption
B. Peripheral neuropathy
C. Hemorrhagic cystitis
D. Heart failure

10. A 60-year-old female without a significant past medical history and only surgical history of bilateral breast implants presents with right-sided breast fullness. Biopsy is taken and histologic examination is consistent with CD30+ anaplastic large cell lymphoma (ALCL) which is ALK(–). The patient undergoes capsular resection with complete resection. Which therapy should the patient receive following resection?

   A. Cyclophosphamide, doxorubicin, vincristine, prednisone (CHOP)
   B. Mogamulizumab
   C. Brentuximab vedotin + cyclophosphamide, doxorubicin, and prednisone (BV + CHP)
   D. Vorinostat
   E. Observation

ANSWERS

1. **B. ALCL, ALK(+).** ALK(+) anaplastic large cell lymphoma (ALCL) has the best overall prognosis of these PTCL subtypes with a 5-year overall survival rate of 70%. Note: The International Prognostic Index (IPI) risk group should also be taken into account and is still prognostic.

2. **C. HTLV-1.** This man most likely has adult T-cell leukemia/lymphoma (ATLL) given his heritage and peripheral blood features; this is associated with human T-cell leukemia virus type 1 (HTLV-1) infection.

3. **D. Mycosis fungoides.** The clinical history and pathology results with epidermotropism and the Pautrier microabscess formation are consistent with mycosis fungoides.

4. **A. Nodal T-follicular helper cell lymphoma, angioimmunoblastic-type (nTFHL-AI).** nTFHL-AI is the most likely diagnosis given the systemic symptoms of arthritis, effusions, B symptoms, and lymphadenopathy, as well as likely hemolytic anemia with an elevated bilirubin and LDH.

5. **D. ALCL, ALK(–).** ALK(–) anaplastic large cell lymphoma (ALCL) has been associated with breast implants. Implant removal and capsulectomy followed by observation are associated with favorable long-term disease-free survival for patients without an associated mass.

6. **C. Topical corticosteroids or radiation.** This patient likely has Mycosis Fungoides (MF). MF limited to the skin should be treated with topical therapies (corticosteroids, mechlorethamine, retinoids, imiquimod) or radiation therapy. The alternative agents listed would be reasonable for advanced-stage MF.

7. **C. Brentuximab vedotin + cyclophosphamide, doxorubicin, and prednisone (BV + CHP).** This patient likely has ALK(–) ALCL. Based on the ECHELON-2 trial, frontline treatment of patients with CD30+ peripheral T-cell lymphoma (PTCL) shows progression-free survival (PFS) and overall survival (OS) benefit with BV + CHP when compared with cyclophosphamide, doxorubicin, vincristine, prednisone (CHOP) therapy. Therefore, BV + CHP is the best first-line option.

8. **B. Biopsy new skin lesion.** Mogamulizumab has been associated with a drug eruption that mimics cutaneous T-cell lymphomas (CTCL). Therefore, lesion should be biopsied to distinguish progression of disease versus drug eruption.

9. **B. Peripheral neuropathy.** Peripheral neuropathy is a common side effect of brentuximab vedotin.

10. **E. Observation.** No additional therapy is needed for ALCL associated with breast implants following surgical removal. If there is incomplete resection, one can consider radiation therapy.

Hodgkin Lymphoma

Radhika Takiar and Yasmin H. Karimi

EPIDEMIOLOGY

1. **How common is Hodgkin lymphoma?**
   - Hodgkin lymphoma accounts for approximately 10% to 12% of all lymphomas in the United States (over 9,000 cases annually).

2. **How is Hodgkin lymphoma classified?**
   - Classic Hodgkin lymphoma (cHL) accounts for 95% of cases. Its histologic subtypes are the following:
     - Nodular sclerosis (70%)
     - Mixed cellularity (25%)
     - Lymphocyte-rich (5%)
     - Lymphocyte-depleted (<1%)
   - Nodular lymphocyte-predominant Hodgkin lymphoma (NLPHL) makes up 5% of "Hodgkin lymphoma" cases. It is immunophenotypically distinct from cHL in that it lacks CD15 and CD30 positivity.
     - It is characterized by an indolent course, late relapses, and is clinically managed like an indolent non-Hodgkin lymphoma (iNHL).

3. **What are the demographics of Hodgkin lymphoma?**
   - It has bimodal age distribution with the first peak around ages 15 to 30 and the second near ages 60 to 65.
   - In cHL there is a slight male predominance, whereas 75% of patients with NLPHL are male.

ETIOLOGY AND RISK FACTORS

1. **What are the risk factors for Hodgkin lymphoma?**
   - Immunosuppression (e.g., solid organ or hematopoietic stem cell transplants)
   - Autoimmune diseases (e.g., rheumatoid arthritis)
   - HIV/AIDS associated with Epstein–Barr virus (EBV)-positive, lymphocyte-depleted subtype
   - Increased incidence in patients with affected family members, but no known genetic predisposition

STAGING

1. Define the staging for Hodgkin lymphoma.

TABLE 21.1 ■ Ann Arbor Staging System

Stage	Description
I	Involvement of single lymph node region or structure (e.g., spleen, thymus, Waldeyer's ring) or a single extranodal site (IE)
II	Involvement of two or more lymph nodes or lymphoid structures on the same side of the diaphragm
III	Involvement of lymph nodes or lymphoid structures on both sides of the diaphragm
IV	Diffuse or disseminated involvement of one or more extranodal organs beyond IE* including any liver or bone marrow involvement, with or without associated lymph node involvement

*Contiguous extranodal extension indicated by "E."

Note: B symptoms (significant unexplained fever, night sweats, or unexplained weight loss exceeding 10% of body weight during the 6 months prior to diagnosis) indicated by "A" (absence) or "B" (presence); bulky disease (mediastinal mass more than one-third the diameter of the thorax or a nodal mass >10 cm) indicated by "X."

SIGNS AND SYMPTOMS

1. What are the common signs and symptoms of Hodgkin lymphoma?

- Most patients present with asymptomatic lymphadenopathy or an incidentally discovered mediastinal mass. Those with a mediastinal mass may present with symptoms of superior vena cava (SVC) syndrome including facial/neck swelling, chest pain, dyspnea, cyanosis, or neurologic symptoms.
- B symptoms include the following:
  - Fever (unexplained, persistent/recurring temperature >38°C)
  - Drenching night sweats
  - Weight loss (>10% over the preceding 6 months), seen in 20% of early- and 50% of advanced-stage disease

2. What is the pattern of disease involvement in Hodgkin lymphoma?

- Cervical nodes are most commonly affected, followed by mediastinal nodes.
  - Spread is generally in a linear fashion to adjacent lymph nodes.
  - Bone marrow involvement is observed in fewer than 5% of cases.

DIAGNOSTIC CRITERIA

1. What is the optimal approach to the diagnosis of Hodgkin lymphoma?

- Excisional lymph node biopsy or core biopsy. Tumor cells in Hodgkin lymphoma are a very small component of malignant cells, with a surrounding reactive milieu of lymphocytes, eosinophils, and fibrosis (sclerosis). Excisional lymph node biopsy is far better at documenting this architecture than core biopsy or fine needle aspiration (FNA). Core biopsy is often necessary due to the location of disease in the mediastinum that is not amenable to excisional biopsy and in these cases several cores are obtained to improve diagnostic yield.

- Clinical staging is done using CT and PET/CT scans, although PET/CT has better accuracy of staging.
- Bone marrow biopsy is no longer required for staging if PET/CT is consistent with marrow involvement. Lack of focal uptake on PET/CT scan is highly sensitive for bone marrow involvement, and in the setting of a negative PET/CT scan bone marrow biopsy results will not change management.

2. How is the diagnosis of cHL made?

- Presence of multinucleate Reed–Sternberg (RS) cells in an appropriate inflammatory background (see Figure 21.1)

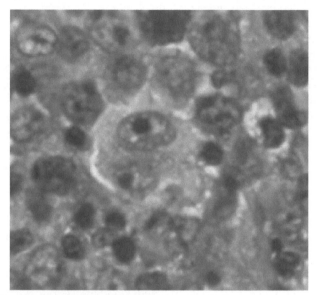

FIGURE 21.1 ■ Reed–Sternberg cell surrounded by inflammatory infiltrate.

- Typical immunophenotype of cHL is CD15- and CD30-positive with absence of the usual B-cell markers CD20 and CD79a, and the common leukocyte antigen CD45.

3. What are the characteristics of PD-L1/PD-L2 expression in Hodgkin lymphoma?

- RS cells typically show overexpression of PD-L1 and PD-L2 on the cell surface, which may contribute to the ineffective but exuberant inflammatory cell background that characterizes the disease.
- Amplification of the 9p24.1 gene locus may lead to increased PD-L1 and PD-L2 expression, as well as increased JAK2 signaling.
- This overexpression of PD-L1 in Hodgkin lymphoma is an attractive target in checkpoint inhibitor therapies noted below.
- PD-L1/PD-L2 expression, while often seen, is not diagnostic of cHL.

4. How is NLPHL diagnosed?

- Presence of lymphocytic and histiocytic cells with "popcorn" appearance, which are cells with multilobulated, vesicular nuclei with prominent nucleoli
  - Typical immunophenotype is CD15 and CD30 negative with positivity for B-cell markers: CD20 and CD79a, and the common leukocyte antigen CD45.

5. **What is the cell of origin of cHL?**
   - Despite their unique immunophenotype, cHL cells have been shown to derive from germinal center B-cells.

INDICATIONS FOR TREATMENT

1. **Who requires treatment for Hodgkin lymphoma?**
   - All patients with cHL are initiated on treatment at the time of diagnosis with curative intent.
     - In contrast, all patients with NLPHL may not require therapy and treatment is determined by stage and symptoms as follows:
       - Radiation with curative intent may be considered for nonbulky stage IA or contiguous stage IIA disease.
       - Immunochemotherapy: For example, R-CHOP (rituximab, cyclophosphamide, doxorubicin, vincristine, and prednisone) or R-ABVD (doxorubicin, bleomycin, vinblastine, and dacarbazine) is considered for certain patients with bulky limited-stage or advanced-stage disease.
       - Observation alone may be considered for some patients, for example patients with completely surgically removed stage IA disease or those with asymptomatic stage III to IV disease.

PROGNOSTIC FACTORS

Treatment for patients with cHL is based on stage and risk assessment. In early-stage disease, risk is broken down into favorable and unfavorable risk stage I to II disease. In advanced stage or stage III or IV disease, the International Prognostication Factor is used.

1. **What are unfavorable factors in early-stage (I–IIA) cHL?**
   - There are multiple different criteria for defining risk in early-stage disease; the two most commonly used are the German Hodgkin's Study Group (GHSG) criteria and the European Organisation for Research and Treatment of Cancer (EORTC) criteria.
   - EORTC defines unfavorable as patients with ≥1 of the following features:
     - Large mediastinal mass (greater than one-third of the mediastinal diameter)
     - Erythrocyte sedimentation rate (ESR) ≥50 mm/hour without or ≥30 mm/hour with B symptoms
     - Involvement of >3 nodal sites
     - Age >50 at diagnosis
   - GHSG defines unfavorable as patients with ≥1 of the following features:
     - Similar to EORTC, although does not incorporate age and defines unfavorable risk as >2 nodal sites involved

2. **What are unfavorable prognostic factors in advanced-stage (IIB–IV) cHL? How does this International Prognostic Factor score impact outcome?**
   - Age >45 years, 1 point
   - Male gender, 1 point
   - Stage IV disease, 1 point
   - Albumin <4 g/dL, 1 point
   - Hemoglobin <10.5 g/dL, 1 point
   - White blood cell count >15,000/mm³, 1 point
   - Lymphopenia with absolute lymphocyte count <600 lymphocytes K/microL, 1 point

TABLE 21.2 ■ Freedom From Progression and Overall Survival as Predicted by the International Prognostic Factor Score

Score	5-Year FFP (%)	5-Year OS (%)
0	84	89
1	77	90
2	67	81
3	60	78
4	51	61
5–7	42	56

FFP, freedom from progression; OS, overall survival.

3. **What are other poor prognostic factors for Hodgkin lymphoma?**
   - In addition to risk stratification above, the following are indicative of higher risk for relapse after treatment of cHL:
     - Positive PET scan after two cycles of ABVD (doxorubicin, bleomycin, vinblastine, and dacarbazine) is strongly associated with inferior 2-year progression-free survival (PFS)
     - Increased density of lymphoma-associated macrophages (CD68-positive cells)
     - Increased metabolic tumor volume on pretreatment PET/CT scan

4. **What is the prognosis for Hodgkin lymphoma?**
   - Cure is obtained in over 80% of all patients.
     - Five-year survival is >90% in early and >75% in advanced-stage disease.

TREATMENT

1. **What is the initial treatment for early-stage (I–IIA) cHL?**
   - Standard of care treatment for early-stage cHL is combined modality therapy with radiation and chemotherapy based on stage and risk factors.
   - In limited-stage, favorable-risk disease, a standard approach is combined modality therapy with two cycles of ABVD with restaging PET/CT followed by 20 Gy of involved site radiation therapy (ISRT), based on the results from the HD-10 trial.
   - Limited-stage, unfavorable-risk disease may be treated with four cycles of ABVD followed by 30 Gy of ISRT based on the GHSG HD-11 trial. An alternative approach, sparing radiation therapy and its potential risks, is six cycles of ABVD alone, in a risk-adapted fashion (if interim PET after two cycles of ABVD is negative; Deauville score [DS] 1–3 per EORTC H10 trial).
   - The Stanford V regimen (doxorubicin, vinblastine, mechlorethamine, etoposide, vincristine, bleomycin, and prednisone) is an alternative to ABVD, although is rarely used due to toxicities and lack of data showing superiority to ABVD.
   - For patients with contraindications to radiation or preference to avoid radiation, studies have evaluated chemotherapy alone options. One such option is ABVD for three cycles followed by interim PET, and if negative (DS 1–2) then no further therapy, based on the RAPID trial. Another option for early-stage disease with B symptoms or extranodal disease is ABVD for two cycles followed by interim PET, and if PET is negative (DS 1–3) then an additional two cycles of ABVD, based on CALGB 50604 trial.

2. **How is advanced-stage (IIB–IV) cHL managed?**
   - One option is ABVD for six cycles with a PET-adapted approach based on the RATHL trial. Patients are given two cycles of ABVD followed by interim PET scan. Those who are PET-negative (DS 1–3) can proceed with AVD (bleomycin omitted) for an additional four cycles. Those who are PET-positive may need to proceed with escalated BEACOPP (bleomycin, etoposide, Adriamycin, cyclophosphamide, vincristine, procarbazine, and prednisone). Outcome appears to be optimized if treatment delays and dose reductions are avoided.
   - To avoid bleomycin, another potential frontline treatment is the A-AVD (brentuximab-vedotin, Adriamycin, vinblastine, and dacarbazine), which was approved based on the results from the ECHELON-1 trial. This was a non–PET-adapted approach that randomized untreated advanced-stage cHL patients to six cycles of ABVD versus A-AVD. The 5-year update demonstrated improvement in PFS with A-AVD compared with ABVD, and more recently presented data showed an overall survival (OS) benefit with A-AVD compared with ABVD (HR 0.59, 95% CI 0.40–0.88, p = .009). Based on these results, A-AVD has become the new standard of care for frontline treatment of advanced-stage cHL.
   - In select patients with high-risk disease (international prognostic score [IPS] ≥4, age <60), an alternative, more intense initial treatment option is escalated BEACOPP (BEACOPPesc; bleomycin, etoposide, Adriamycin [doxorubicin], cyclophosphamide, Oncovin [vincristine], procarbazine, and prednisone). This regimen was studied in the AHL2011 trial where patients received either standard BEACOPPesc for six cycles or a PET-adapted approach with BEACOPPesc for two cycles followed by interim PET. Those who were PET-positive continued BEACOPPesc for four cycles, while those who were PET-negative (DS 1–3) were switched to ABVD for four cycles. A PET-adapted approach has similar PFS to the standard approach, although there was a higher incidence of cytopenias, infections, and risk of secondary hematologic malignancies among the standard treatment arm.
   - Although Stanford V is listed in the National Comprehensive Cancer Network (NCCN) guidelines, this is not frequently utilized in clinical practice due to high rates of both short- and long-term toxicities.
   - Consolidative radiation therapy is an option for patients with residual PET-avid disease on end-of-treatment scans.

RESPONSE-ADAPTED THERAPY

1. **What role does interim PET/CT play in prognosis?**
   - The sensitivity of PET/CT has greatly impacted treatment strategy in Hodgkin lymphoma, with early PET/CT after two cycles of chemotherapy a better predictor of PFS and OS compared with traditional clinical prognostic factors including the IPS.

2. **How are PET/CT findings interpreted?**
   - Fluorodeoxyglucose (FDG) uptake avidity in PET scans for lymphoma tumor masses are scored per the Deauville scoring system:
     - Score 1: no residual uptake above background
     - Score 2: residual uptake less than or equal to the mediastinal blood pool
     - Score 3: residual uptake greater than the mediastinal blood pool but less than or equal to the liver

- Score 4: residual uptake moderately increased compared with the liver
- Score 5: residual uptake markedly increased compared with the liver or new sites of disease
■ Typically, a score of 1 to 3 is considered negative for disease, while scores of 4 and 5 are considered positive. Each trial defines PET negativity slightly differently and should be carefully evaluated when interpreting results. Deauville 4 is often challenging to interpret due to heterogeneity in the degree of change compared with prior scans.

3. **How do early PET/CT results impact treatment course?**
■ A negative PET/CT after two cycles of chemotherapy may allow for an abbreviated number of cycles in early-stage disease and/or omission of bleomycin from ABVD in subsequent cycles, thus sparing potential pulmonary toxicity. Patients receiving ABVD with an interim PET/CT positive for disease may be switched to a more aggressive regimen, such as BEACOPPesc.

SURVIVORSHIP

1. **What is the follow-up required after complete response is obtained with frontline treatment?**
■ After completion of therapy, all patients undergo repeat end-of-treatment imaging to confirm that they are in remission. After this scan, patients are followed clinically with follow-up visits including history and physical examination approximately every 3 to 6 months for 1 to 2 years, then 6 to 12 months for year 3 and annually thereafter.
■ There are no robust data showing improvement in clinical outcomes with routine surveillance imaging and therefore surveillance imaging is often reserved for patients with clinical symptoms and physical exam or labs concerning for relapse.

RELAPSED/REFRACTORY DISEASE

1. **How common is disease relapse in Hodgkin lymphoma?**
■ 10% to 30% of patients achieving an initial complete remission will subsequently relapse, with the rate of relapse being higher among advanced-stage disease (~30%) and lower if early-stage disease (5%–10%).

2. **How is relapsed Hodgkin lymphoma treated?**
■ This is a landscape that is constantly evolving with the introduction of novel agents such as BV (brentuximab vedotin) and immunotherapy into the relapsed setting.
■ Among transplant-eligible patients with late relapses (>12 months), the standard approach would be salvage chemotherapy (platinum- or gemcitabine-based regimens) followed by high-dose chemotherapy and autologous stem cell transplant (ASCT). Salvage chemotherapy followed by ASCT cures around 50% of patients with relapsed cHL.
■ Transplant-eligible patients who relapse earlier (within 12 months) are more likely to have chemorefractory disease and therefore may be better suited for novel agents. Various treatment options exist and should be individualized to patients based on their functional status, underlying comorbidities, and preference.

Options include brentuximab vedotin, pembrolizumab, and nivolumab, either single agent or in combination with chemotherapy or other novel agents.

■ Options for transplant-ineligible patients would be single-agent pembrolizumab (based on KEYNOTE-087) or BV-bendamustine.

3. **What is the role of maintenance therapy following ASCT in Hodgkin lymphoma?**

■ Brentuximab vedotin has been approved as a post-ASCT therapy for patients at high risk of relapse based on the AETHERA trial. High risk of relapse was defined as primary refractory disease, relapse <12 months after frontline therapy, or extranodal relapse. Use of BV maintenance has shown a 5-year PFS benefit among patients with at least two of the high-risk features but has not yet demonstrated an OS advantage. The role of maintenance BV will become unclear as BV is incorporated into frontline therapy based on the ECHELON-1 trial. Current trials are also exploring use of checkpoint inhibitors as consolidation therapy following ASCT.

4. **How is relapse treated following ASCT?**

■ Patients who relapse or progress following salvage chemotherapy or ASCT can be considered for therapy with the following:
  ● Brentuximab-based regimens
  ● Checkpoint inhibitor-based regimens (pembrolizumab or nivolumab)
■ Those achieving a response could be candidates for allogeneic stem cell transplant, although this comes with high rates of graft versus host disease (GVHD).
■ Relapse following multiple lines of therapy may need to be managed with the following:
  ● Clinical trials
  ● Single-agent therapy: lenalidomide, HDAC inhibitor, mTOR inhibitor
  ● Radiation therapy for localized relapses

5. **What is primary progressive/refractory disease?**

■ Primary progressive or refractory Hodgkin lymphoma is defined as disease that progresses or does not respond during initial therapy, or that progresses within 90 days of completing this therapy.
■ Outcomes in these patients have traditionally been very poor with standard chemotherapy approaches as these patients tend to be chemorefractory. The introduction of novel agents for such patients has the potential to improve outcomes on such patients.

NOVEL THERAPIES

1. **What is brentuximab vedotin? What are its usual toxicities?**

■ Brentuximab vedotin is an anti-CD30 monoclonal antibody conjugated to a mitotic spindle inhibitor.
■ Its use has been approved as post-ASCT consolidation therapy for patients at high risk for relapse, and either as single agent or in combination with chemotherapy/immunotherapy for relapsed disease pre-ASCT.
■ Brentuximab is approved for frontline use in stage III/IV Hodgkin lymphoma in combination with traditional chemotherapy (e.g., AVD). Brentuximab should **NOT** be used concurrently with bleomycin due to increased risk for pulmonary toxicity.

- Its main toxicity as a single agent is peripheral neuropathy, although this is often reversible upon discontinuation.
- Cytopenias can also be seen with BV and therefore it is usually given with prophylactic growth factor to minimize risk of infections and complications.

2. **What is the role of checkpoint inhibitor therapy in Hodgkin lymphoma?**
   - Given overexpression of PD-L1/PD-L2 by RS cells, checkpoint inhibitor therapy has proven an attractive treatment option in Hodgkin lymphoma. Anti-PD-1 therapies (e.g., pembrolizumab, nivolumab) have shown efficacy in relapsed disease and are currently being investigated in earlier therapy, including as frontline agents and in combination with brentuximab for relapsed/refractory disease.

SPECIAL CONSIDERATIONS

1. **What are the significant toxicities from treatment?**
   - Pulmonary toxicity (pneumonitis) from bleomycin. PET-adapted approaches have allowed for omission of bleomycin from subsequent cycles of ABVD without compromising efficacy. Bleomycin toxicity is also more common in older adults, particularly with more than two cycles of treatment.
     - Myelosuppression with ABVD. Less than 10% of patients develop febrile neutropenia. It is important (and safe) to maintain dose intensity through neutropenia.
     - Infertility is much more common with BEACOPP regimen compared with ABVD.
     - Cardiac dysfunction results from radiation (e.g., pericarditis, coronary artery disease, and valvular disease) or chemotherapy (e.g., heart failure due to anthracyclines).
     - Secondary malignancies (e.g., breast cancer in females who have received thoracic radiation). Therapy-related myelodysplastic syndrome (MDS) and acute myeloid leukemia (AML) are less common in patients receiving ABVD than in patients who received MOPP (mechlorethamine/vincristine/procarbazine/prednisone) or BEACOPP regimens.

2. **How is disease managed in the older adult?**
   - Given significant risk of therapy-related toxicity from traditional chemotherapy regimens, treatment of older adult patients with Hodgkin lymphoma has begun to focus more heavily on use of brentuximab with regimens such as sequential BV-AVD.

3. **How is NLPHL managed?**
   - Radiation therapy alone for stages IA and IIA
     - Chemotherapy ± radiation for stages IB and IIB or observation for asymptomatic disease
     - Observation may be appropriate for asymptomatic patients with advanced-stage disease that is nonbulky, asymptomatic, and slowly progressive
     - Chemoimmunotherapy (e.g., R-CHOP or R-ABVD) for symptomatic advanced disease

QUESTIONS

1. A 25-year-old female diagnosed with stage IIIA classic Hodgkin lymphoma (cHL) has completed two cycles of treatment with Adriamycin, bleomycin, vinblastine, and dacarbazine (ABVD). An interim PET/CT is performed, with Deauville response score of 2. What is the most appropriate next step in therapy?
   A. No further treatment is recommended.
   B. Continue treatment with four additional cycles of ABVD.
   C. Continue treatment with four cycles of AVD, omitting further bleomycin.
   D. Escalate subsequent treatment to BEACOPP.

2. An otherwise healthy 45-year-old male completed six cycles of Adriamycin, bleomycin, vinblastine, and dacarbazine (ABVD) for stage IV classic Hodgkin lymphoma (cHL). Five years following completion of treatment, he noticed an enlarging cervical lymph node. Biopsy was performed, which confirmed relapse. PET/CT shows diffuse disease. Which of the following is the most appropriate next step in management?
   A. Initiate bleomycin, etoposide, Adriamycin, cyclophosphamide, vincristine (Oncovin), procarbazine, prednisone (BEACOPPesc).
   B. Initiate brentuximab-based regimen.
   C. Initiate salvage chemotherapy with ifosfamide/carboplatin/etoposide (ICE) and plan for autologous stem cell transplant (ASCT).
   D. Proceed to nonmyeloablative allogeneic stem cell transplant.

3. An 81-year-old male is diagnosed with stage IVA classic Hodgkin lymphoma (cHL). He has an Eastern Cooperative Oncology Group (ECOG) performance status of 2. He wishes to pursue therapy for his lymphoma if possible but is concerned with quality of life in the setting of his comorbidities and current frailty. He has a history of hypertension, type 2 diabetes mellitus, and coronary artery disease. Which of the following would be the most reasonable treatment recommendation?
   A. No lymphoma-directed therapy should be offered; patient may be referred to hospice
   B. ABVD for six cycles
   C. BEACOPP for six cycles
   D. Treatment with combination of brentuximab vedotin and AVD

4. A 24-year-old female was diagnosed with stage IIIB classic Hodgkin lymphoma (cHL) with a bulky mediastinal mass. Her treatment comprised six cycles of Adriamycin, bleomycin, vinblastine, and dacarbazine (ABVD) and radiation to the mediastinum. She completed treatment 4 years ago. Long-term surveillance does NOT include which of the following?
   A. Breast MRI or early mammogram
   B. Thyroid function testing
   C. Yearly history and physical exam
   D. Annual PET scan

5. A 20-year-old male diagnosed with stage IVB classic Hodgkin lymphoma (cHL) completed six cycles of ABVD. Six months following completion of treatment, he experiences a biopsy-confirmed relapse of disease. Repeat PET/CT shows involvement of multiple lymph node regions, bone, and liver. What would be the most appropriate next-line therapy?
   A. Salvage chemotherapy followed by autologous stem cell transplant
   B. Workup for allogeneic stem cell transplant
   C. Initiation of pembrolizumab or BV-based regimen
   D. Radiation

6. A 75-year-old male noticed an enlarged lymph node in his neck while shaving. Further imaging revealed right cervical chain lymphadenopathy with no other evidence of disease. Excisional biopsy of a cervical chain lymph node showed popcorn cells that were CD30- and CD15-negative but positive for CD20 and CD79a on immunohistochemistry. He is asymptomatic. The patient has an Eastern Cooperative Oncology Group (ECOG) performance status of 1 to 2. Which of the following would be a reasonable treatment strategy?
   A. Radiation alone
   B. Single-agent rituximab with radiation
   C. Rituximab, cyclophosphamide, doxorubicin, vincristine, and prednisone (R-CHOP)
   D. Rituximab, doxorubicin, bleomycin, vinblastine, and dacarbazine (R-ABVD)

ANSWERS

1. **C. Continue treatment with four cycles of AVD, omitting further bleomycin.** A Deauville score of 2 is considered negative and a good prognostic indicator following initial two cycles of ABVD; however, further therapy is required. As per the RATHL trial (Response-Adapted Therapy for Advanced Hodgkin Lymphoma), bleomycin may be omitted from further cycles of treatment.

2. **C. Initiate salvage chemotherapy with ifosfamide/carboplatin/etoposide (ICE) and plan for autologous stem cell transplant (ASCT).** Standard initial treatment for late relapsed cHL is salvage chemotherapy (such as ICE) followed by ASCT. Re-treating with a combination chemotherapy regimen without ASCT would not be indicated. Brentuximab- based regimens may be better for an early relapse and allogeneic stem cell transplant could be considered in patients relapsing following ASCT.

3. **D. Treatment with combination of brentuximab vedotin and AVD.** The regimen of sequential BV-AVD has been well-studied as upfront therapy for older adult patients with cHL. It is well-tolerated with good response rates and outcomes. Other chemotherapy regimens such as ABVD or BEACOPP have higher toxicities for older adult patients.

4. **D. Annual PET scan.** Because of its high cure rates, long-term follow-up for cHL requires monitoring of a number of possible late complications. Women who received radiation therapy to the chest are at higher risk of developing (often bilateral) breast cancer and require close monitoring with breast MRI or early mammogram. Thyroid function should be monitored as the gland may be affected by mediastinal radiation. After completion of treatment, the National Comprehensive Cancer Network (NCCN) guidelines recommend that a history and physical should be performed every 3 to 6 months for the first 1 to 2 years, then every 6 to 12 months until year 3, and then yearly. Surveillance with PET scan is **NOT** indicated in the absence of clinical concern for relapse.

5. **C. Initiation of pembrolizumab or BV-based regimen.** Given the short time between treatment and relapse, the recommendation would be for a nonchemotherapy-based approach due to concerns for chemorefractory disease. Brentuximab vedotin- and pembrolizumab-based regimens have been approved for use in patients with early relapses. Due to widespread disease, radiation would not be appropriate. Salvage chemotherapy followed by autologous stem cell transplant or allogeneic stem cell transplantation are likely to be less effective given relapse in <12 months.

6. **A. Radiation alone.** The diagnosis in this case is nodular lymphocyte-predominant Hodgkin lymphoma (NLPHL), which typically follows an indolent course. Given its distinct clinical course and immunophenotype, the decision to treat should be approached in a way similar to the indolent non-Hodgkin lymphomas. Given localized stage IA disease, radiation alone would be appropriate. Since he is otherwise asymptomatic without bulky disease, there is no need to add rituximab to radiation or treat with other chemoimmunotherapy regimens.

Other Neoplasms (Histiocytic and Dendritic Cell Neoplasms, Myeloid and Lymphoid Neoplasms With Eosinophilia)

22

James Yoon, Darren King, and Patrick Burke

HISTIOCYTIC DISORDERS

1. **What is a histiocyte?**
   - Histiocyte is a somewhat archaic term used to describe tissue macrophages derived from monocytes. Histiocytic disorders may be benign or malignant, and span a broad range of clinical presentations and pathobiology.

2. **How are histiocytic disorders classified?**
   - The Histiocyte Society classifies histiocytic disorders into five groups, shown in Table 22.1:

TABLE 22.1 ■ Classification of Histiocyte Disorders

Histiocytosis Group	Diseases
"L" group (Langerhans)	■ LCH ■ ICH ■ ECD ■ Mixed LCH/ECD
"C" group (cutaneous/ mucocutaneous)	■ XG family: JXG, AXG, SRH, BCH, GEH, PNH ■ Non-XG family: cutaneous RDD ■ Cutaneous non-LCH with a major systemic component
"R" group (Rosai–Dorfman)	■ Familial RDD ■ Sporadic Rosai–Dorfman disease
"M" group (malignant histiocytoses)	■ Primary malignant histiocytoses ■ Secondary malignant histiocytoses associated with another hematologic neoplasm
"H" group (hemophagocytic lymphohistiocytosis)	■ Primary (inherited) HLH ■ Secondary HLH ■ HLH of unknown origin

AXG, adult xanthogranuloma; BCH, benign cephalic histiocytosis; ECD, Erdheim–Chester disease; GEH, generalized eruptive histiocytosis; HLH, hemophagocytic lymphohistiocytosis; ICH, indeterminate cell histiocytosis; JXG, juvenile xanthogranuloma; LCH, Langerhans cell histiocytosis; PNH, progressive nodular histiocytosis; RDD, Rosai–Dorfman disease; SRH, solitary reticulohistiocytoma; XG, xanthogranuloma.

Source: From Emile J. F. et al. Revised classification of histiocytoses and neoplasms of the macrophage-dendritic cell lineages. *Blood* 2016 127:2672–2681.

3. **What is a Langerhans cell?**
   - Langerhans cells are a subset of dendritic cells localized to the skin and other epithelial mucosa. They are antigen-presenting cells and are morphologically characterized by the presence of "tennis-racket"-shaped Birbeck granules. They proliferate in response to inflammation.

4. **What is Langerhans cell histiocytosis (LCH)?**
   - LCH is a spectrum of disorders ranging from localized, self-resolving lesions to highly morbid/fatal disseminated disease. The disease is characterized by the clonal proliferation and accumulation of a cell population morphologically resembling Langerhans cells (including presence of Birbeck granules); however, LCH is **not** thought to derive from normal Langerhans cell populations. Rather, the immunophenotype of LCH resembles immature myeloid dendritic cells (i.e., CD207-positive).

5. **What is the epidemiology of LCH?**
   - LCH is a rare disease, with case series and epidemiologic studies suggesting a childhood incidence of up to five cases per million and an adult incidence of approximately one to two cases per million. Pulmonary LCH is strongly associated with smoking.

6. **What are the clinical features of LCH?**
   - LCH typically presents as single or multiple lytic bone lesions, with proliferating histiocytes (and reactive lymphocytes, eosinophils, and macrophages) which can infiltrate any organ, including the central nervous system (CNS). Approximately 55% of patients present with disease limited to a single organ (or bone), with the remainder showing multisystem involvement.

TABLE 22.2 ■ LCH Sites of Disease

LCH Organ Site	Clinical Features
Bone	■ Lytic lesions ■ Base of skull lesions may lead to cranial nerve palsies, exophthalmos, or diabetes insipidus
Skin	■ Brown/purple papules ■ Eczematous rash ■ Oral lesions/ulcers/gingivitis
Lymph nodes (approximately 20% of patients)	■ Lymphadenopathy
Bone marrow	■ Cytopenias
liver/spleen	■ Organomegaly ■ Hypersplenism ■ LFT abnormalities
CNS	■ Central diabetes insipidus (posterior pituitary infiltration) ■ Neurodegeneration (ataxia, cognitive decline)

(*continued*)

TABLE 22.2 ■ LCH Sites of Disease (*continued*)

LCH Organ Site	Clinical Features
Gastrointestinal tract	■ Diarrhea
	■ Malabsorption
Lung	■ Dyspnea
	■ Abnormalities
	■ Spontaneous pneumothorax

CNS, central nervous system; LCH, Langerhans cell histiocytosis; LFT, liver function test.

7. **What are "risk organs" in LCH?**
   - ■ High-risk LCH involves the liver, spleen, and bone marrow, and is associated with a high risk of death.

8. **What endocrinopathies may be seen in patients with LCH?**
   - ■ The most common endocrinopathy associated with LCH is central diabetes insipidus (DI) due to infiltration of the posterior pituitary gland. Other endocrinopathies include growth hormone deficiency, hypothyroidism, and hypogonadism.

9. **What other names is LCH known by?**
   - ■ The following disease names are considered archaic and now part of LCH: Hand–Schüller–Christian disease (exophthalmos, DI, and skull lesions), histiocytosis X, Letterer–Siwe disease (lymphadenopathy, rash, hepatosplenomegaly, fever, anemia, and thrombocytopenia), and eosinophilic granuloma of the bone.

10. **How is LCH diagnosed?**
    - ■ Biopsy of a suspected lesion (preferably skin or bone) should show presence of cells positive for CD1a, S-100, and CD207, and/or presence of Birbeck granules.

11. **What is the risk stratification of LCH?**
    - ■ LCH is risk-stratified based on single-organ versus multiorgan involvement, and presence of disease in "risk organs."
      - ● Single-system LCH: unifocal or multifocal disease within a single organ/ system, no involvement of "risk organs"
      - ● Multisystem LCH: disease presence in two or more organ systems or involvement of "risk organs"

12. **How is LCH treated?**
    - ■ LCH treatment depends on the extent and severity of disease. LCH limited to the bone may be treated by local resection/curettage with or without steroid therapy, external beam radiation therapy, bisphosphonates, or chemotherapy. LCH of the skin may be treated by resection, steroids, UVB radiation therapy/ photodynamic therapy, or chemotherapy. Multisystem disease in children is typically treated with a combination of vinblastine and prednisone. In adults, this combination is less tolerated, and single-gent cytarabine or cladribine is often considered. Patients whose disease fails to respond to treatment within 6 weeks have a poor prognosis. End-organ damage (e.g., lung, liver) may warrant solid organ transplant if systemic disease is otherwise well-controlled. Allogeneic hematopoietic cell transplant may be curative; however, its role in

LCH has not yet been firmly established. Participation in clinical trials, especially for multisystem or relapsed/refractory disease, is encouraged.

13. **What other diseases make up the "L" (Langerhans-like) category of histiocytoses?**
   - In addition to LCH, the "L" group of histiocytoses includes indeterminate cell histiocytosis (ICH) and Erdheim–Chester disease (ECD).
     - ICH resembles LCH both clinically and morphologically; however, the clonal cells in ICH show absent CD207 expression, unlike LCH.
     - ECD occurs at a mean age of 50 to 60 years old (3:1 male to female). PET/CT is highly indicative of disease, with the finding of bilateral symmetric cortical osteosclerosis of the diaphyseal and metaphyseal regions of lower extremities. About 50% of patients present with extraskeletal disease. Cardiac involvement and retroperitoneal fibrosis are common. CT of the chest, abdomen, and pelvis including the entire aorta, MRI of the brain, and transthoracic echocardiogram are recommended to complete evaluation for extent of disease.
     - The histologic pattern of ECD on biopsy shows foamy histiocytes infiltrating tissue, typically with fibrosis present and abundant reactive lymphocytes and neutrophils. Unlike LCH, ECD cells do not express CD1a or S-100; however, cases of mixed ECD/LCH components have been described.

14. **What is the role of *BRAF* mutations in the "L" group of histiocytoses?**
   - The *BRAF* V600E mutation has been found to be highly characteristic of "L" group histiocytoses, with case series reporting more than half of LCH cases positive for the mutation and approximately 50% of ECD cases. It is a somatic mutation that causes constitutive activation of downstream mitogen-activated protein kinase (MAPK) pathway proteins. The mutation is associated with increased risk of treatment failure. Single-institution series have noted promising response with vemurafenib. However, the efficacy of targeted therapy in *BRAF*-mutated LCH has not been studied in larger studies.

15. **What are the diseases in the "C" (cutaneous/mucocutaneous) group of histiocytoses?**
   - The "C" group is composed of the following diseases:
     - Xanthogranuloma (XG) family: Juvenile xanthogranuloma (JXG), adult xanthogranuloma (AXG), and solitary reticulohistiocytoma (SRH) are characterized by well-circumscribed dermal nodules sparing the epidermis containing macrophages, foamy cells, lymphocytes, and eosinophils. JXG appears within the first few years as one or several yellow skin nodules, which usually spontaneously resolve. Disease may be extracutaneous or disseminated, however. AXG is typically a persistent, single lesion. SRH lesions show infiltration by oncocytic macrophages and ground-glass giant cells.
     - Non-XG family: This group includes cutaneous Rosai–Dorfman disease (RDD; see Question 17), necrobiotic xanthogranuloma (NXG; characterized by paraproteinemia, large ulcerated plaques commonly in the periorbital and thoracic regions, with associated cardiomyopathy and underlying hematologic malignancies), and multicentric reticulohistiocytosis (MRH; typically affects 50- to 60-year-old women with polyarthritis, associated with malignancy/autoimmune disease, and pathognomonic periungual "coral bead" papules).

16. What are the diseases in the "M" (malignant) group of histiocytoses?

■ The "M" group of histiocytoses include primary malignant histiocytes involving the skin, lymph nodes, gastrointestinal tract, or other locations, and histiocytes secondary to hematologic malignancies. Response to conventional cytotoxic chemotherapy is typically poor. On histology, histiocytes typically express at least some of the following: CD68, CD163, CD4, and lysozyme.

17. What are the diseases in the "R" (Rosai–Dorfman) group of histiocytoses?

■ The "R" group of histiocytoses are divided into sporadic and familial RDD.
  ● Classic sporadic RDD involves the lymph nodes, is usually diagnosed in children, and clinically presents with massive cervical lymphadenopathy, fever, sweats, fatigue, and weight loss. Extranodal disease may involve the skin, bone, CNS soft tissue, and retro-orbital tissue.
  ● Diagnosis is based on biopsy showing histiocytes, which are negative for CD1a and CD207 (unlike LCH). ·
  ● It is associated with autoimmune diseases, including systemic lupus erythematosus, autoimmune hemolytic anemia, and juvenile idiopathic arthritis.
  ● Sporadic RDD usually resolves spontaneously and with good prognosis but with 5% to 11% mortality rate.
  ● Familial RDD may be diagnosed in H syndrome (an inherited condition due to *SLC29A3* mutation associated with hyperpigmentation, hypertrichosis, hepatosplenomegaly, hearing loss, heart abnormalities, hypogonadism, short height, hyperglycemia, and hallux valgus) or autoimmune lymphoproliferative syndrome (ALPS) associated with germline *TNFRSF6* mutation.

18. What are the diseases in the "H" group of histiocytoses?

■ The "H" group of histiocytoses comprises hemophagocytic lymphohistiocytosis (HLH) in its primary and secondary forms.

19. What is HLH?

■ HLH is a rare, highly morbid syndrome characterized by multiorgan system failure in the setting of hyperactivation of the immune system with accumulation of activated macrophages.

20. How is HLH diagnosed?

■ The diagnosis of HLH is clinical, based on meeting five of the eight HLH-2004 diagnostic criteria *or* presence of a defined molecular mutation:
  ● Fever >38.0°C
  ● Splenomegaly
  ● Cytopenias involving at least two lineages (hemoglobin <9 g/dL, platelets <100,000, or absolute neutrophil count <1,000)
  ● Hypertriglyceridemia (fasting triglycerides ≥265 mg/dL) *or* fibrinogen <150 mg/dL
  ● Ferritin ≥500 ng/mL
  ● Hemophagocytosis noted in bone marrow, spleen, or lymph nodes upon biopsy
  ● Low or absent NK-cell activity
  ● Soluble CD25 (soluble interleukin-2 [IL-2] receptor) >2,400 U/mL

21. **What are the causes of acquired HLH syndrome?**
    - Acquired HLH syndrome has been described in the setting of infection (bacterial, fungal, parasitic, or viral, including Epstein–Barr virus, cytomegalovirus, HIV, and influenza), malignancy (hematologic malignancies such as lymphoma or leukemia, as well as solid tumors), during chemotherapy exposure, and in association with autoimmune disorders (including systemic lupus erythematosis [SLE], vasculitis, and adult-onset Still disease). HLH in the setting of an underlying autoimmune disorder is referred to as macrophage activation syndrome (MAS-HLH).

22. **What gene mutations are associated with hereditary HLH?**
    - Hereditary HLH is characterized by the finding of a germline mutation in any one of a number of genes. As further mutations are characterized, many cases of HLH previously described as of "secondary" or "unknown" etiology may now be classified as hereditary HLH.
      - Among the genes with mutations in primary HLH characterized to date are *FHL2, FHL3, FHL4, FHL5, XLP1, RAB27A* (Griscelli syndrome type 2), *LYST* (Chediak–Higashi syndrome), *XLP2, NLRC4, SLC7A7*, and *HMOX1*.
      - Patients with germline mutations predisposing to primary HLH may not present until adulthood, so testing for the above mutations by gene panel is recommended regardless of age at the time of HLH diagnosis

23. **How is HLH treated in the frontline setting?**
    - Frontline treatment of HLH includes treatment of underlying conditions/ infections in the acquired form, as well as use of chemotherapy in both the inherited and acquired forms of the disease. In critically ill patients, early intervention should be considered as distinguishing the etiology of HLH takes time. Standard frontline therapy for both primary and secondary HLH follows the HLH-94 protocol, with use of an 8-week induction course of intravenous etoposide and dexamethasone. Emapalumab, a monoclonal antibody, should be considered in the relapsed/refractory setting.
      - Patients with documented CNS involvement or progressive neurologic symptoms receive intrathecal (IT) methotrexate throughout the treatment course.
      - The role of allogeneic stem cell transplant (SCT) in adults is still not determined but considered in relapsed/refractory disease or in association with underlying malignancy or germline mutation.

DENDRITIC CELL NEOPLASMS

1. **What is a dendritic cell?**
   - Dendritic cells are antigen-presenting cells of the innate immune system and are present in both blood and in tissues.
     - Dendritic cells in tissue are small and have a "star-shaped" appearance due to the presence of dendritic processes, unlike histiocytes/macrophages, which are large, round cells.
     - Circulating dendritic cells do not show dendritic processes and may morphologically resemble monocytes (mDC) or plasma cells (pDC).

2. **What is blastic plasmacytoid dendritic cell neoplasm (BPDCN)?**
   - BPDCN is a rare and aggressive hematologic malignancy of the pDC population characterized by skin disease with or without bone marrow involvement. The disease has undergone many name changes, with "BPDCN" established by the 2008 World Health Organization (WHO) classification system.

3. **What is the epidemiology of BPDCN?**
   - Although data are sparse, case series suggest that BPDCN makes up approximately 0.44% of all hematologic malignancies, with a male to female ratio of 2.5:1. The median age of onset is 60 to 70 years and risk factors are unknown. Of the cases, 10% to 20% may be associated with an antecedent hematologic malignancy (e.g., myelodysplastic syndrome [MDS], chronic myeloid leukemia [CML], or acute myeloid leukemia [AML]).

4. **What are the clinical findings of BPDCN?**
   - Patients typically present initially with skin lesions, which may be solitary or multiple, with variability in size, shape (papules, nodules, or plaques), and color. Cytopenias, lymphadenopathy, and organomegaly are common.

5. **How is BPDCN diagnosed?**
   - The malignant cells in BPDCN obtained via skin or bone marrow biopsy show a characteristic immunophenotype. They are CD4- and CD56-positive, as well as positive for more specific markers of pDCs—CD123 (IL3RA), TCL1, and CD303. Myeloid, monocytic, and T-, or B-lymphoid markers are typically absent. Most cases of BPDCN show clonal chromosomal abnormalities and/or gene mutations; however, none are diagnostic of the disease.

6. **What is the prognosis of BPDCN?**
   - Prognosis of BPDCN is not well-defined but understood to be very poor, with a short overall survival in the range of 1 to 2 years.

7. **How is BPDCN treated?**
   - Tagraxofusp, a CD123-directed cytotoxin consisting of human IL-3 fused to diphtheria toxin, is now recommended induction therapy.
   - Acute lymphoblastic leukemia (ALL), myeloid-, or lymphoma-based regimens are considered to yield lower response rates and poor outcomes.
   - Patients who are elderly or not otherwise candidates for aggressive cytotoxic chemotherapy may receive palliative chemo-radiation therapy (XRT) or steroids for skin lesions, with considerations of low-dose chemotherapy such as oral etoposide or CHOP (cyclophosphamide, doxorubicin, vincristine, and prednisone) with noncurative intent.

8. **What is the role of SCT in the treatment of BPDCN?**
   - Patients who are fit candidates have shown a survival benefit in BPDCN with use of allogeneic SCT, and this is considered the best option for long-term remission in patients achieving complete response (CR) with frontline therapy. The potential role of autoSCT remains unclear.

9. **What are the typical side effects of tagraxofusp?**
   - Typical side effects with tagraxofusp include infusion reactions (amenable to premedication), capillary leak syndrome, transaminitis, thrombocytopenia/neutropenia, hypoalbuminemia, and hyponatremia.

10. **What other dendritic cell neoplasms exist?**
    - There are other, rare dendritic cell neoplasms, including indeterminate dendritic cell tumor (IND-DCT), interdigitating dendritic cell sarcoma (IDCS), and follicular dendritic cell sarcoma (FDCS).

MYELOID/LYMPHOID NEOPLASMS WITH EOSINOPHILIA AND TYROSINE KINASE GENE FUSIONS

1. **What are myeloid/lymphoid neoplasms with eosinophilia and tyrosine kinase gene fusions (MLN-TK)?**
   - An updated group in the WHO 2022 classification, MLN-TKs are myeloid and lymphoid disorders defined by rearrangements in genes involving the tyrosine kinase domain.

TABLE 22.3 ■ Tyrosine Kinase Gene Fusions

TK Fusion	Clinical and Diagnostic Features
FIP1L1-PDGFRA	- A myeloid or lymphoid neoplasm - Prominent eosinophilia (usually) - Elevated tryptase - Presence of *FIP1L1-PDGFRA* fusion or variant fusion involving *PDGFRA* (can perform FISH for *CHIC2* deletion at fusion site)
ETV6-PDGFRB	- Myeloproliferative neoplasm - Prominent eosinophilia (usually) - Neutrophilia or monocytosis (sometimes) - Presence of t(8;12) or demonstration of *ETV6-PDGFRB* or variant fusion involving *PDGFRB*
FGFR1 rearrangement	- Prominent eosinophilia - AML or T-ALL or B-ALL/lymphoma or mixed-phenotype acute leukemia (usually associated with peripheral blood or marrow eosinophilia) - t(8;13) or variant translocation leading to *FGFR1* rearrangement
PCM1-JAK2 (provisional entity)	- A myeloid or lymphoid neoplasm - Prominent eosinophilia (usually) - Presence of t(8;9) or a variant translocation leading to *JAK2* rearrangement

FISH, fluorescence in situ hybridization.

2. **What is the incidence of this group of diseases?**
   - Less than 10% of patients with idiopathic hypereosinophilia are found to have *FIP1L1-PDGFRA* fusion. Data on other specific rearrangements are unknown.

3. **How are MLN-TKs diagnosed?**
   - Patients undergoing workup for eosinophilia in which secondary causes have been ruled out (i.e., diagnosed with primary eosinophilia) should undergo testing for the above fusions/rearrangements given therapeutic and prognostic implications.
   - MLN-TK supersedes other myeloid or lymphoid disorders and systemic mastocytosis when there are overlapping features.

4. How are myeloid/lymphoid neoplasms with eosinophilia treated?

- Patients with disease involving fusions of *PDGFRA* and *PDGFRB* are exquisitely sensitive to imatinib. Diseases with the classic rearrangements can often be treated in the frontline setting with excellent response to imatinib at 100 to 400 mg PO daily.
- Patients with *FGFR1* typically have an aggressive disease course with early progression to AML, and their disease is not responsive to imatinib therapy. Treatment involves cytotoxic agents with goal of CR to be followed by allogeneic hematopoietic cell transplantation (alloHCT) or use of novel FGFR1 inhibitors in the clinical trial setting.
- Patients with *JAK2* rearrangements are typically treated with janus kinase (JAK) inhibitors (e.g., ruxolitinib), often as a bridge to alloHCT given its relatively short duration of response.
- Supportive care (e.g., steroids) is given for end-organ damage (e.g., cardiomyopathy) related to hypereosinophilia.

QUESTIONS

1. An 85-year-old male with congestive heart failure, hypertension, and type 2 diabetes mellitus presents with a painful, ulcerated erythematous plaque measuring 5 × 5 cm to the skin of his right pectoral region. Biopsy of the lesion reveals skin infiltrated by immature-appearing cells which are CD4+, CD56+, and CD123+. Complete blood count (CBC) shows normal peripheral blood counts. Which of the following treatments would be a reasonable management option?
   A. Surgical excision
   B. Chemotherapy with cyclophosphamide, doxorubicin, vincristine, prednisone (CHOP)
   C. Systemic steroids
   D. Local radiation therapy

2. A 35-year-old male with no past medical history presents to the local ED with 3 days of fever to 39°C and significant malaise. Laboratory analysis is notable for a ferritin of 2,000 ng/mL, left upper quadrant tenderness with palpable spleen tip, neutropenia to absolute neutrophil count (ANC) of 800, and thrombocytopenia to a platelet count of 90,000. A bone marrow biopsy is performed, which shows hemophagocytosis. Which of the following additional laboratory abnormalities would be necessary to make a clinical diagnosis of hemophagocytic lymphohistiocytosis (HLH)?
   A. Elevated natural killer (NK) cell activity
   B. Low NK cell activity
   C. Low soluble interleukin-2 level
   D. Elevated antinuclear antibodies (ANA)

3. An otherwise healthy 50-year-old male undergoes routine complete blood count (CBC) at his primary care doctor's office and is found to have an elevated white blood cell (WBC) count to 15,000, with normal hemoglobin and platelet count. Differential shows a hypereosinophilia (75% eosinophils). There is no evidence of end-organ-damage

per chest x-ray (CXR) or troponin. Workup for secondary causes of hypereosinophilia is negative, and the patient is felt to have a primary hypereosinophilia. A bone marrow biopsy is performed with conventional karyotype analysis, fluorescence in situ hybridization (FISH) panel, and next-generation sequencing. Which of the following results would predict that his disease would NOT be responsive to a commercially available tyrosine kinase inhibitor?

A. *PDGFRA* gene rearrangement per karyotype
B. *CHIC2* deletion by FISH
C. *FGFR1* rearrangement per karyotype
D. *PDGFRB* rearrangement per karyotype
E. *JAK2* rearrangement per karyotype

4. A 22-year-old female has been diagnosed with hemophagocytic lymphohistiocytosis (HLH) and is 2 weeks into her induction course with etoposide/dexamethasone with early addition of cyclosporine per HLH-94 protocol. She has never had a lumbar puncture (LP) or shown neurologic symptoms. The patient suffers a generalized tonic-clonic seizure. EEG upon recovery shows nonspecific slow wave. MRI shows decreased signal on T1-weighted images and hyperintense T2 abnormalities in the posterior occipital lobes bilaterally. An LP is performed, with normal cerebrospinal fluid (CSF) analysis. Appropriate antiepileptic therapy has been started. What would be the appropriate next step in management?

A. Administer IT methotrexate.
B. Stop cyclosporine.
C. Continue current treatment.
D. Continue current treatment and begin workup for allogeneic hematopoietic cell transplant.

5. A 45-year-old female treated for blastic plasmacytoid dendritic cell neoplasm (BPDCN) with an ALL induction regimen followed by allogeneic hematopoietic cell transplantation (alloHCT) has relapsed 120 days posttransplant. She has enrolled on a clinical trial to receive a drug-conjugate called tagraxofusp. What is the targeting mechanism of this drug in BPDCN?

A. Binding to CD123 on pDC cell surface
B. Binding to CD4 on pDC cell surface
C. Binding to CD56 on pDC cell surface
D. Binding to CD303 on pDC cell surface

6. A 55-year-old male presents with 3 months of progressive right thigh pain. Plain films reveal a lytic bone lesion to the right femur. A PET/CT is performed, showing fluorodeoxyglucose (FDG)-avidity to the site. No other sites of disease are noted per PET. The patient undergoes extensive workup for plasma cell dyscrasia, which is negative. Ultimately, a biopsy of the right femur lesion is performed. Histology reveals infiltration of the osteolytic lesion by cells with tennis racket-shaped granules, which are positive per immunohistochemistry for CD14. Which of the following would be an appropriate initial treatment strategy?

A. Systemic chemotherapy with vinblastine
B. Systemic chemotherapy with cytarabine
C. Intravenous bisphosphonate therapy
D. Local radiation therapy (XRT) to the femoral lesion

7. **Which of the following is true?**
   A. Langerhans cell histiocytosis (LCH) risk organs are the bone marrow, liver, spleen, and possibly lung.
   B. The M histiocyte group includes familial and sporadic Rosai–Dorfman diseases.
   C. The most common endocrinopathy associated with LCH is primary adrenal insufficiency.
   D. In LCH, biopsy of a lesion demonstrates cells positive for CD1a, negative for S-100, and positive for CD207.

8. **Which of the following is true?**
   A. Patients with *FGFR1* rearrangement and eosinophilia have a higher likelihood of response to imatinib than patients with *PDGFRA* or *PDGFRB* rearrangements.
   B. Clonal eosinophilia can be caused by *PCM1-JAK2* rearrangement.
   C. Patients with *ETV6-PDGFRB* rearrangements have deletion of the *CHIC2* gene.
   D. Patients with *ETV6-PDGFRB* rearrangements and eosinophilia should be treated with a JAK inhibitor.

9. **What of the following is true about hemophagocytic lymphohistiocytosis (HLH)?**
   A. Allogeneic stem cell transplant is indicated in the following situations: relapsed/refractory disease following or during frontline treatment, central nervous system (CNS) involvement, underlying hematologic malignancy, primary HLH due to a germline mutation.
   B. HLH can be due to/co-occur with a variety of infections, malignancy, and autoimmune disease, and can be due to somatic mutations but cannot be due to a germline mutation.
   C. Increased natural killer (NK) cell activity is one of the criteria for diagnosing HLH.
   D. Low triglyceride is one of the criteria for diagnosing HLH.

ANSWERS

1. **D. Local radiation therapy.** This is an older adult patient with multiple comorbidities with blastic plasmacytoid dendritic cell neoplasm (BPDCN). He has an isolated skin lesion and no evidence (yet) of hematologic involvement. Prompt palliative benefit would be expected with radiation therapy to the isolated skin lesion, with the understanding that the disease will likely progress in the near future. Given sensitivity to radiation therapy, surgical excision would not be recommended. Given age and comorbidities, chemotherapy with CHOP and systemic steroids would likely have increased morbidity risk.

2. **B. Low NK cell activity.** HLH is associated with low to absent NK cell activity, which is one of the eight diagnostic criteria for the disease. Elevated soluble IL-2R level is another diagnostic criterion. Elevated ANA may suggest a secondary etiology of the HLH but is not a diagnostic criterion.

3. **C. *FGFR1* rearrangement per karyotype.** The above gene rearrangements are associated with myeloid/lymphoid neoplasms with eosinophilia, which is in the differential for any patient with primary hypereosinophilia. *PDGFRA* and *PDGFRB* rearrangements are sensitive to imatinib, with *CHIC2* deletion by FISH a surrogate marker for *PDGFRA* rearrangement. Disease with *JAK2* rearrangement is sensitive to ruxolitinib, although duration of response is limited. Disease with *FGFR1* rearrangement is not sensitive to imatinib. Clinical trial development of *FGFR1* inhibitors is ongoing.

4. **B. Stop cyclosporine.** The MRI findings are consistent with a diagnosis of posterior reversible encephalopathy syndrome (PRES), with negative CSF arguing against HLH involvement of the central nervous system (CNS) and precluding need for IT methotrexate course. PRES has been associated with HLH treatment and remains unclear whether it is related to the disease itself or to the treatment modalities used. There is a suggestion that cyclosporine may increase the risk of developing PRES and is therefore recommended to be held. Current treatment of HLH is tending to not include frontline use of cyclosporine. Transplant is not indicated at this time without further information regarding the patient's disease (e.g., primary vs. secondary), but she would not appear to have CNS involvement of HLH as an indication to proceed for transplant.

5. **A. Binding to CD123 on pDC cell surface.** All of the above choices are markers found on plasma cells (pDC) and in BPDCN. CD123 is interleukin-3A (IL-3A) receptor and is the target of the drug tagraxofusp, which is diphtheria toxin conjugated to recombinant IL-3A.

6. **D. Local radiation therapy (XRT) to the femoral lesion.** All of the above choices are therapies used in the management of Langerhans cell histiocytosis (LCH), including bone involvement. Given the unifocal nature of the patient's disease, however, systemic treatment could most likely be avoided with use of localized XRT alone.

7. **A. Langerhans cell histiocytosis (LCH) risk organs are the bone marrow, liver, spleen, and possibly lung.** The R histiocyte group includes familial and sporadic Rosai–Dorfman diseases, while the M group contains primary malignant histiocytoses and secondary malignant histiocytoses associated with another hematologic neoplasm. The most common endocrinopathy associated with LCH is central diabetes insipidus. In LCH, biopsy of a lesion demonstrates cells positive for CD1a, positive for S-100, and positive for CD207.

8. **B. Clonal eosinophilia can be caused by *PCM1-JAK2* rearrangement.** Patients with *FGFR1* rearrangement and eosinophilia have a lower likelihood of response to imatinib than patients with *PDGFRA* or *PDGFRB* rearrangements. Patients with *FIP1L1-PDGFRA* rearrangements have deletion of the *CHIC2* gene. Patients with *ETV6-PDGFRB* rearrangements and eosinophilia are treated with imatinib.

9. **A. Allogeneic stem cell transplant is indicated in the following situations: relapsed/refractory disease following or during frontline treatment, central nervous system (CNS) involvement, underlying hematologic malignancy, primary HLH due to a germline mutation.** HLH can be due to germline mutations. Decreased NK cell activity is one of the criteria for diagnosing HLH. Hypertriglyceridemia is one of the criteria for diagnosing HLH.

Marcus Geer, Samuel Reynolds, and Matthew J. Pianko

Hematologic Emergencies

TUMOR LYSIS SYNDROME

1. **What is tumor lysis syndrome (TLS)?**
   - TLS is a clinical syndrome associated with the release of intracellular products into the systemic circulation following spontaneous or induced tumor cell death.
   - TLS is associated with risk of renal injury from precipitation of uric acid/phosphate crystals and electrolyte abnormalities.

2. **What are the risk factors for TLS?**
   - Highly proliferative malignancies, including acute lymphoblastic leukemia, Burkitt lymphoma, diffuse large B-cell lymphoma (DLBCL), and small cell lung cancer
   - High tumor burden (e.g., hyperleukocytosis)
   - High sensitivity to cytotoxic chemotherapy; that is, rapid cell turnover and/or death
   - Preexisting hyperuricemia, renal insufficiency, and hypovolemia

3. **What are the key laboratory findings associated with TLS?**
   - High: potassium, phosphate, uric acid, lactate dehydrogenase (LDH)
   - Low: calcium (formed by complexes between intracellular phosphate binding with free calcium)
   - Acute renal failure (defined as serum creatinine >1.5x the institutional upper limit of normal)

4. **What are the clinical manifestations of TLS?**
   - Nausea, vomiting, diarrhea, lethargy
   - Muscle cramps, paresthesias, tetany
   - Confusion, hallucinations, seizures, syncope
   - Cardiac arrhythmias, heart failure
   - Sudden death

5. **What is the recommended management of TLS?**
   - Aggressive intravascular volume reexpansion with intravenous fluid (IVF); diuresis may be utilized as needed to maintain adequate fluid balance
   - Electrolyte repletion/removal; renal replacement therapy PRN

- Urate-lowering therapy; options include the following:
  - Allopurinol
    - Analogue of hypoxanthine (a natural purine base), which competitively inhibits xanthine oxidase
    - Decreases formation of new uric acid, does not reduce preexisting uric acid
    - Renal dose adjustment required due to risk of cutaneous hypersensitivity reaction
    - Requires renal dose adjustment
    - Reduces degradation of other purines; caution advised accordingly when cotreating with 6-mercaptopurine, azathioprine
    - Adjust doses of medications also metabolized by the cytochrome P450 system
  - Febuxostat
    - Alternative xanthine oxidase inhibitor
    - Can be used in the instance of allopurinol allergy or another contraindication to allopurinol (severe drug interaction)
  - Rasburicase
    - Recombinant urate oxidase, which enzymatically converts uric acid into allantoin, a more soluble substance than uric acid
    - Acutely decreases serum concentration of uric acid but may require repeated dosing
    - Cannot be used in pregnant women or in glucose-6-phosphate-dehydrogenase (G6PD) deficiency (causes severe hemolysis and methemoglobinemia)
    - Nonpurine selective xanthine oxidase inhibitor
    - Following use of rasburicase, follow-up uric acid blood samples must be obtained on ice to inhibit enzyme activity in order to accurately measure uric acid.
  - General recommendations
    - Allopurinol should be used as frontline therapy; may start at 600 mg on day 1, 300 mg twice daily on Days 2 to 3, 300 mg daily thereafter
    - Assess for the indication for rasburicase:
      - Uric acid <9: rasburicase not indicated
      - Uric acid 9 to 12: consider avoiding rasburicase; continue IVF, urate-lowering therapy
      - Uric acid 12 to 15: rasburicase 3 mg intravenously (IV) once
      - Uric acid >15: rasburicase 6 mg IV once

HYPERLEUKOCYTOSIS AND LEUKOSTASIS

1. **What is hyperleukocytosis?**
   - White blood cell (WBC) counts >100×10^9/L
   - Seen in 5% to 20% of patients with acute leukemia
   - Risk factors: young age, monocytic differentiation subtypes, certain cytogenetic abnormalities

2. **What is leukostasis?**
   - Increased serum viscosity due to elevated number of WBCs, which are less deformable compared with red blood cells (RBCs) and which induce endothelial expression of adhesion molecules

- Aggregation of blasts leads to vascular occlusion, end-organ compromise (see clinical signs below)
- Associated with high risk of early mortality

3. **What are the clinical signs of leukostasis?**
   - Pulmonary: dyspnea, hypoxia ± diffuse alveolar infiltrates
   - Neurologic: headache, visual changes, confusion, somnolence, and coma
   - Less common: electrocardiographic evidence of myocardial ischemia or right ventricular overload, renal insufficiency, priapism, acute limb ischemia, and bowel infarction
   - Can manifest in acute myeloid leukemia (AML) with WBC count as low as $50 \times 10^9/L$ but is more common when it exceeds $100 \times 10^9/L$
   - Leukostasis less likely in acute lymphocytic leukemia (ALL), chronic myeloid leukemia (CML), and chronic lymphocytic leukemia (CLL).

4. **What is the treatment for leukostasis?**
   - Aggressive hydration with IVF
   - Cytoreductive measures:
     - Induction chemotherapy (preferred)
     - Hydroxyurea (cannot be given to women who are pregnant or breastfeeding)
     - Leukapheresis: limited and conflicting data on its benefits; contraindicated in acute promyelocytic leukemia (APL) due to increased risk of hemorrhage in the setting of disseminated intravascular coagulation (DIC).
   - During treatment:
     - Avoid blood transfusions, particularly red cell products, if possible due to the induction of increased whole blood viscosity.
     - Monitor for/manage tumor lysis and DIC.

URGENT/EMERGENT MANAGEMENT OF ACUTE LEUKEMIA

1. **What are the clinical signs/symptoms of newly diagnosed acute leukemia?**
   - Bone marrow failure: anemia (fatigue, shortness of breath), bleeding (petechiae, bruising), recurrent infections due to neutropenia (± fever)
   - Tissue infiltration by leukemic blasts: gums, skin, meninges (most commonly associated with monocytic phenotype)
   - DIC (seen most frequently in patients with APL)
   - Leukostasis (as previously discussed)

2. **What tests do you immediately obtain in a patient whom you suspect has a new diagnosis of acute leukemia?**
   - Preparation of a peripheral blood smear, key to evaluate for presence of blasts with Auer rods, which may suggest APL
   - Complete blood count (CBC) with differential
   - Comprehensive metabolic panel, uric acid, phosphorus, and LDH
   - Evaluation for coagulopathy and DIC: coagulation studies, including prothrombin time (PT), international normalized ratio (INR), and partial thromboplastin time (PTT), fibrinogen
   - Flow cytometry for peripheral blood immunophenotyping

3. **What are the recommended immediate interventions for a patient with a new diagnosis of AML?**
   - Consider urate-lowering therapy as TLS prophylaxis, for example, allopurinol
     - Consider rasburicase if significantly elevated serum uric acid levels as per previously noted guidelines (or as per institutional practice)
   - Hydroxyurea if leukoreduction is needed
   - Leukapheresis if there is concern for leukostasis
   - All-trans retinoic acid (ATRA) if concern for APL, histologically indicated by the following:
     - Presence of large bundles of Auer rods, "sliding plates" appearance of bilobed nuclei typical of APL but not specific
     - Hypogranular variant exists that is without significant Auer rods
   - Supportive care if there is evidence of DIC
     - For example, transfusion of cryoprecipitate for hypofibrinogenemia or fresh frozen plasma for elevated PTT or INR with bleeding

FEBRILE NEUTROPENIA

1. **What is febrile neutropenia?**
   - Fever: Per the Infectious Diseases Society of America (IDSA) guidelines, single temperature higher than 38.3°C (101.3°F) or sustained temperature higher than 38°C (100.4°F) for more than 1 hour
   - Neutropenia: absolute neutrophil count (ANC) <500 or ANC <1,000 with predicted decline to <500 in 48 hours

2. **What are the signs and symptoms of febrile neutropenia?**
   - Signs and symptoms apart from fever may be minimal, even absent.
   - Presentation is largely dependent on the nature of any underlying infection and the culprit organism and host immune status.

3. **What should the evaluation of febrile neutropenia include?**
   - Evaluations include a thorough physical exam with particular attention to skin, sinuses, mouth/oropharynx, lungs, abdomen, perirectal area (avoid digital rectal exam), and indwelling catheters or other hardware.
   - Laboratory studies include CBC with differential, comprehensive metabolic panel, two sets of blood cultures (peripheral and from indwelling catheter or port if applicable), urinalysis with culture, and other site-specific cultures as applicable (stool, skin lesions, etc.).
   - Ideally, cultures should be obtained prior to initiating antibiotics but do not delay antimicrobial therapy for critically ill/hemodynamically unstable patients.
   - Radiologic studies include routine chest x-ray and additional imaging for localizing symptoms as warranted.

4. **What are the classic associated pathogens in febrile neutropenia?**
   - Infectious source identified in approximately only 30% of patients

- Bacterial pathogens MOST common
  - Initial increasing trend toward gram-positive organisms (*Staphylococcus* and *Streptococcus*) since 1980s has started to swing toward gram-negative organisms, given the rise of multidrug resistance
  - Gram-negative bacilli are common, particularly *Pseudomonas aeruginosa*.
- Fungal and viral pathogens also common; invasive fungal infections especially prevalent in high-risk neutropenia (includes duration for >7 days, concomitant hypotension)
- Empiric treatment must provide broad coverage against gram-negative organisms, including *Pseudomonas*. Gram-positive and anaerobic coverage should also be offered if clinical evidence suggests such or if risk factors of concomitant infection are present.

5. **What is the treatment for febrile neutropenia?**
   - See algorithm in Figure 23.1.
   - For select patients with anticipated brief neutropenia (<7 days), few to no comorbidities or symptoms, outpatient therapy (ciprofloxacin and amoxicillin/clavulanate) with close monitoring may be acceptable based on institutional policy on a case-by-case basis. This is not commonly offered.
   - High-risk patients require inpatient hospitalization with empiric broad-spectrum IV antibiotics.
   - For uncomplicated infections, monotherapy with broad-spectrum beta-lactams with pseudomonal coverage is as effective as combined therapy.
     - Cefepime, piperacillin-tazobactam, imipenem, meropenem, and ceftazidime are all reasonable first-line options.
     - Best choice is based on institutional/regional susceptibilities.
   - Combination therapy should be used in the setting of severe sepsis/septic shock or in areas with high prevalence of multidrug resistant (MDR) gram-negative rod-based organisms.
     - Typically use a beta-lactam plus an aminoglycoside or fluoroquinolone.
   - Role of vancomycin:
     - Should NOT be used initially unless one or more of the following applies:
       - Clinically suspected catheter-related infection
       - Gram-positive bacteria identified on blood culture while susceptibilities are pending
       - Known colonization with methicillin-resistant *Staphylococcus aureus* (MRSA)
       - Severe mucositis or soft tissue infection
       - Severe sepsis or septic shock
   - Role of antifungal therapy:
     - Should be initiated for persistent fever after 4 to 7 days of broad-spectrum therapy
   - Duration of antibiotics:
     - Documented infection: Treat for standard duration indicated for specific infection and/or until neutropenia resolves, whichever is longer.
     - Undocumented infection: Treat until fever disappears and ANC of greater than 500 for at least 24 hours.

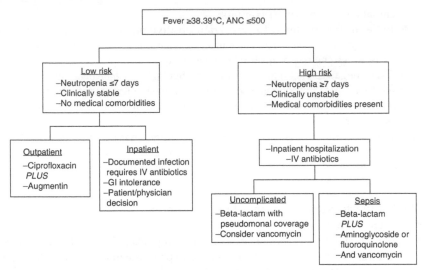

FIGURE 23.1 ■ Algorithm for treatment of febrile neutropenia.

ANC, absolute neutrophil count; GI, gastrointestinal; IV, intravenous.

CHEMOTHERAPY EXTRAVASATION

1. **What is extravasation of chemotherapy?**
   - Unintended leakage of chemotherapy drug into extravascular space
   - Vesicants cause tissue necrosis; irritants cause inflammation only

2. **What are the common vesicant and irritant chemotherapeutic drugs?**

TABLE 23.1 ■ Management of Chemotherapy Extravasation

Vesicant	Commonly Used Treatments
Anthracyclines	■ Dexrazoxane
■ Daunorubicin, doxorubicin, epirubicin, idarubicin, mitomycin C	■ Topical DMSO
	■ Topical cooling
Vinca alkaloids	■ Subcutaneous hyaluronidase
■ Vincristine, vinblastine, vinorelbine	■ Topical warming
Irritant	**Commonly Used Treatments**
Taxanes*	■ Topical cooling
■ Docetaxel, paclitaxel	■ Subcutaneous hyaluronidase
Platinums*	
■ Carboplatin, cisplatin	
■ Oxaliplatin	■ Sodium thiosulfate/topical warming
Epipodophyllotoxins	
■ Etoposide, teniposide	■ Topical warming
Topoisomerase I inhibitors	
■ Irinotecan, topotecan	■ Topical cooling

*May have vesicant properties at high volume/concentration, but generally act as irritants.

DMSO, dimethylsulfoxide.

TOXICITIES OF IMMUNE EFFECTOR CELL THERAPIES

1. **How are they defined?**
   - Chimeric antigen receptor (CAR) T-cells and bispecific T-cell engagers (BITEs) are associated with unique immunologic toxicities.
   - Immunologic toxicities result from rapid expansion of immune cells targeting cancer-associated antigens with increased expression of proinflammatory cytokines.
   - Immunologic toxicities tend to occur shortly after initial infusion of the product and resolve with appropriate management.
   - Symptoms of toxicities may be severe, requiring ICU level of care, and can be fatal.
   - Rates of toxicities vary between diseases and therapies.

2. **What are the symptoms of cytokine release syndrome (CRS)?**
   - CRS is accompanied by fever by definition.
   - Other associated symptoms include constitutional symptoms, dyspnea/hypoxia manifesting as pulmonary infiltrates requiring supplemental oxygen, hypotension, cardiac arrhythmias, and other organ dysfunction.

3. **What is the management of CRS?**
   - Low-grade CRS can be managed with antipyretics and supportive care.
   - Tocilizumab, an interleukin-6 (IL-6) receptor antagonist is the only FDA-approved therapy for CRS.
   - High-dose steroids are commonly used in the management of CRS.
   - Other therapies, including anakinra (IL-1 antagonist), tumor necrosis factor (TNF) alpha inhibitors, and siltuximab (IL-6 antagonist), are undergoing further evaluation.

4. **What are the symptoms of immune effector cell-associated neurotoxicity syndrome (ICANS)?**
   - ICANS typically manifests following onset of CRS but can rarely present independently.
   - ICANS symptoms can be very heterogeneous and include encephalopathy, confusion, hallucinations, word finding difficulties, headache, tremors, changes in handwriting, seizures, cerebral edema, and death.

5. **What is the management of ICANS?**
   - There are no FDA-approved therapies for ICANS.
   - High-dose steroids are the backbone of treatment.
   - There is no consensus on the most appropriate second-line therapy, and options include tocilizumab, anakinra, TNF-alpha inhibitors, and siltuximab, among others.

Supportive Care

ANTIMICROBIAL PROPHYLAXIS

1. **What antimicrobial precautions should be instituted in patients with neutropenia?**
   - Limit exogenous pathogen exposure.
     - High-efficiency particulate air (HEPA)-filtered room
     - No sick visitors

- Avoidance of raw fruits or vegetables or live plant exposure
- Prohibiting smoking, including tobacco and marijuana
- Handwashing

2. **What antimicrobial prophylaxis is recommended?**
   - Acyclovir antiviral prophylaxis is recommended.
   - Antibiotic prophylaxis with a fluoroquinolone is recommended if ANC is $<0.5 \times 10^9/L$ >7 days.
   - Antifungal prophylaxis with either posaconazole or voriconazole is recommended against invasive mold infections and *Candida* spp. Fluconazole would only target *Candida* and would not be adequate in this patient population, with prolonged neutropenia.
   - Prophylaxis for pneumocystis pneumonia (PJP) is recommended for patients receiving induction chemotherapy for ALL, a purine analogue such as fludarabine or who will be on the dose equivalent of ≥20 mg of prednisone/day for ≥1 month. Consider PJP prophylaxis in patients on multiple immunosuppressive agents or with potential for prolonged lymphopenia with absolute lymphocyte count (ALC) ≤ 0.5. Appropriate choices include trimethoprim-sulfamethoxazole, pentamidine inhalation, dapsone (check G6PD), and atovaquone.

CHEMOTHERAPY-INDUCED NAUSEA AND VOMITING

1. **What are the types of chemotherapy-induced nausea and vomiting (CINV)?**
   - Acute: up to 24 hours after chemotherapy, mediated by 5-HT3 release from enterochromaffin cells
   - Delayed: more than 24 hours after chemotherapy, mediated by NK_1 receptors
   - Anticipatory: occurs on the day of or some hours before the anticipated chemotherapy; typically triggered by taste, odor, sight, and distressing thoughts/anxiety

2. **What is the emetogenicity of various chemotherapeutic agents?**

TABLE 23.2

	Risk of Emesis (Without Antiemetics)			
	High >90%	Moderate 31%–90%	Low 10%–30%	Minimal <10%
IV agents	Carmustine	Alemtuzumab	Bortezomib	Cladribine
	Cisplatin	Azacytidine	Carfilzomib	Bevacizumab
	Cyclophosphamide ≥1,500 mg/m²	Bendamustine	Cytarabine ≤1,000 mg/m²	Bleomycin
		Cabazitaxel		Busulfan
	Dacarbazine	Carboplatin	Docetaxel	Cetuximab
	Dactinomycin	Clofarabine	Eribulin	Fludarabine
	Mechlorethamine	Cyclophosphamide ≤1,500 mg/m²	Etoposide	Rituximab
	Streptozotocin		5-Fluorouracil	Vinblastine
		Cytarabine >1,000 mg/m²	Gemcitabine	Vincristine
				Vinorelbine

(continued)

TABLE 23.2 (*continued*)

	Risk of Emesis (Without Antiemetics)			
	High >90%	Moderate 31%–90%	Low 10%–30%	Minimal <10%
IV agents (continued)		Daunorubicin*	Ixabepilone	
		Denileukin diftitox	Methotrexate (>1,000 mg/m²)	
		Doxorubicin*	Mitomycin	
		Epirubicin*	Mitoxantrone	
		Idarubicin*	Paclitaxel	
		Ifosfamide	Panitumumab	
		Irinotecan	PEG-liposomal doxorubicin	
		Melphalan	Pemetrexed	
		Oxaliplatin	Romidepsin	
		Pralatrexate	Temsirolimus	
		Temozolomide	Topotecan	
			Trastuzumab	
			Vorinostat	
PO agents	Hexamethyl-melamine	Altretamine	Axitinib	6-Thioguanine
	Procarbazine	Busulfan	Bexarotene	Chlorambucil
		Crizotinib	Capecitabine	Erlotinib
		Cyclophosphamide	Cetuximab	Gefitinib
		Imatinib	Dasatinib	Hydroxyurea
		Lomustine	Estramustine	Melphalan
		Temozolomide	Etoposide	Methotrexate
		Tretinoin	Everolimus	Regorafenib
		Vandetanib	Fludarabine	Sorafenib
		Vinorelbine	Lapatinib	
			Lenalidomide	
			Nilotinib	
			Panitumumab	
			Pazopanib	
			Sunitinib	
			Tegafur uracil	
			Thalidomide	
			Topotecan	
			Vemurafenib	
			Vorinostat	

*When combined with cyclophosphamide, these anthracyclines have high emetic risk.

3. **What antiemetic agents are available?**
   - Serotonin (5-HT$_3$) receptor antagonists
     - First-generation: dolasetron, granisetron (transdermal patch option), ondansetron (oral dissolving tablet option), tropisetron
     - Second-generation: palonosetron (higher affinity for receptor and longer half-life)
     - Oral and IV forms similarly effective
     - Side effects: headache, diarrhea, transient transaminitis, and EKG changes; prolonged QT interval seen primarily with dolasetron; Constipation with the 5-HT$_3$ receptor antagonists can be severe
   - NK$_1$ receptor antagonists
     - Aprepitant and its prodrug fosaprepitant
     - Potential drug interaction: moderate inhibitor of CYP3A4
   - Steroids
     - Dexamethasone and methylprednisolone equally effective in both oral and parenteral formulations
     - Side effects: insomnia, mood changes, irritability, and hyperglycemia
   - Dopamine (D$_2$) receptor antagonists
     - Prochlorperazine, promethazine, haloperidol, and metoclopramide
     - Side effects: sedation, extrapyramidal reactions, anticholinergic effects, EKG changes (haloperidol, droperidol), hypotension with rapid IV administration (phenothiazines)
   - Benzodiazepines
     - Lorazepam and alprazolam
     - Side effects: dose-related sedation and delirium (especially in older adult patients); benzodiazepines can potentiate the sedating effects of opioids and should be used with caution in patients receiving concomitant opioids
   - Cannabinoids
     - Dronabinol and nabilone
     - Side effects: sedation, confusion, dizziness, short-term memory loss, euphoria/dysphoria, ataxia, dry mouth, and orthostatic hypotension
   - Antihistamines
     - Diphenhydramine and hydroxyzine
     - Are not useful for CINV, but helpful for motion sickness
     - Side effects: sedation, dry mouth, visual changes, mydriasis, decreased gastrointestinal (GI) motility, urinary changes, and increased heart rate
   - Neuroleptics
     - Olanzapine
     - Useful for both acute and delayed CINV refractory to other treatments; may also be considered as earlier line therapy in the presence of severe symptoms

4. How do you prevent nausea and vomiting?

TABLE 23.3 ■ Prevention of Chemotherapy-Induced Nausea and Vomiting

Prophylaxis Recommended					
High		Moderate		Low	
Acute	Delayed	Acute	Delayed	Acute	Delayed
5-HT3RA + dex + aprepitant ± lorazepam	Dex + aprepitant ± lorazepam	Anthracycline/ cyclophosphamide 5-HT3RA + dex + aprepitant ± lorazepam Others: 5-HT3RA ± dex ± lorazepam	Aprepitant ± dex ± lorazepam	Dex ± lorazepam prochlorperazine ± lorazepam Metoclopramide ± lorazepam	None

5-HT3RA, serotonin receptor antagonist; dex, dexamethasone.

5. How do you treat breakthrough and refractory CINV?
- Avoid repeated dosing of agents that were given for prophylaxis and already failed.
- Consider adding prochlorperazine, metoclopramide, a benzodiazepine, or a neuroleptic (e.g., olanzapine).

6. What are nonpharmacologic measures for antiemetic prophylaxis?
- Ginger capsules or chews (prior to and during treatment cycle)
- Cognitive distraction (e.g., playing video games during treatment)
- Systematic desensitization (visualization and learned relaxation techniques)
- Hypnosis
- Acupuncture
- Transcutaneous electrical nerve stimulation
- Mindfulness through guided meditation

CANCER-ASSOCIATED VENOUS THROMBOEMBOLIC DISEASE

1. What are the risk factors for venous thromboembolism (VTE)?
- Clinical/medical factors
  - Active cancer, particularly advanced stage (i.e., metastatic disease)
  - Various higher risk cancer types: brain, pancreas, stomach, bladder, gynecologic, lung, lymphoma, myeloproliferative neoplasms, kidney
  - Bulky regional lymphadenopathy with extrinsic vascular compression
  - Hematologic predisposition: inherited and/or acquired hypercoagulable states
  - Medical comorbidities: infection, renal failure, pulmonary disease, heart failure
  - Older age
- Modifiable risk factors
  - Tobacco smoking
  - Obesity
  - Poor activity/exercise

- Treatment-associated risk factors
  - Major surgery
  - Indwelling central venous catheter(s)
  - Certain chemotherapeutic agents, that is, thalidomide/lenalidomide/poma-lidomide, especially in combination with dexamethasone
  - Exogenous hormonal therapy, including oral contraceptives and tamoxifen/raloxifene

TABLE 23.4 ■ Khorana Predictive Model for Chemotherapy-Associated VTE

Patient Characteristics	Risk Score
■ Site of primary cancer	2
• Very high risk (stomach, pancreas)	
• High risk (lung, lymphoma, gynecologic, renal, bladder, testicular)	
■ Prechemotherapy platelet count ≥350/microL	1
■ Hemoglobin <10 or use of erythropoietin stimulating agent (ESA)	1
■ Prechemotherapy leukocyte count >11 × 10⁹/L	1
■ BMI >35	1

Total Score	Risk Category	Approximate Risk of Symptomatic VTE
0	Low	0.3%–0.8%
1, 2	Intermediate	1.8%–2.0%
3 or higher	High	6.7%–7.1%

BMI, body mass index; ESAs, erythropoietin stimulating agents; VTE, venous thromboembolism.

2. When is inpatient pharmacologic VTE prophylaxis contraindicated?

- Absolute contraindications
  - Recent central nervous system (CNS) bleed
  - Intracranial or spinal lesion at high risk for bleeding
  - Major active bleeding, that is, >2 U packed red blood cells (PRBC) transfused in the past 24 hours
- Relative contraindications
  - Thrombocytopenia (<50,000)
  - Severe platelet dysfunction
  - Recent major surgery at high risk for bleeding

PAIN MANAGEMENT

1. What are the critical features of a comprehensive pain assessment?

- Interview the patient to characterize the distribution, quality, severity, and timing of the pain; discuss pain radiation if present. Identify factors that provoke or alleviate pain. If multiple sources of pain are present, each should be characterized separately.
- Identify psychosocial factors that may interfere with treatment of pain.
  - Concurrent mood disorders
  - Fear of addiction or death

- Social, financial, and spiritual stressors
- Prior abuse of alcohol, tobacco, opioids, or other substances
- Inspect and palpate the site of pain. Rule out referred pain or neurologic deficits.
- Reassess the patient regularly, especially when there is any change in quality or severity of pain, or more frequent use of as-needed opioid medications.
- Severe, uncontrollable pain is a medical emergency, specifically as it may indicate an acute underlying process such as fracture or deep tissue infection.

2. What is an appropriate approach to cancer pain management?

- Determine the likely mechanism of the pain. Many patients with cancer have pain that is not cancer-related and should NOT be treated with opioids.
- Determine if the patient is a good candidate for opioids. Patients should be able to take the medication responsibly. Patients with prior history of polysubstance abuse should be provided opioids in smaller quantities (1–2 weeks at a time) and be under close supervision/guidance with staff members.

TABLE 23.5 ■ Approach to Cancer Pain Management

		Immediate Prognosis	
		Good	Poor
Severity of cancer pain	Mild	NSAID and/or acetaminophen PRN	Dose-find with strong, short-acting opioid PRN; rotate to strong, short-acting PRN + long-acting opioid over time
	Moderate–severe	Strong, short-acting opioid PRN only	

3. What are opioid equivalences as compared with single-dose morphine?

TABLE 23.6

Drug	Parenteral Dose (mg)	Oral Dose (mg)	Factor (IV ≥ PO)	Peak	Duration of Action (Hours)	Starting IV Dose	Starting PO Dose
Morphine*	10	30	3	PO: 1.5–2 hr IV: 20 min	3–4	2–4 mg every 2–4 hr	15 mg immediate release every 4 hr
Hydromorphone	1.5	7.5	5	PO and IV: 1 hr	2–3	0.2–2 mg every 2 hr	2–4 mg every 4–6 hr
Fentanyl	100 mcg	–	–	IV: 1–5 min Transdermal: 24 hr	1–3	0.25–1 mcg/kg PRN	Transdermal: 12–25 mcg/hr every 72 hr
Levorphanol	2	4	2	PO: 1 hr IV: 20 min	3–6	1 mg every 3–6 hr	2 mg every 6–8 hr
Oxycodone	–	15–20	–	1–2 hr	3–5	–	5–10 mg every 4–6 hr

(continued)

TABLE 23.6 (continued)

Drug	Paren-teral Dose (mg)	Oral Dose (mg)	Factor (IV ≥ PO)	Peak	Duration of Action (Hours)	Starting IV Dose	Starting PO Dose
Hydrocodone	–	30–45	–	2 hr	3–5	–	5–10 mg every 4–6 hr
Oxymorphone	1	10	10	PO: 1 hr	3–6	0.5 mg every 4 hr	5–10 mg immediate release every 4 hr
Codeine	–	200	–	1.5 hr	3–4	–	30–60 mg every 4 hr
Tramadol	–	50–100	–		3–7	–	50–100 mg every 4–6 hr

*The conversion ratio of methadone to oral morphine equivalents is dose-dependent

4. What factors should guide opioid selection?

- Choice of opioid depends on the severity of the pain as well as the patient's past trials of opioids. Generally speaking:
  - Short-acting opioids are indicated for intermittent or breakthrough pain.
  - Long-acting opioids are indicated when the patient's short-acting opioids are being used in a continuous manner and are no longer providing adequate relief.
- Compounded opioids should be avoided in patients whose pain condition is likely to worsen over time as there is a ceiling level, preventing upward titration.
- Using long- and short-acting combinations with the same base opioid is recommended to make dose adjustments easier by providing overlapping analgesia.
- First-line:
  - Mild pain: hydrocodone
  - Moderate to severe pain: oxycodone or morphine
- Some situations merit specific opioids:
  - Poor compliance or mild cognitive impairment: transdermal fentanyl patch
  - Intractable constipation: transdermal fentanyl
  - Neurotoxicity: hydromorphone, oxycodone, or methadone
  - Renal impairment: buprenorphine, fentanyl, and methadone (if patient is not on dialysis); avoid morphine due to risk of metabolite accumulation
  - Liver impairment: oxycodone
  - Opioid tolerance: hydromorphone
  - Complex pain (with heavy neuropathic component): methadone

5. How do you initiate short-acting opioids?

- For patients who are opioid-naïve, begin opioids at the lowest recommended dose (see Table 23.6); consider even lower doses for older patients or patients with renal or liver disease.
  - Effectiveness of a given dose can be gauged within 1 hour of taking an oral opioid and 15 minutes of taking an IV opioid.

- For ambulatory patients with pain but not in crisis, start opioids as above and have them keep a diary, with short interval follow-up. When pain control is not achieved, increase dose in increments by 30% to 50%.
- For ambulatory patients in a pain crisis, start opioids as recommended above, have them keep a diary, and reassess within 24 hours. If pain is not controlled, increase dose by 100% and reassess again within 24 hours.
- Patients with malabsorption, intractable vomiting, or whose pain cannot be controlled at home with oral opioids should be admitted to the hospital for IV treatment.
- Consider early palliative care consultation for optimization of pain relief and quality of life throughout oncology care

6. How do you initiate long-acting opioids?
- Patients should not be started on a long-acting opioid without "dose finding" with a short-acting opioid first to determine the total daily dose (TDD). Consider using the same opioid in long- and short-acting forms for ease of dose adjustment.
- Once the TDD is known, divide the TDD by the number of times the patient will be taking the long-acting opioid per day. For example, for BID long-acting morphine, 50% of the TDD should be given in the morning and 50% of the TDD should be given in the evening.
- When converting a patient from one opioid to another (e.g., morphine to oxycodone), calculate the TDD of the initial opioid and convert to the equivalent TDD of the replacement opioid using the equianalgesic doses (see Table 23.3). Account for incomplete cross-tolerance by decreasing the TDD of the new opioid by 25% to 50%. Then, convert into long- and short-acting forms as indicated by pain control needs.

7. What is the appropriate dosing for breakthrough pain medication?
- Once patients are on a long-acting opioid, the short-acting breakthrough opioid should be dosed at 10% to 20% of the TDD.
  - For example, if a patient is taking 40 mg long-acting oxycodone twice daily, then an appropriate dose of breakthrough medication would be 5 to 10 mg oxycodone every 4 hours as needed.
- Oral opioids may be safely dosed as often as every 1 to 2 hours during a pain crisis.
  - Titration of medications during an inpatient stay is common.
  - Short-acting opioids given orally reach peak effect at 1 hour and last no more than 4 hours.

8. What are the common side effects of opioids?
- Constipation is very common across all opioids and does not improve with long-term dosing.
- Prevent constipation in patients on opioids by administering a motility agent (bisacodyl or senna) daily.
  - Titrate the dose every 2 to 3 days for a bowel movement at least once every 48 hours.
  - Avoid constipating agents (e.g., fiber, anticholinergics, haloperidol, calcium channel blockers, iron, anticonvulsants, ondansetron).
- Other side effects include delirium, myoclonus, urinary retention, sedation, nausea and vomiting, pruritus, and respiratory depression. Tolerance develops over time for all these effects, **except delirium, myoclonus, and urinary retention;** these side effects and hypersensitivity reactions often require hospitalization and switching to a different opioid.

9. **What are the risks of long-term opioid use?**
   - Addiction: Malingering for opioids is rare in patients with active cancer but can be seen among patients whose cancers are in remission, especially those with a preceding history of polysubstance abuse. Every effort should be made to titrate patients entirely off opioids once their cancer is in remission to prevent addiction.
   - Dependence: This manifests as withdrawal symptoms (nausea, chills, sweats) at cessation or dose reduction.
   - Tolerance: Patients taking opioids regularly develop tolerance; providers should expect that TDD will go up over time, even when disease is stable.
   - Hyperalgesia: This is increased pain sensitivity that develops with regular, long-term opioid use; precise mechanism is poorly understood; escalating the opioid dose may paradoxically increase the level of pain. Gradually reduce dose as tolerated.

10. **How does one terminate opioid therapy?**
    - Decrease TDD by 10% to 20% daily or more slowly if withdrawal develops.
    - Treat withdrawal: loperamide (for diarrhea), prochlorperazine (for nausea/vomiting), and clonidine (for sweats).

11. **What are examples of adjuvant analgesics?**
    - Anticonvulsant medications
      - Gabapentin, pregabalin, lamotrigine, topiramate, carbamazepine, valproic acid, and phenytoin
    - Antidepressants
      - Serotonin-norepinephrine reuptake inhibitor (SNRI), selective serotonin reuptake inhibitor (SSRI), and tricyclic antidepressant (TCA)
      - Useful as singular agents in patients without cancer
      - SNRIs such as duloxetine frequently utilized when the predominant aspect of pain is neuropathic
      - For patients with cancer, generally added once opioids have been initiated; patients should be monitored for anticholinergic side effects; avoid TCA use in the older adults.
    - Bisphosphonates
      - Pamidronate, ibandronate, and zoledronate
      - Effective for treating bone pain related to metastases (e.g., in multiple myeloma)
      - Also used to decrease the incidence of myeloma-related skeletal events in patients with existing skeletal lesions and those who are at increased risk for skeletal events (e.g., baseline osteopenia/osteoporosis)
      - Local anesthesia (e.g., lidocaine patch)
      - Effective for treating localized, superficial neuropathic and somatic pain syndromes
    - Corticosteroids
      - Effective for pain and weakness associated with nerve impingement or bony metastases
    - Antispasmodics (e.g., dicyclomine)
      - Effective for visceral pain
    - Interventional pain clinic
      - Institution-dependent; various modalities, including nerve/plexus blocks, infusion pumps, stimulation units, kyphoplasty/vertebroplasty, may be employed

12. **What are examples of nonpharmacologic pain therapy?**
    - Acupuncture
    - Relaxation/biofeedback
    - Recreation/art/music therapy
    - Transcutaneous electrical nerve stimulation
    - Myofascial trigger release
    - Massage
    - Behavioral counseling

CANCER CACHEXIA

1. **What is cancer cachexia?**
    - Cancer cachexia is characterized by loss of appetite, chronic nausea, fatigue, and weight loss, ≥5% decrease over 6 months. It is thought to be secondary to the following:
      - Proinflammatory cytokines (TNF, IL-1, IL-6, interferon [IFN]) lead to hypermetabolism and anorexia (from changes in ghrelin, leptin, and serotonin production and neuromodulation).
      - Tumor production of proteolysis-inducing factor and lipid-mobilizing factor causes fat and muscle loss.
      - Inefficient energy metabolism and insulin resistance lead to further lean body mass depletion.
    - Cancer cachexia is an independent predictor of early mortality.

2. **What are the appropriate interventions for anorexia/cachexia?**
    - Treat reversible causes.
      - Nausea and vomiting
      - Xerostomia, mucositis, dental caries/other issues, dysgeusia
      - Dysphagia, early satiety, bowel obstruction, constipation, pain with eating
      - Depression, anxiety
    - Identify endocrine abnormalities and treatment if present
    - Review and eliminate medications that interfere with appetite, provided that disease-modifying therapies (e.g., chemoimmunotherapy) are not withheld.
    - Identify food insecurity and other socioeconomic factors that may contribute to poor food intake; manage if present.
    - Nutritionists should be involved early and often to help identify barriers to increased intake or recommend dietary modifications.
    - Caloric supplementation:
      - Increased intake does not result in improved survival or tumor response.
      - Enteral feeding is preferred (less infection risk, decreased catabolic hormones, improved wound healing, shorter hospital stays, and maintenance of gut integrity).
      - Parenteral nutrition is rarely indicated unless patient is NPO for extended periods of time (e.g., during critical illness).
    - Pharmacologic interventions:
      - Metoclopramide helps treat nausea as well as delayed gastric emptying in patients who complain of early satiety. Monitor for extrapyramidal side effects (EPS).
      - Glucocorticoids help increase appetite but should only be utilized for short periods of time due to various long-term effects, including hyperglycemia and adrenal insufficiency.

- Megestrol is a synthetic progesterone formulation and is rarely effective if the patient has not responded to steroids in the past.
  - Do not administer megestrol concurrently with steroids.
  - Caution is advised in advanced malignancy as megestrol can increase the risk for thromboembolic disease.
- Mirtazapine may be utilized as an appetite stimulant.
- Dronabinol is not effective for increasing appetite in cancer patients.

DYSPNEA

1. **What is an appropriate approach to the management of dyspnea?**
   - First assess and identify for potentially reversible causes.
     - Infection: targeted antibiotics
     - Anemia: RBC transfusion
     - Bronchospasm: stabilization of airway, administration of bronchodilator
     - Pneumothorax: chest tube placement
     - Pulmonary embolism: anticoagulate if possible
     - Mechanical airway obstruction: stabilization of airway, consideration for bronchoscopy for mass identification; consideration for bronchodilators, antimuscarinics
     - Effusions (pleural and pericardial): evaluate with ultrasonography/echocardiography; drain if indicated
   - Relieve symptoms.
     - Nonpharmacologic
       - Fans (for patients without chronic obstructive pulmonary disease [COPD] or coronary artery disease [CAD]), cooler temperatures, stress management, and relaxation therapy
       - Supplemental oxygen for hypoxia (SaO_2 <90%) or subjective short-term palliation
       - Emotional, psychosocial, and educational support; utilize social workers, patient care advocates if needed
     - Pharmacologic
       - Low-dose opioids to reduce air hunger; morphine effective for symptomatic relief in this setting
       - Anxiolytics to reduce the anxiety that coexists with dyspnea (use with caution in patients who are taking concomitant opioids)
       - Expectorants (e.g., guaifenesin) to thin secretions
       - Antitussives (e.g., dextromethorphan, codeine, and hydrocodone) to reduce frequency of cough
       - Anticholinergics (e.g., atropine and hyoscine) to control secretions; avoid as concurrent therapy with other anticholinergics (e.g., long-acting muscarinic receptor antagonists) to prevent toxicity
     - Noninvasive positive pressure ventilation continuous positive airway pressure (CPAP) and bilevel positive airway pressure (BiPAP)

PSYCHIATRIC SYNDROMES

1. **What are the common psychiatric syndromes seen in cancer patients?**
   - Adjustment disorder
   - Major depression
   - Anxiety

- Delirium
- Drug toxicity

2. **What is adjustment disorder?**
   - Time-limited, maladaptive reaction to a specific stressor (e.g., cancer diagnosis and treatment)
   - Onset within 3 months of stressor, duration <6 months
   - Lack neurovegetative signs and suicidal ideation
   - Treatment directed at crisis intervention, brief psychotherapy, and symptom management

3. **What are the diagnostic criteria for major depressive disorder (MDD)?**
   - MDD is characterized by persistent low mood or anhedonia plus five of the following for at least 2 weeks:
     - Sleep disturbance
     - Loss of interest
     - Feelings of hopelessness, helplessness, or guilt
     - Low energy
     - Poor concentration
     - Appetite disturbance
     - Psychomotor retardation/agitation
     - Suicidal or homicidal ideation
   - Screen using the patient health questionnaire (PHQ)-2, assess and track symptoms using the PHQ-9
   - Consider pseudo-depression (see the following section)

4. **What are some causes of pseudo-depression?**
   - Uncontrolled pain
   - Hypothyroidism
   - Medications (steroids, certain chemotherapies such as interferon)
   - Metabolic abnormalities (electrolytes, B_{12}, or folate deficiency)
   - Organic brain disease (metastatic brain involvement, endocrinopathies, etc.)
   - Dementia
   - Substance abuse
   - Adjustment disorder
   - Fatigue
   - Personality disorders

5. **What is the treatment of MDD?**
   - Psychotherapy
   - Pharmacotherapy
     - SSRIs and SNRIs are especially useful in patients who also have neuropathic pain. It can take up to 8 weeks to see full benefit, and dosage escalations are commonly needed to reach desired therapeutic effect.
     - Methylphenidate has a shorter duration of action, but should be avoided in anyone who has insomnia, agitation, active CAD, or anxiety.
     - TCAs should be avoided in patients over age 65.
     - Mirtazapine is effective and should be considered for patients with cancer-associated anorexia and/or insomnia.
     - Antidepressants should be continued for 12 months from the point of remission if first episode of MDD.

6. What are commonly used antidepressants?

TABLE 23.7

Class	Name	Dose Range (mg)	Side Effects
SSRI	Fluoxetine	5–60	GI distress (denoted hereafter by "GI symptoms"), weight changes, sleep disruption, sexual dysfunction, dry mouth, hyponatremia, serotonin syndrome (if combined with other medications
	Paroxetine	10–60	
	Sertraline	12.5–200	
	Citalopram	10–60	
	Escitalopram	5–40	
Mixed agents	Venlafaxine	18.75–300	GI symptoms, sexual dysfunction, anticholinergic effects, hypertension with doses >225 mg, reduces hot flashes
	Bupropion	37.5–450	GI symptoms, tremor, lowers seizure threshold
	Duloxetine	20–60	GI symptoms, headache, dizziness; also indicated for neuropathic pain
	Mirtazapine	7.5–45	Sedation, dry mouth, increased appetite and weight gain
	Trazodone	25–200	Sedation, orthostatic hypotension, priapism
Tricyclic antidepressants	Amitriptyline	25–150	Dry mouth, sedation, weight gain, GI symptoms, EKG changes, orthostatic hypotension, anticholinergic effects
	Nortriptyline	25–150	
	Desipramine	25–150	
	Doxepin	25–150	
Psychostimulants	Methylphenidate	2.5–60*	Hypertension, tachycardia, anxiety
	Dextroamphetamine	10–60	

*For off-label use in depression, maximum dose is 20 mg and sustained release product is not recommended. For stimulant use, maximum daily dose is 60 mg.

SSRI, selective serotonin reuptake inhibitor.

7. What is the management of anxiety?
- Rule out reversible causes, manage as indicated.
  - Metabolic disturbances (e.g., hypercalcemia, hypoglycemia, and carcinoid syndrome)
  - Medications (e.g., thyroxine and phenothiazines)

- Nonpharmacologic treatment
  - Behavioral therapy, psychotherapy
- Pharmacologic treatment
  - Antidepressants (e.g., SSRIs and mixed agents)
  - Neuroleptics (e.g., Haloperidol and atypical antipsychotics) for severe and persistent anxiety
  - Other drugs: buspirone, propranolol (for autonomic symptoms), sedative hypnotics (for insomnia, avoid routine use)

8. What is delirium?
- Acute state characterized by inattention, fluctuating courses of cognitive impairment, perceptual disturbances, delusions, mood changes, and disruption of sleep–wake cycle
- May be hyperactive (agitated) or hypoactive

9. What is the management of delirium?
- Identify and treat precipitating factors
  - Direct CNS causes:
    - Brain solid tumor, metastases
    - Seizures
  - Indirect causes:
    - Metabolic encephalopathy
    - Electrolyte imbalance
    - Medications (steroids, narcotics, anticholinergics, antiemetics)
    - Infection
    - Hematologic abnormalities, including severe anemia and/or leukostasis
    - Nutritional deficiencies
    - Paraneoplastic syndromes
- Pharmacologic treatment:
  - Neuroleptics (e.g., haloperidol)
    - Side effects: sedation, EPS, hypotension, QT prolongation
  - Atypical neuroleptics (e.g., olanzapine, quetiapine, and risperidone)
    - Side effects: sedation, weight gain, metabolic syndrome, QT prolongation
  - Benzodiazepines (e.g., lorazepam, midazolam)
    - Should be avoided in patients with delirium
  - Palliative sedation (only for terminal delirium, with patient and/or surrogate consent)
    - Consider morphine, lorazepam
- Environmental modification:
  - Keep the environment calm and quiet with adequate indirect light during daytime hours.
  - Provide glasses or corrective lensing and hearing aids to maximize sensory perception.
  - Consider the use of night lights to combat nighttime confusion.
  - Use music which has an individual significance to the confused and agitated client to prevent the increase in or decrease agitated behaviors.
  - Minimize nighttime noises and television.

QUESTIONS

1. A 28-year-old otherwise healthy male presents with malaise and fever, and a routine complete blood count (CBC) reveals elevated white blood cells (WBCs) of 20 × 10⁹/L, a hemoglobin of 8.3 g/dL, and a platelet count of 58 × 10⁹/L. A peripheral smear reveals large, immature-appearing WBCs that are concerning for acute leukemia. Flow cytometry yields the diagnosis of acute lymphoblastic leukemia (ALL). After a thorough evaluation has been obtained, it is recommended that he begin induction chemotherapy with a pediatric-inspired protocol. What atypical infection does he require prophylaxis for?
   A. HIV
   B. Hepatitis C
   C. Pneumocystis pneumonia
   D. *Neisseria meningitidis*

2. You are attending on the inpatient hematology/oncology service and are taking care of a 66-year-old female with diffuse large B-cell lymphoma (DLBCL) status post her first cycle of R-CHOP chemotherapy. She presented 4 days ago with fever (Tmax 101.2°F) and was found to be neutropenic with absolute neutrophil count (ANC) of 0.4 × 10⁹/L. She complained of general malaise and myalgias but did not have any localizing symptoms. Chest x-ray and urinalysis at the time of admission were unremarkable. After blood cultures were obtained, she was started on empiric therapy with piperacillin-tazobactam. Vancomycin was then added given that she does have a port in place. It is now day 5 and she is still persistently febrile with Tmax of 100.9°F. Her vitals are otherwise stable and she continues to not have any localizing symptoms. Her cultures have thus far been negative. Her ANC is now 0.25 × 10⁹/L. What medication changes would you consider making next?
   A. Discontinue piperacillin-tazobactam and start meropenem.
   B. Add amikacin.
   C. Discontinue vancomycin and start daptomycin.
   D. Add fluconazole.

3. A 60-year-old male with history of stage 3 chronic kidney disease secondary to a history of poorly controlled type 2 diabetes as well as essential hypertension is started on "7+3" induction chemotherapy with daunorubicin and cytarabine for a newly diagnosed acute myeloid leukemia with t(8;21). His baseline labs include a white blood cell (WBC) count of 65 × 10⁹/L, hemoglobin of 8.9 g/dL, platelet count 45 × 10⁹/L, serum sodium of 138 mmol/L, serum potassium of 4.3 mmol/L, serum creatinine of 1.7 mg/dL, serum calcium of 9.7 mg/dL, serum phosphorus of 5.0 mg/dL, and serum albumin of 3.8 g/dL. He has already been started on intravenous (IV) fluids and allopurinol. 24 hours later, you note an improvement in his WBC to 25 × 10⁹/L, but his serum creatinine is now 3.5 mg/dL, serum potassium 6.0 mmol/L, serum calcium 7.4 mg/dL, and serum phosphorus 6.2 mg/dL. He continues to have adequate urine output and his physical exam does not reveal signs

of fluid overload. You check a serum uric acid, which was not checked at baseline, and it is 14 g/dL. What intervention should you consider?

A. Administer a 1-L bolus of normal saline.

B. Administer rasburicase.

C. Consult nephrology for initiation of dialysis.

D. Add febuxostat.

4. You are asked to evaluate a 35-year-old female in the ED. She is otherwise healthy and has no medical problems. Her only medication is a daily multivitamin. She presented for evaluation in the ED as she noted the development of a petechial rash in her bilateral lower extremities. She has also noted that her current menstrual cycle is characterized by significantly heavier bleeding without any personal history of menorrhagia. Routine blood work in the ED revealed a white blood cell (WBC) count of 8.5 × 10⁹/L, hemoglobin of 6.3 g/dL, and platelet count of 38 × 10⁹/L. Coagulation tests reveal that she has an elevated PTT and PT, as well as a low fibrinogen at 82 mg/dL. A serum pregnancy test is negative. You reveal the peripheral blood smear and see the presence of large, immature-appearing WBC with many dense blue cytoplasmic granules. The nuclei also appear to be bilobed. In addition to initiating supportive care, what other treatment would you recommend STAT?

A. Hydroxyurea

B. All-trans retinoic acid (ATRA)

C. Daunorubicin and cytarabine

D. Dexamethasone

5. A 63-year-old otherwise healthy female is referred to you for a new diagnosis of standard-risk immunoglobulin G (IgG) kappa multiple myeloma. This was recently diagnosed after she experienced pain in her right arm after a mechanical fall. An x-ray obtained at the time revealed the presence of a lytic lesion in her right humerus, which prompted further evaluation. A skeletal survey done as part of her evaluation revealed additional lytic lesions in her calvarium, left humerus, and right iliac bone. She is currently without any pain and does not use any analgesics. You recommend initiation of treatment with lenalidomide, bortezomib, and dexamethasone. In addition to discussing venous thromboembolism (VTE) prophylaxis and shingles prophylaxis, what other supportive measures would you recommend at this time?

A. Radiation to bone lesions

B. Prophylactic intravenous immunoglobulin (IVIG) infusions given her increased risk for infection

C. Initiation of bisphosphonates

D. Instruct to avoid exercise given that she has lytic lesions

6. You are seeing a 25-year-old female with hemoglobin SS disease. She is currently on oxycodone 5 mg as needed for pain control and is compliant with her hydroxyurea and folic acid supplementation. Her pain has been managed well as an outpatient and she is rarely admitted for pain crises. She reports that she is needing the oxycodone six times a day, which controls her pain at a 3/10 and which she states is

tolerable. She is on an appropriate bowel regimen and is not having any constipation. She is concerned about the frequency at which she is needing to take the oxycodone, especially as she wakes up at night to take her medication, and is inquiring regarding long-acting pain medication. You recommend:

A. MS Contin 30 mg every 12 hours with 5 mg oxycodone PRN for breakthrough
B. Oxycontin 15 mg every 12 hours
C. Oxycontin 15 mg every 12 hours with 5 mg oxycodone PRN for breakthrough
D. Oxycontin 30 mg every 12 hours with 5 mg oxycodone PRN for breakthrough

7. You are called by the ED to evaluate a 57-year-old, otherwise healthy male who was brought in for evaluation of progressive confusion. According to his wife, her husband had complained of a worsening generalized headache since yesterday and found him acutely confused this morning. He has no history of alcohol or substance abuse and had otherwise not had any complaints prior to this. In the ED, a routine complete blood count (CBC) showed a white blood cell (WBC) count of 112×10^9, hemoglobin of 11 g/dL, and platelet count of 89×10^9. The preliminary differential on the CBC reports 63% blasts. A CT of the head without contrast does not reveal any acute intracranial process. When you evaluate the patient at the bedside, he is difficult to arouse, unable to follow commands, and unable to cooperate with a neuro exam. His vital signs are otherwise stable. You review his peripheral smear under the microscope and the blasts appear to be consistent with acute myeloid leukemia (AML), without features to suggest acute promyelocytic leukemia (APL). In addition to recommending aggressive intravenous (IV) hydration, what other intervention should you consider for this patient at this time?

A. MRI of the brain with gadolinium
B. Administering hydroxyurea
C. Performing a lumbar puncture
D. Initiation of leukapheresis

8. You are seeing your patient who was recently diagnosed with stage III diffuse large B-cell lymphoma (DLBCL) receiving chemotherapy with R-CHOP. She is a 62-year-old female whose only other medical problem was a history of anxiety. She was very apprehensive to initiate chemotherapy given her concerns for side effects. You had received several calls given her concerns about nausea that were controlled with prochlorperazine and ondansetron. She is now in your office for evaluation prior to cycle 2 of chemotherapy. She states that she tolerated cycle 1 better than anticipated; no fevers, chills, and some mild fatigue that improved on its own. She did not have any emesis, and nausea was well controlled with around-the-clock prochlorperazine and ondansetron. She states that she is continuing to take those medications given her fear of nausea. Her chief concern today is constipation, reporting not having had a bowel movement for 3 days.

She states that this is very atypical for her. She does not take any opiate medications. In addition to her antiemetics, her only other medications are prednisone (as part of R-CHOP) and alprazolam. She has not noticed any significant change in her diet. Her vital signs are stable and her physical exam is otherwise benign. What is the most likely cause of her constipation?

A. Ondansetron
B. Large bowel obstruction
C. Side effect of chemotherapy
D. Alprazolam

ANSWERS

1. **C. Pneumocystis pneumonia.** The patient is receiving induction chemotherapy for ALL, which incorporates long-term use of high-dose steroids, especially in the pediatric-inspired protocols. Therefore, prophylaxis for pneumocystis pneumonia is indicated.

2. **D. Add fluconazole.** The patient is persistently febrile despite being on appropriate broad-spectrum antibiotics. It is appropriate to consider adding antifungal coverage in this patient given her increased risk for fungemia.

3. **B. Administer rasburicase.** The patient has evidence of tumor lysis syndrome with a rise in serum potassium and phosphorus, as well as a decrease in serum calcium. He is also noted to have a very elevated serum uric acid. His rising creatinine suggests that he is developing renal impairment, likely secondary to tumor lysis syndrome, compounded by poor baseline renal function. At this time, administering additional intravenous fluid (IVF) or adding febuxostat is not likely to significantly improve his renal function. He does not have any obvious indication for dialysis, although a nephrology consultation should be considered if his renal function continues to deteriorate. Administering rasburicase should be considered in this patient to reduce serum uric acid, thereby limiting further damage to the renal tubules.

4. **B. All-trans retinoic acid (ATRA).** The patient presents with classic findings suspicious for acute promyelocytic leukemia (APL), including the finding of disseminated intravascular coagulation (DIC) on blood work, as well as blasts with bilobed nuclei and cytoplasm filled with dense granules, which are likely Auer rods. The initiation of timely therapy is crucial for the outcomes of these patients. In addition to treating the DIC, the patient should also be started on ATRA. She should have a thorough evaluation, including diagnostic testing that will confirm the diagnosis of APL, but one should not wait for the results of these studies prior to initiation of ATRA.

5. **C. Initiation of bisphosphonates.** Initiate bisphosphonates following dental evaluation. Bisphosphonates are indicated to decrease the incidence of myeloma-related skeletal events, especially as this patient already has known lytic lesions. Radiation is currently not indicated as the patient is asymptomatic; should the patient develop significant pain associated with her bone lesions, radiation can certainly be considered. While patients with multiple myeloma are considered immune-compromised, there is no role for treatment with intravenous immunoglobulin (IVIG) (which is sometimes considered in chronic lymphocytic leukemia [CLL]). Finally, there is no evidence to suggest that exercise increases the risk of adverse skeletal events, especially as this patient will be starting on a bisphosphonate.

6. **C. Oxycontin 15 mg every 12 hours with 5 mg oxycodone PRN for breakthrough.** To convert from short-acting opioids to long-acting opioids, you calculate the total daily dose (TDD) and divide it by the frequency

at which it will be taken. In the example of this patient, her TDD of oxycodone is 6 × 5 mg = 30 mg. Oxycontin is prescribed every 12 hours, so her a.m. and p.m. doses should be 15 mg. While BID oxycontin may be sufficient for her pain control, breakthrough short-acting pain medications at 10% to 20% of her TDD are still recommended. Finally, if possible, the long-acting and short-acting formulation should be of the same opioid.

7. **D. Initiation of leukapheresis.** This patient's altered mental status is likely due to leukostasis which he is at risk for given his elevated WBC in the setting of likely a new diagnosis of AML. Signs and symptoms of leukostasis are attributable to increased viscosity and resultant vascular occlusion. It is important to avoid leukapheresis in patients with APL as this increases their risk for hemorrhage. Patients receiving leukapheresis should be monitored closely given the risk for development of disseminated intravascular coagulation (DIC).

8. **A. Ondansetron.** Ondansetron is a first-generation 5-HT3 receptor antagonist. This class of drugs is very effective for the treatment of chemotherapy-induced nausea and vomiting (CINV). However, a known side effect is constipation, which can be severe. It is very important when starting patients on these medications to educate them on preventing constipation (i.e., increased fiber intake, appropriate bowel regimen). In the case of this patient, she is continuing to take her ondansetron well after the expected time frame of CINV and it is important to discuss with her how to appropriately take this drug.

Transfusion Medicine: Indications for Using Blood Products and Risks Associated With Blood Products

Laura Cooling

Pretransfusion Testing and Compatibility

- A type and screen has three components: ABO type, RhD type, and antibody screen.
- A type and screen sample is good for only 3 days. A current type and screen is required to dispense blood products for transfusion.

ABO BLOOD GROUP

- ABO are carbohydrate antigens expressed by glycoproteins and glycolipids on red cells and other tissues.
- The *ABO* gene codes for a glycosyltransferase that adds either a galactose (B antigen) or N-acetylgalactosamine (GalNAc; A antigen) to the H (O) fucose antigen precursor (Table 24.1). Group O is autosomal-recessive due to null *ABO* alleles.
- ABO antibodies are naturally occurring IgM against the missing group A or group B antigen on RBC (Table 24.2). ABO antibodies are capable of fixing complement with hemolysis.
- ABO typing requires testing red cells for A and B antigens and plasma for ABO antibodies.
- The RBC and plasma typing must agree for a valid ABO type. Patients with missing or extra reactivity are supported with group O RBC pending investigation and resolution in the laboratory. Cold autoantibodies, ABO-mismatched stem cell transplants, and intravenous immunoglobulin (IVIg) can cause ABO discrepancies.

TABLE 24.1 ■ ABO Antigen Structure and Expression on Red Cells

ABO Antigen	Dominant Sugar	Structure	RBC Expression
H	Fucose	**Fucose** (1,2) Galactose-	Group O
B	Galactose (Gal)	**Galactose** (1,3) Galactose- ↑ (1,2) Fucose	Group B, AB
A	N-acetylgalactosamine (GalNAc)	**GalNAc** (1,3) Galactose- ↑ (1,2) Fucose	Group A, AB

RBC, red blood cell.

ABO COMPATIBILITY BY BLOOD COMPONENT

- Donor RBC must be compatible with patient plasma (Table 24.2).
- Donor plasma (fresh frozen plasma, FFP) must be compatible with patient red cells.
- Whole blood must be the same ABO type (identical) as patient ABO.
- Donor platelets (PLT): ABO compatibility is preferred but not required. When possible, it should be the same ABO type as the patient. PLT in additive solution (PAS-PLT) has minimal donor plasma, ABO titers <1:8, and can be considered "plasma compatible."
- Donor cryoprecipitate: ABO compatibility is preferred but not required.

TABLE 24.2 ■ ABO Reactions and Blood Product Compatibility

Patient Testing			Blood Product Compatibility		
ABO Type	RBC Antigen	Plasma Antibody	RBC	FFP	WB
A	A	Anti-B	A, O	A, AB	A
B	B	Anti-A	B, O	B, AB	B
AB	A, B	None	A, B, AB, O	AB	AB
O	H	Anti-A, Anti-B	O	O, A, B, AB	O

FFP, fresh frozen plasma; RBC, red blood cell; WB, whole blood.

Rh BLOOD GROUP

- The Rh system contains two related genes, RHD and RHCE, that are inherited as a haplotype and show ethnic differences between Blacks, Whites, and Asians. There are >50 Rh antigens.
- Rh-positive red cells express the RhD protein. There is <u>NO</u> RhD protein on Rh-negative red cells. Only 15% Whites, 8% Blacks, and 1% Asians are Rh-negative.
- RhD-negative individuals are at risk of making anti-D if exposed to Rh-positive red cells. Rh-negative women receive prophylactic RhIG to prevent anti-D formation during pregnancy.
- Extended Rh phenotyping refers to typing for C,c,E,e antigens on RhCE protein.
- RHD and RHCE genes can recombine to form hybrid RHD-RHCE alleles, also known as partial D phenotypes. Partial D phenotypes are not uncommon in Black populations. Patients with partial D can make alloantibodies to missing, high-incidence Rh antigens and require Rh-negative RBC. In some cases, donor RBC must be matched for Rh at the molecular level.
- The weak D phenotype arises from point mutations that decrease RhD expression. Most weak D phenotypes can be transfused with Rh-positive RBCs.

RhD COMPATIBILITY FOR TRANSFUSION

- Rh compatibility required only for RBC transfusions and products >2 mL RBC contamination
- RhD-negative patients = Rh-negative RBC
- RhD-positive patients = Rh-positive or Rh-negative RBC
- Partial D = Rh-negative RBC (may require molecular-matched donor RBC)

- Confirmed weak D = Rh-positive or Rh-negative RBC
- Rh-positive RBC administered to Rh-negative males and postmenopausal women in trauma/massive transfusion scenarios

ANTIBODY SCREEN

- Purpose: Identify red cell alloantibodies in patient plasma that could react with donor RBC.
- Method: Patient plasma is incubated against two to three group O red cells, followed by addition of antihuman globulin (AHG). The antibody screen is an indirect antiglobulin test (IAT).
- The antibody screen may be positive due to RBC alloantibodies, autoantibodies, and drug-associated antibodies. A positive screen requires antibody identification using at least 10 group O phenotyped red cells.
- Significant RBC alloantibodies cause hemolysis, hemolytic disease of the fetus and newborn (HDFN), and shortened red cell survival. Common blood group facts are listed in Table 24.3.
- Several therapeutic drugs used in hematology can cause a positive antibody screen (Table 24.4).

TABLE 24.3 ■ Some Clinically Relevant RBC Antibodies

Blood Group	Comments
Rh (RhD, RhCE)	Rh antibodies are clinically significant.
	Anti-C, Anti-E are common in Blacks, who tend to be Dce (Ro) Rh phenotype.
	Recombinant RhD and RhCE alleles are not uncommon in Blacks.
	Rh null is rare with stomatocytes, mild hemolytic anemia.
Kell (KEL)	Only 10% of the population is K1-positive. Anti-K1 is a common alloantibody.
	Anti-K1 can cause a reticulocytopenic HDFN in pregnancy.
	Kell glycoprotein is linked to Kx protein in red cell membrane. Loss of Kx is associated with McLeod phenotype, acanthocytosis, chronic granulomatous disease, and neuromuscular disorders.
Kidd (Jk^a, Jk^b)	Clinically significant, including intravascular hemolysis (*Kidd Kills*).
	Rapid evanescence and may disappear within months after transfusion.
	It is the most common cause of delayed hemolytic transfusion reactions.
Duffy (Fy^a, Fy^b)	Clinically significant (*Duffy Dies*).
	Most Blacks type Duffy null (Fy [a-b-]) but are genetically Fy^b+, due to an erythroid-specific mutation in a GATA promoter. Duffy null is associated with benign ethnic neutropenia and *Plasmodium vivax* resistance.
MNS (MN, SsU)	Reside on glycophorin A and B.
	Antibodies against S,s,U antigens are clinically significant.
	1% of Blacks are U-negative and require rare blood.

(continued)

TABLE 24.3 ■ Some Clinically Relevant RBC Antibodies (*continued*)

Blood Group	Comments
Dombrock (Do)	Antibody can be clinically significant with hemolysis, short RBC survival.
	Anti-Dombrock antibodies are found in highly alloimmunized patients and difficult to identify (e.g., sickle cell patients).
I	Common, low-titer IgM isoagglutinin. High-titer anti-I is seen in cold autoimmune hemolytic anemia.
P	Auto-anti-P is seen in PCH. Auto-P in PCH is a biphasic hemolysin and diagnosed with the Donath–Landsteiner test.

HDFN, hemolytic disease of the fetus and newborn; IgM, immunoglobulin M; PCH, paroxysmal cold hemoglobinuria; RBC, red blood cell.

TABLE 24.4 ■ Hematologic Drugs That Cause a Positive Antibody Screen

Drug Class	Comments
Anti-CD36 (Daratumumab)	CD36 weakly expressed on red cells; antibody identification requires DTT-treated panel cells for testing; patients should be Kell (K1) phenotyped prior to starting drug
Anti-CD47	CD47 on RBC and platelets; associated with hemolytic anemia and thrombocytopenia
Checkpoint inhibitors (anti-PD1, PDL1, CTLA-4)	Stimulate autoantibodies, autoimmune hemolytic anemia; also associated with ITP and hemophagocytic syndrome
Gamma globulin (IVIG)	Passive infusion of ABO antibodies, other alloantibodies
RhIG	Passive infusion of anti-D

CTLA-4, cytotoxic T-lymphocyte-associated antigen 4; DTT, dithiothreitol; ITP, idiopathic thrombocytopenia purpura; PD-1, programmed cell death protein; PDL1, programmed death-ligand 1.

Red Blood Cell Crossmatching

- ABO/Rh compatibility and crossmatching are necessary for RBC and any blood components containing >2 mL red cell contamination (granulocytes, bone marrow, pooled PLTs).
  - Positive history/presence of alloantibodies: antigen-negative, IAT-crossmatch RBC
  - No history/evidence of alloantibodies: confirm ABO compatibility only using electronic crossmatch (barcodes on blood units) or immediate-spin crossmatch (patient plasma against donor RBC).

- Emergency release refers to release of RBC before completion of full testing due to urgent medical need.

EXTENDED ANTIGEN MATCHING

- Match donor RBC beyond ABO and RhD antigens.
  - Known red cell·alloantibodies requiring antigen-negative RBC
  - Prophylactic matching to prevent alloimmunization in sickle cell disease and thalassemia.
    - Minimum matching Rh (DCcEe) and Kell (K1)
    - Extended match for Duffy (Fy), Kidd (Jk), and Ss in high-risk patients

BLOOD COMPONENTS

BLOOD COMPONENT COLLECTION AND STORAGE

- Blood products can be processed from whole blood donations or by single donor apheresis. Human leukocyte antigen (HLA) PLTs, granulocytes, and peripheral blood stem cells can only be collected by apheresis.
- Blood products have different storage requirements (Table 24.5). Most RBCs today are stored in additive solutions and can be stored for 42 days at 1°C to 6°C.
- FFP outdates within 24 hours of thawing. FFP can be relabeled "thawed plasma" and stored for 5 days at 4°C. Thawed plasma inventories are used in trauma and massive transfusion.
- Cryoprecipitate is manufactured by thawing FFP at 4°C. Several units (5–10) of cryoprecipitate are pooled to achieve a therapeutic dose of fibrinogen in adults.
  - Calculate the amount of cryoprecipitate to pool based on patient weight and plasma volume.
  - Fibrinogen dose = (desired increase in fibrinogen [mg/dL]) x (mL plasma volume ÷ 100 [mL/dL])
    Plasma volume = (70 mL/kg) x patient weight (kg) × (1 – hematocrit [Hct])
    Number of cryo units pool = fibrinogen dose (mg) ÷ 250 (estimated mg fibrinogen per unit).
- PLTs can be single donor by apheresis or isolated from whole blood using buffy coat or PLT-rich plasma methods (random PLTs).
- Apheresis PLTs contain >3 x 10^{11} PLT per unit.
- Whole blood-derived PLT contains >5.5 × 10^5 PLT per unit.
  - A standard adult dose is 5 pooled PLT units (United States) or 4 units (Canada).
  - Pooling under closed sterile conditions by the blood supplier has a 5-day outdate (prepooled PLT). Pooled PLTs prepared by hospital blood banks expire within 4 hours.
- PLTs are stored at room temperature with agitation to promote gas exchange. PLTs can be stored for 5 days or up to 7 days, if units are tested daily for bacteria after day 4 of storage.
- Granulocytes are stored at room temperature without agitation and outdates in 24 hours.

TABLE 24.5 ■ Blood Product Storage and Contents

Component	Collection	Storage Temperature	Storage Outdates	Content Per Unit
RBC	Whole blood Apheresis	1–6°C	42 days*	~200 mL packed RBC
FFP/FP-24	Whole blood apheresis	≤ –18°C	1 year (24 hours thawed)	1 unit/mL factors
Platelets	Whole blood apheresis	22°C–24°C	5 days	>3 × 10^{11} PLT
Cryoprecipitate	FFP thawed at 4°C overnight	≤ –18°C	1 year (6 hours thawed)	~80–120 U FVIII >150 mg fibrinogen ~20%–30% FXIII ~40%–70% vWF
Granulocytes	Apheresis	22°C–24°C	24 hours	>1 × 10^{10} neutrophil
Stem cells (cryopreserved)	Bone marrow apheresis	–150°C	>10 years	>2 × 10^6/kg recipient for transplant

*Depends on the anticoagulant used. RBC in CPD (21 days, 80% Hct), RBC in CPDA (35 days), and RBC in additive solutions (AS; e.g., Adsol) are 42 days (55%–65% Hct).

CPD, citrate phosphate dextrose; CTPDA, citrate phosphate dextrose adenine; FFP, fresh frozen plasma; FVIII, factor 8; FXIII, Factor 13; Hct, hematocrit; PLT, platelet; RBC, red blood cell; vWF, von Willebrand factor.

ADULT BLOOD PRODUCT DOSING

- Blood transfusion must be tailored to the patient. Some general guidelines used in clinical practice are shown in Table 24.6.
- Fluids compatible with blood products are saline, plasmanate, and 5% albumin. Do not infuse blood products with hypotonic solutions, Ringer's (contains calcium), 5% dextrose, and drugs.
- Unless active bleeding, prophylactic PLT transfusion is contraindicated in TTP, HIT, posttransfusion purpura (PTP), and ITP. In PTP and ITP, transfusion to raise PLT count is futile and may delay recovery (PTP). In TTP and HIT, PLT transfusion rarely increases PLT count and may provoke thrombotic events.

TABLE 24.6 ■ Common Clinical Indications and Dosing for Blood Products in Adults

Product	RBC	Platelets	FFP/Plasma	Cryoprecipitate
Indication	Hgb <7 inpatient Hgb <8 outpatient Hgb <10–11 ECMO, congenital heart disease	PLT <10K prophylactic PLT <20K risk bleeding due to infection, DIC, etc. PLT <30K defibrotide PLT <50 bleeding PLT <80–100K ECMO, cardiovascular surgery, neurosurgery	PT >1.5× normal *and* active bleeding *or* bleeding risk due to procedure TTP apheresis	Low fibrinogen (<100 mg/dL) Historically, FXIII deficiency vWF deficiency

(continued)

TABLE 24.6 ■ Common Clinical Indications and Dosing for Blood Products in Adults (*continued*)

Product	RBC	Platelets	FFP/Plasma	Cryoprecipitate
Dose	1 unit	1 apheresis unit	10–20 mL/kg	Pool 5–10 units
Routine	3–4 mL/min	10 mL/min	10 mL/min	10 mL/min
Infusion	1.5–2 hr/unit	20–30 min/unit	20–30 min/unit	15 min/pool unit
Response	1 g Hgb/unit RBC	25K-50K increase PLT at 1-hour posttransfusion	↑ clotting factors >20%	10-unit pool will ↑ fibrinogen 50–100 mg/dL

DIC, disseminated intravascular coagulation; ECMO, extracorporeal membrane oxygenation; FFP, fresh frozen plasma; Hgb, hemoglobin; HIT, heparin-induced thrombocytopenia; ITP, idiopathic thrombocytopenia purpura; PLT, platelet; PT, prothrombin time; PTP, post-transfusion purpura; RBC, red blood cell; TTP, thrombotic thrombocytopenia purpura; vWF, von Willebrand Factor; VXIII, factor 13.

BLOOD PRODUCT MODIFICATIONS

1. Leukoreduction (LR)
■ LR is the removal of residual donor white blood cell (WBC) in cellular components (RBC, PLT) by filtration.
■ LR is defined as less than 5 million WBC per unit. Current filters decrease WBC $< 10^5$ to 10^6/unit.
■ LR-RBC and LR-PLT are "CMV-safe" for cytomegalovirus (CMV)-negative patients.
■ LR decreases the risk and incidence of HLA alloimmunization and febrile reactions.

2. Irradiation
■ Irradiation prevents transfusion-associated graft versus host disease (TA-GVHD) due to engraftment of residual donor WBC in cellular components (RBC, PLT). FFP and cryo are not irradiated.
■ Indications for irradiation:
  ● Hematologic malignancy
  ● Hematopoietic stem cell transplantation (HSCT)
  ● Fludarabine, antithymocyte globulin (ATG), other lymphodepleting chemotherapy
  ● Other malignancy receiving multiagent, high-dose chemotherapy
  ● Aplastic anemia
  ● Congenital cellular immunodeficiency
  ● Premature, low birthweight infants
  ● HLA-matched PLTs
  ● Directed-donor blood (RBC, PLT) from first-degree relatives
  ● Granulocytes
■ Solid organ transplant patients, most nonheme cancers, hemoglobinopathy, and HIV patients do not require irradiated blood products. Stem cells for transplant must NOT be irradiated.
■ Irradiation damages RBC membranes and decreases storage time and survival. Irradiation should not be used in sickle cell and other patients requiring lifelong transfusion support unless indicated.

3. **Pathogen reduction (PR)**
   - PR treatment inactivates DNA to prevent transfusion-transmitted diseases (TTD), including bacteria, viruses, and parasites. PR also inactivates donor WBC and is equivalent to irradiation to prevent TA-GVHD. PR is limited to PLTs, plasma and cryoprecipitate at this time. PR-RBC is in clinical trials.

4. **Washed products**
   - Wash RBC and PLT to remove donor plasma in limited situations. Washed components are considered no longer sterile and have shortened outdate (RBC = 24 hours; PLTs <4 hours).
   - Indications for washed RBC or PLT:
     - Severe congenital immunglobulin A (IgA) deficiency (IgA <0.5 mg/dL)
     - Repeated severe allergic reactions despite aggressive premedication
     - RBC transfusion in posttransfusion purpura (PTP)—PLT transfusion should be avoided
     - Directed-donor maternal PLT in neonatal alloimmune thrombocytopenia (NAIT)

SPECIALTY PRODUCTS

1. **Granulocytes**
   - Granulocytes are collected by apheresis from steroid ± granulocyte colony stimulating factor (G-CSF)-stimulated volunteer donors.
   - Granulocytes must be ABO/Rh-, crossmatch-, and CMV-compatible with the patient.
   - Granulocytes must be irradiated. Granulocytes must not be leukoreduced.
   - Granulocyte indications:
     - Severe neutropenia (absolute neutrophil count [ANC] <500/microL) with expectation of marrow recovery *and* either
       - Documented persistent bacteremia despite antibiotic treatment for >48 to 72 hours, *or*
       - Documented fungal infection
     - Severe resistant bacterial infection in patients with congenital neutrophil defects
   - High risk for stimulating HLA and granulocyte-specific alloantibodies and severe pulmonary reactions, especially in HLA alloimmunized patients and patients on intravenous (IV) antifungal medication

2. **PLT refractoriness**
   - Persistent failure to respond to PLT transfusion as measured by the 1-hour posttransfusion corrected count PLT increment (CCI). Most PLT refractoriness is nonimmune (50%) or mixed nonimmune and immune (25%).
   - Laboratory studies: 1-hour posttransfusion PLT counts, class 1 HLA antibody screen percent panel reactive antibody (%PRA). The patient's HLA type or a PLT crossmatch using patient serum against donor PLTs. If the PLT crossmatch is positive with a negative HLA-PRA, consider testing for PLT-specific antibodies.
   - Diagnosis of PLT refractoriness:
     - CCI <7 in three consecutive transfusions or majority of five transfusions. The CCI includes the PLT posttransfusion increment, patient size (body surface area, [BSA]), and the number of PLTs transfused.

$$CCI = \frac{(\text{Post-PLT count} - \text{Pre-PLT count}) \times (\text{Patient BSA, M}^2)}{(\text{Total number of PLT transfused } [\times 10^{11}])}$$

Example: A large patient (BSA = 2.5 m^2) was transfused with 1-unit apheresis PLT containing 3.3×10^{11} PLT, with a rise in PLT count from 5K/mcL to 17K/mcL at 1-hour posttransfusion. The CCI = (17 − 5) × 2.5 divided by 3.5. The CCI = 8.6, which is a good response to transfusion.

- HLA-selected PLTs: Limited HLA antibodies (HLA-PRA <70%–80%) can receive PLTs that are negative for specific HLA antigens (HLA antigen-negative). Severe HLA alloimmunization requires HLA-matched PLTs, which are limited <3% of HLA-typed apheresis donors.
- Crossmatched PLTs: Patient plasma is crossmatched against donor apheresis PLTs by microtiter or flow cytometry methods. Crossmatched PLTs are as efficacious as HLA-selected PLTs and helpful as a bridge while awaiting HLA testing. Drugs (ATG, anti-CD47), HLA, PLT, and ABO antibodies can result in a positive PLT crossmatch.

ADVERSE EVENTS FROM TRANSFUSION

Acute transfusion reactions occur during or within 4 to 6 hours of transfusion.

1. **Acute hemolytic transfusion reaction (AHTR)**
   - AHTR is complement-mediated intravascular hemolysis usually due to ABO as a result of mislabeled specimen. Rarely, AHTR can occur with PLTs (group O PLT to group A patient).
   - Incidence is 1:40,000, fatal 1:1.8 million.
   - Symptoms include fever (typically within 15 minutes and >2°C rise in temperature), chills, nausea, pain at the flank/chest/abdomen or IV site, hypotension, anxiety, and hemoglobinuria. In anesthetized patients, hemoglobinuria and hypotension may be the only signs of AHTR.
   - Potential complications include acute kidney injury (30%), disseminated intravascular coagulation (DIC; 8%), shock, and death.
   - Diagnostic laboratory studies include direct antiglobulin test (DAT), lactate dehydrogenase (LDH), haptoglobin, bilirubin (direct, indirect), urinalysis for hemoglobinuria, peripheral blood smear, and complete blood count (CBC). The DAT may be negative in the setting of brisk hemolysis. Renal function and coagulation studies should also be followed.
   - Diagnosis requires both laboratory findings and exclusion of nonimmune causes for hemolysis.
   - Treatment is normal saline to maintain urine output of 100 mL/hour for the first 24 hours. Diuretics may be used to promote diuresis. Blood products may be required for DIC and bleeding. Heparin (5,000 U bolus) has been used in severe DIC with refractory bleeding in this setting.

2. **Febrile nonhemolytic transfusion reaction (FNHTR)**
   - FNHTR is defined as >1°C in temperature above 37°C with no other identifiable cause for fever.
   - Incidence is 0.1% to 1%. It is most common with RBC and PLT transfusion due to passive infusion of WBC-derived cytokines during storage. It is a diagnosis of exclusion.
   - Treatment is antipyretics. Patients with repeated FNHTR will benefit from premedication. Risk may be decreased with prestorage-leukoreduced RBC and PLT

3. Allergic transfusion reaction
- Incidence is 1% to 3% mild reactions and 1:20,000 to 50,000 anaphylactic reactions.
- It is most common with plasma and PLTs. Atopic patients are at increased risk.
- It is usually due to patient antibodies against protein alloantigens or soluble substances in donor plasma. PLTs also release cytokines (RANTES) during storage that promote allergic reactions.
- Mild allergic reactions include rash, urticaria and pruritus usually located on the face, trunk, and extremities.
- Severe allergic reactions include angioedema, nausea/vomiting, abdominal pain, diarrhea, bronchospasm, hypotension, shock, and death. There is no fever (COLD SHOCK).
- Mild reaction treatment includes antihistamines. Unit can be restarted if symptoms resolve.
- Severe reaction treatment includes antihistamines and steroids, supplemental O_2, and fluids as necessary. Escalation to beta-agonists and epinephrine as needed. Do not restart unit.
- Anaphylactoid reactions should be evaluated for possible severe congenital deficiencies in IgA (IgA <0.05 mg/dL) and haptoglobin (rare, Asians). Severe IgA deficiency requires washed RBC and PLT. IgA-deficient plasma is only available through rare donor registries.

4. Transfusion-associated circulatory overload (TACO)
- TACO has an incidence of 1% and is higher in at-risk populations.
- TACO is more likely to occur with RBC transfusion and massive transfusion scenarios. Risk factors are older age, severe anemia, heart failure, renal insufficiency, and large volume transfusion.
- Symptoms include dyspnea, cough, orthopnea, tachycardia, hypertension, and headache.
- Diagnosis is by chest x-ray, positive fluid balance, and elevated B-type natriuretic peptide (BNP) from pretransfusion (>1.5 increase, BNP >100 pg/mL).
- Treatment includes diuretics, sitting the patient upright, and supplemental O_2 as appropriate. For subsequent transfusions, decrease volume and infusion rates (1 mL/kg/hour), and prophylactic diuretic use.

5. Transfusion-related acute lung injury (TRALI)
- Incidence 1:190,000; mortality as high as 10%
- Acute, noncardiogenic, pulmonary edema within 6 hours of transfusion
- New bilateral pulmonary edema, hypoxemia (PaO_2/FiO_2 <300 mmHg, SpO_2 <90%), no evidence of elevated left hypertension and exclusion of other causes of acute respiratory distress syndrome (ARDS)
- Multiple etiologies:
  - Infusion of HLA (class 1 or 2) or granulocyte-specific donor antibodies reactive against recipient WBC and pulmonary endothelium
  - Oxidation of RBC and PLT membranes with generation of bioactive phospholipids (PAF-like) capable of activating neutrophils
  - PLT–neutrophil interaction with formation of neutrophil extracellular traps (NET)
  - Patient risk factors: infection/pneumonia, recent surgery, and G-CSF; underlying patient morbidities may prime neutrophils and increase risk for TRALI (two-hit hypothesis)

- Treatment is supportive, including possible intubation. It usually resolves within 48 to 72 hours. Diuretics should be avoided since patients are intravascularly depleted with third spacing of fluids.
- Blood supplier should be notified in suspected TRALI cases. It requires investigation of the donor and quarantine of all other components from that donor located at other hospitals.
- Mitigation: Historically, TRALI is associated with multiparous female donors. Currently, all FFP is from male donors only. PLT donors are screened for history of pregnancy or transfusions, followed by HLA antibody testing.

6. Hypotensive reaction
- This is an abrupt decrease in systolic blood pressure (>30 mmHg) within 15 to 30 minutes of starting a transfusion. Patient may have concurrent hypoxia, fever, flushing, and abdominal pain.
- Symptoms resolve within minutes of stopping transfusion, with no further intervention. Blood must NOT be restarted due to risk of recurrent symptoms.
- Etiology is accumulation of bradykinin in the unit. Angiotensin-converting enzyme (ACE) inhibitors may increase risk.
- Hypotensive reactions are also seen in apheresis, extracorporeal membrane oxygenation (ECMO), and cardiac bypass due to bradykinin generation in the circuit. Blood pressure recovery can be prolonged in these settings.

7. Septic reaction/bacterial contamination
- PLTs are most susceptible to bacterial growth because they are stored at room temperature.
  - Contamination is usually by gram-positive skin organisms (*Streptococcus, Staphylococcus, Cutibacterium*).
  - Contamination is linked to older units near outdate (>4 days).
  - Symptoms range from asymptomatic to febrile reactions.
- RBC units are rarely linked to septic reactions due to 4°C storage.
  - Contamination is by gram-negative organisms, especially *Yersinia, Serratia,* and *Pseudomonas*.
  - Septic reactions are more common in older units (>25 days old).
  - Symptoms are endotoxic shock with high fever (>2°C), dyspnea, hypotension, and shock.
  - Septic RBC transfusion reactions have a high morbidity and mortality rate.
- Colonized indwelling catheter central venous catheter (CVC), peripherally inserted central catheter (PICC): There is risk of bacteremia with infusion of blood products through colonized line. It is more common than contamination of blood products.
- Diagnosis is by Gram stain and positive culture of transfused unit. Same organisms should be isolated from the patient. If blood is transfused through indwelling catheter (CVC), exclude line contamination. New posttransfusion elevated WBC and procalcitonin can be early indicators.
- Treatment is supportive and by broad-spectrum antibiotics to cover gram-positive (PLTs) and gram-negative (RBC) organisms pending bacterial identification and sensitivity testing.
- Suspected bacterial contamination must be reported immediately to the blood supplier. Other blood components from the donor/donation must be removed and quarantined.

■ Mitigation measures to prevent bacterial contamination include donor history and physical, skin decontamination prior to phlebotomy, delayed LR to allow neutrophils to phagocytize bacteria, 7-day culturing of apheresis PLTs, and now PR.

DELAYED TRANSFUSION COMPLICATIONS OCCURRING DAYS TO YEARS AFTER TRANSFUSION

1. Red cell alloimmunization
■ Formation of new red cell alloantibodies (7–14 days)
■ Restimulation of preexisting, evanescent alloantibodies (<7 days; e.g., anti-Kidd [Jk]-"Kidd Kills" recur within 48 hours of transfusion)
■ Delayed hemolytic transfusion reaction (DHTR); hemolysis usually extravascular
■ Hyperhemolysis rare; known risk in highly alloimmunized sickle cell and thalassemia patients; characterized by brisk hemolysis, reticulocytopenia, and post-transfusion hemoglobin lower than pretransfusion hemoglobin; additional RBC transfusion can exacerbate hemolysis and is discouraged

2. PLT alloimmunization
■ HLA alloimmunization
■ PLT-specific alloantibodies
● PTP: onset of severe thrombocytopenia 7 to 14 days after transfusion; treated with IVIG; prophylactic PLT transfusion contraindicated unless bleeding; apheresis contraindicated
● NAIT: fetal thrombocytopenia due to maternal alloantibodies; mother treated with IVIG during pregnancy
● HPA-1A (PL^{A1}) most common PLT-specific alloantibody in Whites; anti-CD36 more common in Asians and Blacks due to CD36 deficiency
■ HLA and PLT-specific antibodies: can cause immune PLT refractoriness

3. TA-GVHD
■ Rare; prevented by irradiation (RBC, PLT) in at-risk individuals (see the "Irradiation" section)

4. Iron overload
■ Risk >15 to 20 units of RBC transfused; patients require chronic RBC transfusion support.
■ Monitor serum ferritin. Total iron stores are monitored based on liver iron by MRI, where T2* >20 msec at risk for cardiac dysfunction.
■ Treatment is iron chelation and phlebotomy.

5. TTD
■ All blood donors are screened for TTD at every donation (Table 24.7).
● Donor History Questionnaire (DHQ)
● Donor laboratory testing by PCR/NAT (nucleic acid testing) or serology (antibody, Ab) for HIV, HCV, HBV, HTLV, syphilis, *Trypanosoma cruzi*, West Nile virus, Zika virus, and *Babesia* (PCR in 14 states designated as endemic areas)

TABLE 24.7 ■ Donor Testing for Infectious Disease and Residual Risk

Potential TTD	Donor Testing	Estimated Residual Risk
HIV (1, 2)	HIV Ab, HIV PCR	1:1.5 million
HCV	HCV-NAT, anti-HCV	1:1.1 million
HBV	HBSAg, anti-HBc, HBV-NAT	1:1.2 million
CMV	Anti-CMV	<1:1 million
HTLV (1,2)	Anti-HTLV-1/2	<1:1 million
West Nile virus	PCR	Rare
Zika virus	PCR	Rare
Trypanosoma cruzi	Anti-T. cruzi	1:42,000
Syphilis	RPR	Rare
Bacteria	Culture (platelets)	1:100,000 apheresis platelet with no pathogen reduction
CJD, vCJD	None	Rare, no cases in the United States
Babesia	(endemic areas)	1:18,000–1:100,000
Malaria	None	Rare

Ab, antibody; CJD, Creutzfelt-Jakob disease; HBV, hepatitis B virus; HCV, hepatitis C virus; HTLV, human T-cell leukemia virus; NAT, nucleic acid test; PCR, polymerase chain reaction; RPR, rapid plasma reagin; TTD, transfusion-transmitted disease; vCJD, variant CJD.

- Additional mitigation strategies to prevent TTD:
  - Leukoreduction (CMV-safe)
  - Testing PLTs for bacterial contamination during storage
  - Pathogen reduction (PR-PLTs, PR-RBC in trial)
  - Pooled plasma derivatives (IVIG, albumin): require donor testing and DHQ at donation, plus several viral inactivation steps during manufacturing

APHERESIS

- Apheresis refers to centrifugal separation and collection of blood components. Apheresis is used for therapeutic indications and donor blood collection (Table 24.8).
- Acid-citrate-dextrose (ACD-A) is the standard anticoagulation used during the procedure.
- Indications for apheresis are available from the American Society for Apheresis (ASFA).

TABLE 24.8 ■ Apheresis Procedures

Procedure	Description	Indications
Therapeutic plasma exchange	Removal of patient plasma and replacement with 5% albumin or plasma	TTP, CAPS, hyperviscosity, some autoimmune disorders, acute humoral rejection

(continued

TABLE 24. 8 ■ Apheresis Procedures (*continued*)

Procedure	Description	Indications
Plasmapheresis	Removal of plasma with no replacement fluids	Donor apheresis
Red cell exchange	Removal of patient red cells and replacement with donor RBC	Sickle cell disease ■ Chronic exchange ■ Acute chest, stroke
Plateletpheresis	Removal of patient (or donor) platelet; no replacement fluids	Apheresis platelets Thrombocytosis (>1 million platelet/mcL)
Leukocytapheresis	Removal of patient (or donor) leukocytes; no replacement fluids	Hyperleukocytosis with hyperviscosity (e.g., AML), granulocyte collection, stem cell collection, MNC collection (CART)
Photopheresis	Collection and UV irradiation of patient MNC, followed by reinfusion	Cellular GVHD following stem cell or solid organ transplant, including bronchiolitis obliterans in lung transplant, Sézary syndrome

AML, acute myeloid leukemia; CAPS, catastrophic antiphospholipid syndrome; CART, chimeric antigen receptor T-cell; GVHD, graft-versus-host disease; MNC, mononuclear cell; RBC, red blood cell; TTP, thrombotic thrombocytopenia purpura.

COMPLICATIONS OF APHERESIS

1. **Citrate toxicity/hypocalcemia**
   - Perioral and extremity paresthesia, feelings of "vibrating", chills, abdominal pain/cramping, carpopedal spasm/tetany, lightheadedness, hypotension, prolonged QTc, arrhythmia
   - Risk of citrate toxicity highest in leukapheresis and therapeutic plasma exchange (TPE) using plasma replacement
     - Leukapheresis involves processing 2 to 3 blood volumes and 1 to 2 L citrate anticoagulant.
     - Plasma also contains citrate (1 gm/unit FFP).
   - Treatment: pause procedure, administer calcium (IV better than oral); if symptoms persist despite calcium replacement, check ionized Ca++ and magnesium levels
   - Prevention: Prophylactic calcium replacement through separate IV line; common practice in leukapheresis and TPE using plasma replacement; may be necessary in some patients undergoing TPE with albumin replacement: albumin also binds calcium ions

2. **Hypotension due to fluid shifts, citrate, dilutional anemia, vasovagal reactions, and ACE inhibitors/hypotensive reaction (should be held 24 hours prior to apheresis)**

3. **Coagulopathy due to citrate, loss of clotting factors (TPE), and PLTs**
   - Average PLT loss is 20% per procedure for TPE and 30% to 50% for leukapheresis.
   - Clotting factors should recover within 24 to 48 hours after apheresis and normal liver function.

4. **Transfusion reaction when using plasma or RBC replacement fluids**

5. **Venous access complications**

6. **Ethylene oxide (ETO) hypersensitivity reaction (rare)**
   - Acute allergic reaction within 15 to 20 minutes of starting the procedure; ETO used to sterilize apheresis kits can elute during saline priming of tubing sets
   - Atopic individuals and patients/donors with history of repeated apheresis procedures at risk
   - Treat per allergic reactions; double-prime apheresis tubing and premedicate for future procedures

7. **Air embolism (rare)**
   - Risk with all rapid infusion devices including apheresis
   - Acute pain, cough, cyanosis, arrythmia, shock, and cardiac arrest
   - Patient placed head-down on the left side to dislodge air from pulmonary valve

QUESTIONS

1. **A 65-year-old woman with acute myeloid leukemia is undergoing induction chemotherapy. She is requiring both red blood cell (RBC) and platelet transfusion support. The patient has persistently low platelet counts (platelet 3000/microL) despite twice a day platelet transfusion. Which of the following is an appropriate next step?**
   A. Order a 1-hour post-platelet count after each subsequent platelet transfusion.
   B. Order crossmatched platelets.
   C. Order HLA-selected platelets.
   D. Request that the patient's daughter donate apheresis platelets for their mother (directed-donor platelets).

2. **A 25-year-old patient with sickle cell disease is admitted with an acute pain crisis. She is treated with hydration, opioids for pain control, and was transfused 2 units of red blood cell (RBC) for hemoglobin (Hgb) of 6.5 g/dL. She is group B+ with a history of an anti-Fyᵃ alloantibody. Transfused RBCs were B+, matched for Rh, K, Fy(a) antigens (negative for C, E, K, Fyᵃ), and crossmatch-compatible by the indirect antiglobulin test (IAT). Her hemoglobin rose to 8.5 g/dL posttransfusion but then abruptly decreased (Hgb=5 gm/dL) 3 days later with worsening hemolysis. Which of the following actions is contraindicated in this clinical setting?**
   A. Order a direct antiglobulin test (DAT, direct Coombs) and repeat type and screen.
   B. Order a reticulocyte count and hemoglobin electrophoresis.
   C. Administer steroids.
   D. Order emergency transfusion of 2 units, ABO/Rh-compatible RBC to correct her anemia.

3. Which of the following blood products should be irradiated?
   A. Red blood cells (RBCs) for a kidney transplant recipient
   B. RBC for a sickle cell patient
   C. HLA-matched platelets for a cardiac surgery patient
   D. Plasma for an aplastic anemia patient

4. A 25-year-old, group A, Rh-negative male presented with petechiae and nosebleeds approximately 4 weeks after infection with Covid-19. His complete blood count (CBC) showed a normal white blood cell (WBC) count, hemoglobin, low platelets (5000/microL), and markedly elevated reticulated platelets (% immature platelet fraction [IPF] = 30%). He was subsequently diagnosed with acute idiopathic thrombocytopenia purpura [ITP] and treated with steroids and high-dose intravenous immunoglobulin (IVIG; 2 gm/kg over 2 days). On hospital day 4, he required 2 units of group AB apheresis platelets for a severe nosebleed. On hospital day 5, his laboratories showed a decrease in hemoglobin (Hgb 14 → 11 gm/dL), haptoglobin <10 gm/dL, indirect bilirubin of 11 gm/dL, and positive DAT (immunoglobulin G [IgG] = 3+, C3 = 2+). What is the most likely cause of hemolysis in this patient?
   A. Platelet transfusion
   B. High-dose IVIG
   C. Disseminated intravascular coagulation (DIC)
   D. Steroid-induced hypertension

5. A 40-year-old group O, cytomegalovirus (CMV)-negative man with acute myeloid leukemia (AML) is admitted for a haploidentical, related stem cell transplant. His transplant course has been complicated by delayed engraftment with prolonged pancytopenia and *Aspergillus* pneumonia. The transplant team has requested granulocyte transfusions. Which of the following is NOT true regarding granulocyte transfusion in this patient?
   A. The donor must be ABO/Rh-compatible and the granulocyte product must be crossmatched with the patient.
   B. The granulocyte donor may be either CMV-negative or CMV-positive.
   C. Granulocytes must be irradiated.
   D. Granulocytes are stored at room temperature and must be infused within 24 hours of collection.

6. A 45-year-old man with confusion, microangiopathic hemolytic anemia, and low ADAMTS13 activity (<5%) was admitted for thrombotic thrombocytopenia purpura (TTP) and therapeutic plasma exchange. During his second procedure, he developed nausea and complained that his legs felt "funny and numb." What is the most logical next step in managing the patient?
   A. Administer intravenous (IV) fluids for hypovolemia.
   B. Order a brain MRI for a possible stroke.
   C. Pause the procedure and administer calcium.
   D. Reassure the patient that his symptoms are due to TTP and will resolve with time.

ANSWERS

1. **A. Order a 1-hour post-platelet count after each subsequent platelet transfusion**. The patient may be either refractory to platelets or have platelet consumption with short survival. A poor 1-hour post-transfusion corrected platelet count increment (CCI <7) after three successive or the majority of five platelet transfusions will confirm platelet refractoriness. The next steps could include a trial of either crossmatched platelets or HLA-selected platelets, if the patient has known HLA antibodies. If the patient is highly HLA alloimmunized (percent reactive antibody [PRA] >80%), a trial of HLA-matched platelets is appropriate. It is not appropriate for her daughter to donate directed-donor platelets. Her daughter is a potential donor for any future haploidentical stem cell transplant. In addition, her daughter cannot support her platelet transfusion needs due to donor limits on the number and frequency of platelet donations per year (24/year). Finally, if the patient is HLA-alloimmunized, she was likely sensitized during pregnancy and her daughter is HLA-incompatible.

2. **D. Order emergency transfusion of 2 units, ABO/Rh-compatible RBC to correct her anemia**. This patient likely has hyperhemolysis. A characteristic finding is a posttransfusion hemoglobin that is lower than the pretransfusion hemoglobin. Ordering a DAT and type and screen is appropriate since hyperhemolysis may be triggered by a delayed hemolytic transfusion reaction due to a new red cell alloantibody (>7 days posttransfusion) or an amnestic response with reemergence of an alloantibody (<7 days). In addition, hyperhemolysis is often associated with a fall in reticulocyte count. A hemoglobin electrophoresis often shows hemolysis of the patient's RBC with a rise in HgbA (donor RBC). Further RBC transfusions can worsen hyperhemolysis and are discouraged. RBC transfusions should only be administered for hemodynamic instability after approval by a hematologist.

3. **C. Human leukocyte antigen (HLA)-matched platelets for a cardiac surgery patient.** HLA-matched platelets must be irradiated due to the risk of transfusion-associated graft versus host disease (TA-GVHD), regardless of the patient's underlying diagnosis. Although aplastic anemia patients are at risk for TA-GVHD and should receive irradiated cellular components (RBC, platelets), plasma and cryoprecipitate are acellular and do not need irradiation. Organ transplant recipients, most adult solid organ cancers, and sickle cell patients are not at risk for TA-GVHD. Furthermore, in sickle cell disease, irradiation may lead to decreased RBC survival due to damage and increasing stiffness of RBC membranes.

4. **B. High-dose IVIG.** IVIG contains ABO antibodies and can lead to ABO-mediated intravascular hemolysis. Group A and AB patients receiving high-dose IVIG are most susceptible. Hemolysis has been reported after transfusion of ABO plasma-incompatible platelet transfusions; however, the platelets transfused were group AB, which lacks ABO antibodies and is plasma-compatible with the patient (group A). DIC and severe hypertension are not associated with positive DAT.

5. **B. The granulocyte donor may be either CMV-negative or CMV-positive.** The recipient is CMV-negative and at risk for transfusion-associated cytomegalovirus infection (TA-CMV). Because granulocytes cannot be leukoreduced to make them "CMV-safe," the donor must also be CMV-negative. Granulocytes contain >10^8 lymphocytes and must be irradiated. Granulocytes contain >2 mL red blood cells (RBC) and must be ABO/Rh- and crossmatch-compatible with the patient.

6. **C. Pause the procedure and administer calcium.** Citrate is used for anticoagulation during apheresis and is also present in plasma (1 g citrate per unit). Citrate symptoms are those of hypocalcemia due to chelation of calcium ions. Treatment is calcium replacement (IV preferred). The procedure is typically paused for a short period to allow distribution of calcium and metabolism of citrate.

Introduction to Bone Marrow Transplantation

25

Marcus Geer and Monalisa Ghosh

1. **What are the indications for hematopoietic stem cell transplantation?**
   - Blood-forming stem cells can be used for treatment of hematologic malignancies such as myeloproliferative neoplasms, myelodysplastic syndrome, acute leukemia, and relapsed lymphomas. They can also be used for treatment of aplastic anemia and bone marrow failure syndromes.

2. **What do the terms *allogeneic stem cell transplantation* and *autologous stem cell transplantation* mean?**
   - Allogeneic: Allogeneic stem cell transplantation refers to transplantation where the donor cells **do not** come from the recipient. This strategy is commonly utilized in the setting of diseases such as myelodysplastic syndrome or acute leukemia, among others. The goal of this approach is to use the donor immune system to achieve a so-called graft versus leukemia effect to detect and kill malignant cells.
   - Autologous: Autologous stem cell transplantation refers to transplantation where the transplanted cells are harvested from the recipient. This strategy is used when the goal is to deliver high-dose chemotherapy to the patient with subsequent transplantation utilized to rescue the hematopoietic system. Graft versus leukemia effect is not the goal of this transplantation approach. This treatment is used in multiple myeloma, difficult-to-treat lymphomas, and sometimes testicular cancer.

3. **What are the sources of stem cells and progenitor cells for hematopoietic stem cells (HSC) transplantation?**
   - Donor sources
     - Bone marrow or peripheral blood stem cells (PBSCs) can be obtained from matched sibling, matched unrelated, or haploidentical donors.
     - Umbilical cord blood can be obtained from donors.
   - Bone marrow
     - Collection of stem cells from the bone marrow is a more invasive procedure compared with collection of stem cells from other sources.
     - Engraftment usually occurs between 18 and 21 days after transplantation.
     - Collection process:
       - Collection occurs in the operating room under general anesthesia.
       - Both posterior iliac crests are used to collect 50 to 100 aspirations on each side.
       - The goal is to collect at least 2×10^8 nucleated marrow cells per kilogram body weight of the recipient.
   - Peripheral blood
     - Collection of stem cells from peripheral blood is as less invasive procedure than collection of stem cells from bone marrow.

- Engraftment usually occurs between 12 and 15 days after transplantation when using fully human leukocyte antigen (HLA)-matched donors. Engraftment occurs a few days later when using a haploidentical donor.
- Peripheral blood grafts contain more T-cells than bone marrow collections.
- Collection process:
  - Granulocyte colony-stimulating factor (G-CSF) at a dose of 10 mcg/kg once daily is usually used to mobilize HSCs from the bone marrow.
  - PBSCs are collected by apheresis starting on day 5 of G-CSF injections.
  - The adequacy of the collection is determined by measuring the absolute number of CD34+ cells per kilogram of recipient body weight.
  - The minimal acceptable dose is usually $>2 \times 10^6$ CD34+ cells per kilogram of recipient body weight for adults (maximum of $8–9 \times 10^6$ CD34+ cells per kilogram of recipient body weight).
  - The optimal dose is $\geq 4 \times 10^6$ CD34+ cells per kilogram of recipient body weight.
  - Some studies have shown that doses of $>8 \times 10^6$ CD34+ cells per kilogram are associated with high rates of chronic graft versus host disease (GVHD) in matched sibling donor allogeneic transplants.
  - There is no evidence of additional benefit from doses $>9 \times 10^6$ CD34+ cells per kilogram in matched unrelated donor allogeneic transplants.
  - Higher doses of CD34+ cells are associated with earlier engraftment.
  - Lower doses of CD34+ cells are correlated with delayed platelet recovery.
  - If insufficient numbers of CD34+ cells are collected, then plerixafor (CXCR4 antagonist) can be used for further mobilization.
- Umbilical cord blood
  - Collection and procurement of umbilical cord blood is the easiest among the available graft options.
  - Engraftment time is variable but is generally longer than engraftment after using bone marrow or PBSC sources. Platelet recovery often takes longer.
  - It contains fewer T-cells than PBSC collections. Often, only a 4/6 HLA match is needed.
  - The risk of infection is higher because immune cells from umbilical cord blood (UCB) are immunologically naïve and CD8+ T-cell recovery is delayed compared with patients receiving bone marrow or PBSC transplant.
  - Collection process:
    - Umbilical cord blood is rich in HSCs.
    - Cells are collected from umbilical blood vessels in the placenta during delivery, then cryopreserved for future use.
    - Each collection tends to have a relatively smaller number of HSCs compared with other sources. Therefore, to obtain enough HSCs for an adult, two sources of cord blood are usually needed.
    - The optimal collection is approximately 2.5×10^7 total nucleated cells per kilogram of recipient body weight or $\geq 2 \times 10^5$ CD34+ cells per kilogram of recipient body weight.
    - If there is HLA mismatch, then higher cell doses are needed.
      - 5/6 HLA match: $>4 \times 10^7$ nucleated cells per kilogram of recipient body weight
      - 4/6 HLA match: $>5 \times 10^7$ nucleated cells per kilogram of recipient body weight

- Comparison of stem cell sources
  - Engraftment
    - PBSCs engraft more rapidly than bone marrow.
    - Engraftment time is variable for umbilical cord stem cells.
  - GVHD
    - PBSC collections can have 10-fold higher amounts of T-cells than marrow collections.
    - GVHD, especially chronic GVHD, occurs at higher rates in allogeneic transplants using PBSCs than in allogeneic transplants using bone marrow.
    - Umbilical cord collections have fewer T-cells. Rates of GVHD are lower than in transplants using PBSCs.
  - Graft versus tumor effect
    - There is increased graft versus tumor effect in allogeneic transplants using PBSCs than in allogeneic transplants using bone marrow due to the increased number of T-cells in PBSC collections.
  - Survival
    - Overall, there is not much evidence of difference in survival rates in patients receiving transplants with bone marrow versus PBSCs or umbilical cord blood cells.

4. How do the recipient and donor cells interact?

- Recipient immune system
  - If the recipient's immune system is intact, the recipient T-cells and NK cells will reject the allograft (donor cells).
  - Pretransplant conditioning of the recipient with chemotherapy and/or radiation plus posttransplant immunosuppression is used to keep the recipient's immune system from rejecting the allograft.
- Allograft
  - Donor T-cells help facilitate HSC engraftment.
  - Depletion of T-cells from the allograft results in increased rates of graft rejection and decreased graft versus tumor effect.
- HLA matching
  - HLAs are encoded on chromosome 6.
    - Major histocompatibility complex (MHC)
      - Class I
        - HLA-A, HLA-B, HLA-C
        - Present on all cells
      - Class II
        - DR, DQ, DP, DM, DO
        - Present on immune antigen-presenting cells
    - Minor histocompatibility antigens
      - Also play a role in alloimmune response
  - The chance that a full sibling matches to a recipient is slightly less than 25%.
  - Matched unrelated donors:
    - Match at HLA-A, HLA-B, HLA-C, DRB1, and DQB1
    - More likely to be a mismatch at minor histocompatibility antigens
      - Increased risk of GVHD
      - Increased chance of graft-versus-tumor (GVT)

- Graft versus tumor effect
  - Graft T-cells and NK cells recognize residual host tumor cells and eradicate them.
    - CD8+ cytotoxic T-cells recognize tumor antigens in the context of MHC class 1 antigens.
    - CD4+ T-cells recognize tumor-associated antigens in the context of MHC class II antigens.
      - Th1 cytokines, such as IFN-γ and IL-2, upregulate the expression of class I MHC antigens and promote expansion and activation of CD8+ cytotoxic T-cells.
    - NK cells recognize stress ligands and cells lacking MHC expression.
  - T-cell depletion of allograft increases the rate of relapse.
  - Donor lymphocyte infusions consisting primarily of T-cells are often used to treat relapsed malignant disease after allogeneic transplantation.
- GVHD
  - GVHD develops dues to a complex interaction of donor T-cells in the allograft and host antigens.
  - T-cells in the allograft target the MHC molecules of the recipient.
  - T-cells in the allograft become activated by antigen-presenting cells, T-cell receptor and MHC interactions, and interaction with vascular endothelial cells.
  - Damage to host tissues from chemotherapy and radiation helps potentiate the activation of donor T-cells.
  - Activated T-cells and other immune cells release inflammatory cytokines such as tumor necrosis factor-alpha, IL-6, and IL-1, which mediate the graft versus host reaction, leading to tissue damage and inflammation.
  - GVHD can be treated with suppression of the host immune system and activated T-cells by using immunosuppressive and T-cell targeted drugs.

QUESTIONS

1. **A 40-year-old man presents for consideration of allogeneic stem cell transplant for high-risk acute myeloid leukemia. Which of the following factors would increase his risk of developing graft versus host disease (GVHD) following transplant?**
   A. Peripheral blood stem cell graft
   B. Use of a matched unrelated donor
   C. Use of a multiparous female donor
   D. Use of myeloablative conditioning regimen
   E. All of the above

2. **Which of the following factors is least likely to influence selection of a stem cell donor?**
   A. Cytomegalovirus (CMV) seronegative
   B. Advanced age
   C. ABO mismatch
   D. Human leukocyte antigen (HLA) compatibility

3. A 56-year-old woman of Hispanic ethnicity presents for discussion of allogeneic stem cell transplant for refractory acute lymphoblastic leukemia. She has no eligible sibling donors. An unrelated donor is available that is an 7/8 human leukocyte antigen (HLA) match. Abatacept is chosen for graft versus host disease (GVHD) prophylaxis. What is the target of abatacept?
   A. PDL1
   B. ROCK2
   C. CD80/CD86
   D. IL-1

4. Compared with other allogeneic stem cell donor sources, use of umbilical cord blood is associated with:
   A. Higher rates of graft versus host disease
   B. Longer duration of neutropenia
   C. Lower overall survival
   D. Higher rates of infection related mortality

5. A 34-year-old patient is receiving total body irradiation as part of myeloablative conditioning prior to allogeneic stem cell transplantation for acute myeloid leukemia. Which of the following is true regarding the use of total body irradiation (TBI)?
   A. Use of TBI is associated with lower rates of acute graft versus host disease (GVHD).
   B. Doses up to 18 Gy are generally well-tolerated.
   C. Lung shielding eliminates the risk of irreversible lung injury.
   D. Tolerability is improved with dose fractionation.

6. A 28-year-old patient is undergoing an allogeneic hematopoietic stem cell transplant for refractory Hodgkin lymphoma. Which donor/recipient serologic pairing confers the highest risk of cytomegalovirus (CMV) reactivation?
   A. CMV−/CMV−
   B. CMV−/CMV+
   C. CMV+/CMV−
   D. CMV+/CMV+

7. Which of the following methods of donor stem cell collection results in a product with the most T-cells?
   A. Bone marrow aspiration
   B. Peripheral blood apheresis
   C. Umbilical cord blood collection

8. The human leukocyte antigens (HLAs) are encoded on chromosome 6 and include class I (HLA-A, B, C) and class II (HLA-DR, DQ, DP, DM, DO) molecules. The chance that a full sibling is an exact HLA match is approximately:
   A. 12.5%
   B. 25%
   C. 50%
   D. 75%
   E. 100%

ANSWERS

1. **E. All of the above.** Compared with bone marrow or umbilical cord blood grafts, peripheral blood stem cell grafts contain a higher proportion of donor lymphocytes, increasing the risk of subsequent GVHD. Use of matched unrelated donors, especially when sex-mismatched with a multiparous female donor to a male recipient, confers higher risk than a related counterpart. Use of myeloablative conditioning causes increased tissue damage and antigen exposure, making it more likely to trigger a subsequent GvHD response.

2. **C. ABO mismatch.** ABO and Rh mismatch between donor and recipient is not prohibitive to moving forward with stem cell transplant. Use of ABO-mismatched grafts are associated with increased risk of hemolytic reactions and red cell aplasia. Use of an HLA-matched graft from a younger donor has been shown to have a linear relationship with improved outcomes.

3. **C. CD80/CD86.** Abatacept (CTLA4-IgG) was initially approved for management of rheumatologic diseases and acts by interrupting the costimulatory signaling between CD28 and CD80/CD86. Following the ABA2 study, abatacept obtained Food and Drug Administration (FDA) approval for GvHD prophylaxis to be given in combination with methotrexate and a calcineurin inhibitor.

4. **B. Longer duration of neutropenia.** Use of umbilical cord blood grafts is associated with higher rates of graft failure and longer cytopenias compared with bone marrow and peripheral blood grafts. Given the longer rates of neutropenia, there is a corresponding increase in the number of infections posttransplant. However, there is not an increase in infection-related mortality, and overall survival of patients is similar to other donor sources.

5. **D. Tolerability is improved with dose fractionation.** Total body irradiation-based conditioning is associated with a higher degree of tissue damage, which contributes to increased rates of GVHD and other transplant-related complications. Doses of 10 to 14 Gy are typically used in clinical practice. Mitigation efforts such as hyperfractionated dosing and lung shielding have improved tolerability, but there remains a significant risk for organ toxicity.

6. **C. CMV+/CMV−.** CMV serologic status of both the donor and the recipient is incorporated into the selection of potential stem cell donors given the significant risk of CMV reactivation posttransplant. Recipient CMV seropositivity with a naïve donor immune system confers the greatest risk for reactivation; however, prophylactic antiviral letermovir can be used to reduce the risk pharmacologically.

7. **B. Peripheral blood apheresis.** Peripheral blood collections have 10-fold higher amounts of T-cells than marrow collections. Umbilical cord blood has fewer T-cells compared with peripheral blood collections. The higher

amounts of T-cells are thought to contribute to higher rates of graft-versus-host disease (GVHD) seen in donations from peripheral blood collections compared with bone marrow collections.

8. **B. 25%.** Each individual has two HLA haplotypes. Thus, offspring from two individuals have a 25% chance of sharing the same two haplotypes, 50% chance of sharing one haplotype, and 25% of sharing no haplotypes.

Hematopoietic Cell Transplant in the Management of Hematologic Disease

26

Samuel B. Reynolds and Mary Mansour Riwes

1. What are the different types of hematopoietic cell transplantation (HCT) and how are they subclassified?

TABLE 26.1

Modality	**Autologous**
	Collection of patient's own hematopoietic stem cells for later transplant into the same patient
	Allogeneic
	Transplantation of stem cells from an HLA-matched donor
	Syngeneic
	Transplantation of stem cells from an HLA-identical donor, i.e., monozygotic twins

Allogeneic HCT only:

Donor source	**Matched related**
	Achieved when a related donor is at least an 8/8 HLA match with recipient (meaning identical HLA-A, HLA-B, HLA-C, and HLA-DRB1 loci). Please note that the HLA-DQB1 and HLA-DP1 loci may also be present for a 10/10 or 12/12 match, respectively.
	Matched unrelated
	Unrelated donor is at least an 8/8 HLA match with the recipient; commonly abbreviated as "MUD."
	Mismatched
	Donor is less than an 8/8 HLA match with the recipient.
	Haploidentical
	A related donor is mismatched at as many as 3/6 HLA loci (HLA-A, HLA-B, and HLA-DR).
	Umbilical cord blood
	Stem cells collected from umbilical cord and placenta after an infant is born. Immaturity of this immune environment allows for level of HLA mismatch that would otherwise be prohibitive from other sources. Requires at least 4/6 HLA match, including at loci HLA-A, HLA-B, and HLA-DRB1; ≥4/8 match with HLA-A, HLA-B, HLA-C, and HLA-DRB1 is also acceptable.

(continued)

TABLE 26.1 *(continued)*

Stem cell source	**Peripheral blood stem cells** Stem cells are collected from donor using peripheral blood pheresis. Stem cells are mobilized using either a chemokine-based, chemotherapy-based regimen, or a combination of both. **Bone marrow** Hematopoietic stem cells are collected directly from the bone marrow, generally in the operating room under general anesthesia. Preprocedure mobilization is not typically employed.
Preparative regimen	**Myeloablative** Conditioning regimen is expected to destroy stem cells with usually irreversible and often fatal pancytopenia unless rescued with HCT. A commonly used regimen is total body irradiation ≥5 Gy in a single dose of busulfan >8 mg/kg (myeloablative regimens containing busulfan are generally >8 mg/kg). **Nonmyeloablative** Conditioning regimen with less cytopenia but with significant lymphopenia; does not require stem cell rescue. One example: fludarabine 30 mg/m²/day and cyclophosphamide 750 mg/m²/day 4–7 and 5 days prior to transplant (respectively) with total body irradiation (TBI) ≤2 Gy. **Reduced intensity** Intermediate between myeloablative and nonmyeloablative. For example, busulfan ≤8 mg/kg or melphalan ≤140 mg/m².

HCT, hematopoietic cell transplantation; HLA, human leukocyte antigen; TBI, total body irradiation.

2. **How many HCTs occur in the United States yearly?**
   - Between 2016 and 2020, nearly 66,000 autologous and over 45,000 allogeneic transplants were performed in the United States.
   - Among allogeneic transplants, unrelated donors were the most common, followed by human leukocyte antigen (HLA)-matched siblings and other related donors.

3. **What are the indications for an autologous stem cell transplant?**
   - Malignant (cancerous) conditions
     - Myeloma
       - Again between 2016 and 2020, over 38,000 autologous stem cell transplants were performed for myeloma in the United States.
       - Evidence supports autologous HCT following induction chemotherapy for all eligible patients with symptomatic myeloma, both for standard and high-risk disease. Melphalan is a commonly used conditioning regimen.
     - Other plasma cell dyscrasias
       - Autologous HCT can also be considered for AL amyloidosis and plasma cell leukemia.
     - Non-Hodgkin lymphoma
       - Autologous HCT is offered for relapsed *diffuse large B-cell lymphoma* (DLBCL), although there is no evidence for its use in first complete remission (CR) in DLBCL.

- Common conditioning regimens include BEAM (BCNU, etoposide, cytarabine, and melphalan) and cyclophosphamide/total body irradiation (TBI).
- Autologous HCT is recommended as consolidative therapy for fit patients with aggressive stage II bulky to stage IV *mantle cell lymphoma*. There is no consensus regarding its use in the relapsed setting; routine use is not currently recommended.
- Autologous HCT is recommended as consolidative therapy for fit patients with *peripheral T-cell lymphoma* (PTCL) in first CR, although there is still debate in this setting as well. It is not recommended in patients with PTCL not otherwise specified (NOS) with low or low/intermediate International Prognostic Index (IPI) scores.
- Autologous HCT can be considered for relapsed *follicular lymphoma* on an individualized basis.
- Hodgkin lymphoma
  - Autologous HCT is recommended for *relapsed* and *refractory* disease. Its impact on progression-free survival is established but is still under investigation for overall survival benefit.
  - Common conditioning regimens include BEAM or cyclophosphamide/TBI.
- Relapsed germ cell tumors
  - Autologous HCT can be considered for certain individuals with relapsed metastatic germ cell tumors and is typically preceded by intensive chemotherapy, such as combination paclitaxel, ifosfamide, and cisplatin.
- Acute promyelocytic leukemia (APL)
  - Consolidative therapy with an autologous HCT is still the standard of care for fit patients with relapsed APL in a molecular remission after repeat induction therapy (in CR2).
- Benign (noncancerous) conditions
  - Autoimmune conditions
    - Autologous HCT is being investigated for a variety of nonmalignant conditions, including dermato- and polymyositis, scleroderma, and systemic lupus erythematosus.

4. What are the indications for an allogeneic stem cell transplant?
- Malignant
  - Acute myeloid leukemia (AML)
    - Allogeneic HCT is recommended as the standard of care for eligible patients with AML with intermediate- or high-risk features in CR1.
    - Allogeneic HCT can also be considered for certain patients in CR3+ or not in remission with minimal disease at the time of transplant.
  - APL
    - Allogeneic HCT is recommended for patients with APL not in molecular remission after induction therapy in CR2. It can also be considered for relapsed disease after prior autologous HCT.
  - Acute lymphoid leukemia (ALL)
    - Allogeneic is generally considered standard of care in CR1 for eligible high-risk patients as well as all eligible patients in CR2.
    - Another challenge (and ongoing area of research) is that risk stratification systems are constantly evolving. In general, consider allogeneic HCT in CR1 for patients with Philadelphia chromosome or Philadelphia chromosome-like positivity and patients with t(4;11).

■ Relapses are more common in both CR1 and CR2 when measurable residual disease (MRD) is present.
- Myelodysplastic disease/myeloproliferative neoplasms
  - Allogeneic HCT is recommended for eligible patients with intermediate- or high-risk disease by the Revised International Prognostic Scoring System (IPSS-R^2). Various factors considered in this scoring include the presence of cytopenias, poor-risk cytogenetics, and marrow blast percentage.
- Chronic myeloid leukemia (CML)
  - The routine employment of allogeneic transplant in CML has been supplanted by first-, second-, and third-generation tyrosine kinase inhibitors (TKIs). It is now considered standard of care only for patients presenting in accelerated or blast phase or for those refractory to or intolerant of TKIs.
- Chronic lymphocytic leukemia (CLL)
  - Allogeneic HCT can be considered for transplant-eligible patients with CLL and high-risk features such as del(17p)/TP53 as second-line management for relapsed or refractory disease after prior venetoclax or Bruton Tyrosine Kinase (BTK) inhibitor-containing therapies.
  - For eligible patients without del(17p)/TP53 mutations, again with venetoclax or BTK inhibitor-refractory disease, allogeneic HCT can be employed as fourth-line therapy.
- Myeloma
  - Allogeneic HCT is still considered experimental as an upfront treatment strategy in patients with myeloma, for example in younger patients with high-risk cytogenetics. It can also be considered in eligible patients with refractory disease or in those who have progressed despite autologous HCT.
- Non-Hodgkin lymphoma
  - Allogeneic HCT is still under investigation in this subgroup but can be considered for relapsed follicular following salvage autologous HCT or as fourth-line therapy in large B-cell or mantle lymphoma. It may also be considered in relapsed/refractory PTCL.
- Hodgkin lymphoma
  - Allogeneic HCT can be considered for relapsed/refractory disease, even in patients who have undergone autologous HCT.
■ Benign
- Aplastic anemia
  - Allogeneic HCT, utilizing bone marrow from an available related donor, should be considered as the upfront standard of care for eligible young patients (≤40 years old) with a new diagnosis of acquired severe aplastic anemia (ASAA). If urgent transplantation is needed, cells from a matched unrelated donor (MUD) may be utilized.
  - Allogeneic HCT can be considered after failure of immunosuppressive therapy for older patients (40–60 years old). Selected patients in this age range with an available matched related donor can also be transplanted.
- Congenital marrow failure syndromes
  - Allogeneic HCT can be considered for patients with a variety of congenital marrow failure syndromes, including Fanconi anemia (although nonhematologic manifestations may persist) and dyskeratosis congenita.
  - Conditioning must be carefully considered in these patients due to their disease-associated comorbidities.

- Hemoglobinopathies
  - Allogeneic HCT can be considered for selected patients with sickle cell disease who have an available matched related donor. Transplantation is generally reserved in more severe disease, including in patients who have experienced acute chest syndrome, stroke, retinopathy, or damage to other end organs. Antithymocyte globulin is commonly added to conditioning regimens.
  - Indications for patients without a related donor generally become more stringent, such as those with recurrent stroke despite an adequate transfusion strategy.
  - Allogeneic HCT remains under development for thalassemia.

5. What is the Hematopoietic Comorbidity Index (HCT-CI)?

- The HCT-CI was developed as a risk assessment tool in patients undergoing (or being evaluated for) HCT and focuses specifically on various cardiac, gastrointestinal, and pulmonary comorbidities.
- The generated numerical score provides an estimate of a patient's anticipated outcomes with hematopoietic transplant. A score of 12, for example, corresponds with a high-risk for nonrelapse mortality following allogeneic HCT, a 2-year nonrelapse mortality of 41%, and a 2-year overall survival of 34%.

TABLE 26.2 ■ Hematopoietic Comorbidity Index (HCT-CI) by Individual Organ/Tissue-Specific Comorbidities

Comorbidity	Definition	HCT-CI Score
Arrhythmia	Atrial fibrillation or flutter, supraventricular tachycardia, sick sinus syndrome, heart block, any ventricular arrhythmia	1
Cardiovascular comorbidity	CAD, CHF, MI, or EF ≤50% or SF ≤26	1
Inflammatory bowel disease	Crohn's or ulcerative colitis	1
Diabetes	Presence of diabetes, steroid-induced hyperglycemia	1
Cerebrovascular disease	TIA, SAH, cerebral thrombosis, embolism, hemorrhage	1
Psychiatric	Depression, anxiety requiring treatment or psychiatric consultation	1
Hepatic comorbidity, mild	Chronic hepatitis, bilirubin >ULN, to 1.5 × ULN, or AST/ALT >ULN to 2.5 × ULN	1–3
Hepatic comorbidity, moderate/severe	Cirrhosis, bilirubin >1.5 × ULN, or AST/ALT >2.5 × ULN	1
Infection	Documented infection, FUO, pulmonary nodules suspicious of fungal pneumonia	1
Rheumatologic	SLE, RA, polymyositis, mixed CTD, polymyalgia rheumatica	2

(continued)

TABLE 26.2 ■ Hematopoietic Comorbidity Index (HCT-CI) by Individual Organ/Tissue-Specific Comorbidities (*continued*)

Comorbidity	Definition	HCT-CI Score
Peptic ulcer	Gastric ulcer, duodenal ulcer requiring treatment	2
Moderate/severe renal failure	Cr >2 mg/dL, on dialysis or prior renal transplant	2
Moderate pulmonary	DL_{co} and/or FEV_1 >65%–80% or dyspnea or slight activity	2
Severe pulmonary	DL_{co} and/or FEV_1 ≤65 or dyspnea at rest or requiring oxygen	3
Primary solid tumor	Excluding nonmelanoma skin cancer	3
Heart valve disease	Excluding mitral valve prolapse	3

ALT, alanine transaminase; AST, aspartate aminotransferase; CAD, coronary artery disease; CHF, congestive heart failure; Cr, creatinine; CTD, connective tissue disorder; DLco, diffusing lung capacity corrected; EF, ejection fraction; FEV_1, forced expiratory volume in 1 second; FUO, fever of unknown origin; HCT-CI, Hematopoietic Comorbidity Index; MI, myocardial infarction; RA, rheumatoid arthritis; SAH, sub-arachnoid hemorrhage; SF, shortening fraction; SLE, systemic lupus erythematosus; TIA, transient ischemic attack; ULN, upper limit of normal.

QUESTIONS

1. A 58-year-old man is diagnosed with stage III mantle cell lymphoma. He is treated with six cycles of R-CHOP (rituximab, cyclophosphamide, doxorubicin, vincristine, and prednisone) chemotherapy, which he tolerated well. Imaging suggests that he is in complete remission (CR). He has two human leukocyte antigen (HLA)-matched sisters. Which of the following would you offer at this time?
   A. Rituximab maintenance
   B. Allogeneic hematopoietic cell transplant (HCT) utilizing one of his HLA-matched siblings
   C. Observation
   D. High-dose chemotherapy and autologous HCT

2. A 28-year-old man with no prior medical history is diagnosed with Philadelphia chromosome-like acute lymphoid leukemia (ALL). He begins induction chemotherapy and achieves a complete hematologic remission. What is the most appropriate consolidative therapeutic approach?
   A. Allogeneic hematopoietic cell transplant (HCT) using his identical twin brother
   B. POMP (6-mercaptopurine, vincristine, methotrexate, prednisone) maintenance chemotherapy
   C. Matched unrelated allogeneic HCT
   D. High-dose chemotherapy and autologous HCT

3. **A 77-year-old woman with a history of type 2 diabetes mellitus, previously treated breast cancer, and depression is diagnosed with high-risk myelodysplastic syndrome (MDS). Her marrow blast percentage is 3%, she has multiple cytopenias with red blood cell transfusion dependency, an Eastern Cooperative Group performance status (ECOG PS) of 1 as well as intermediate-risk cytogenetics; her Revised International Prognostic Scoring System (IPSS-R^2). The patient has a human leukocyte antigen (HLA)-matched related sibling. What would you recommend?**
   A. Treatment with 5-azacitidine
   B. Treatment with 3 + 7 standard induction chemotherapy
   C. Reduced-intensity allogeneic hematopoietic cell transplant (HCT)
   D. Lenalidomide

4. **A 60-year-old man is diagnosed with stage IV, double-hit diffuse large B-cell lymphoma (DLBCL). After treatment with multiagent chemotherapy, he achieves complete remission based on imaging. What further therapy do you recommend at this time?**
   A. Allogeneic hematopoietic cell transplant (HCT) using a matched unrelated donor
   B. Rituximab maintenance
   C. Observation
   D. High-dose chemotherapy and autologous HCT

5. **Which of these patients would not be recommended to undergo an allogeneic hematopoietic cell transplant (HCT) in first complete remission?**
   A. Fit 45-year-old man with acute myeloid leukemia (AML) demonstrating t(8;21)
   B. Fit 45-year-old man with AML demonstrating normal karyotype and *FLT-3 ITD* mutation
   C. Fit 45-year-old man with relapsed acute promyelocytic leukemia (APL) who has not achieved complete molecular remission after repeat induction
   D. Fit 45-year-old man with a history of testicular cancer for which he received chemotherapy, now with AML

6. **A 43-year-old man with high-risk acute myeloid leukemia (AML) achieves complete remission following induction chemotherapy. He has a human leukocyte antigen (HLA)-matched sibling. His Hematopoietic Comorbidity Index (HCT-CI) is 0. What would you recommend for consolidation therapy?**
   A. Autologous stem cell transplant
   B. High-dose cytarabine chemotherapy for four cycles
   C. Matched related allogeneic stem cell transplant with fludarabine and cyclophosphamide (nonmyeloablative regimen)
   D. Matched related allogeneic stem cell transplant with busulfan and cyclophosphamide conditioning (myeloablative regimen)

7. A 49-year-old woman with inv(16) acute myeloid leukemia (AML) is treated with standard induction chemotherapy, 3 + 7, and achieves complete remission. She receives four cycles of high-dose cytarabine consolidation. Unfortunately, 14 months after completing therapy, she suffers a relapse. She undergoes repeat induction chemotherapy using fludarabine, cytarabine, granulocyte colony-stimulating factor (G-CSF), and idarubicin, and achieves a second complete remission. What should now be offered to consolidate her remission?
   A. Allogeneic stem cell transplant
   B. Autologous stem cell transplant
   C. High-dose cytarabine chemotherapy
   D. Hypomethylating agent for four cycles

ANSWERS

1. **D. High-dose chemotherapy and autologous HCT.** Autologous stem cell transplant (SCT) is recommended in first CR for eligible patients with mantle cell lymphoma. Rituximab maintenance can be considered post-HCT but should not be chosen in place of HCT for eligible patients. Allogeneic HCT is reserved for patients with mantle cell lymphoma who have primary refractory or relapsed disease. Observation alone would be insufficient for this patient.

2. **C. Matched unrelated allogeneic HCT.** Philadelphia chromosome-like ALL is considered a poor prognostic feature. As such, allogeneic HCT is recommended in first complete remission (CR1). Syngeneic HCT, that is, using his identical twin brother, is not recommended when transplant is utilized for malignant conditions as there is a higher risk of relapse. POMP maintenance and autologous HCT are both inappropriate choices for this high-risk disease in a transplant eligible, fit young man.

3. **A. Treatment with 5-azacitidine.** Despite having high-risk MDS, the patient is elderly with significant comorbidities giving her a Hematopoietic Comorbidity Index (HCT-CI) score of 5. The HCT-CI was developed to assess relevant comorbidities in allogeneic HCT patients and allow for appropriate risk assessment prior to transplant. It considers such factors as hepatic disease, pulmonary disease, cardiac disease, psychiatric disturbance, prior malignancy, and irritable bowel disease (IBD), among others. A score of 5 is considered high risk for nonrelapse mortality, with an estimated 2-year nonrelapse mortality of 41% versus a 2-year overall survival of only 34%. Therefore, allogeneic HCT would not be recommended. Lenalidomide could be considered for the 5q minus syndrome, which this patient does not have. 5-azacytidine has been demonstrated to improve survival in patients with high-risk MDS.

4. **C. Observation.** At this time, there is insufficient evidence to suggest upfront autologous HCT for patients with DLBCL, even those with adverse prognostic features such as double hit. Autologous HCT would be recommended in the setting of relapsed disease. Allogeneic HCT is rarely considered for patients with primary refractory DLBCL, which this patient fortunately does not have. There is no role for rituximab maintenance in DLBCL.

5. **A. Fit 45-year-old man with acute myeloid leukemia (AML) demonstrating t(8;21).** This patient has a core-binding factor leukemia, which is considered favorable risk disease. These patients should undergo consolidation with chemotherapy alone, and allogeneic HCT should be reserved only relapsed disease upon achievement of second complete remission (CR2). All of the other patients listed have an indication to proceed with allogeneic HCT at this time.

6. **D. Matched related allogeneic stem cell transplant with busulfan and cyclophosphamide conditioning (myeloablative regimen).** Patients with high-risk AML who are fit are recommended to undergo allogeneic

stem cell transplant in first complete remission to minimize risk of disease relapse and improve overall survival. Given his low HCT-CI, the recommendation would be for a myeloablative over a nonmyeloablative conditioning regimen for improved leukemia-free survival.

7. **A. Allogeneic stem cell transplant.** For young, fit patients who have a late relapse from initial AML therapy, treatment options include clinical trials or chemotherapy followed by an allogeneic stem cell transplant. This patient is young and should be considered for an allogeneic stem cell transplant in second complete remission.

Samuel B. Reynolds and Mary Mansour Riwes

MARROW ENGRAFTMENT FAILURE

1. **What is graft failure and how common is it?**
   - Graft failure is the term used when donor stem cells are not engrafted within the host marrow and are failing to produce the elements necessary for hematopoiesis. This may be demonstrated by either of the following:
     - Primary graft rejection: failure of the donor stem cells to ever engraft; defined by absolute neutrophil count (ANC) <0.5 × 10⁹, with platelets <20 × 10⁹/L and hemoglobin <8 g/dL at day +28
     - Secondary graft rejection: loss of donor cells after initial engraftment; ANC <0.5 × 10⁹ not related to relapse
   - The causes of graft failure may be rejection, an immunologic phenomenon, or other causes including infection and various medications
   - The risk of graft rejection is related to the degree of human leukocyte antigen (HLA) incompatibility and donor-specific HLA antibodies. Other contributing factors include the use of cryopreservation (which increase risk) and conditioning regimen (various regimens increase or decrease risk depending on disease state).
   - Graft failure remains relatively rare, although the incidence is estimated at as much as 11% of transplant recipients.

GRAFT-VERSUS-HOST DISEASE

1. **What is graft-versus-host disease (GVHD)? How common is it?**
   - GVHD is a phenomenon whereby immunocompetent donor CD8+ lymphocytes respond to polymorphic HLAs present in immunodeficient host tissues. The outcome is an immune response directed against resident host tissues, including the skin, intestine, lungs, and liver. The interactions between donor lymphocytes and polymorphic HLAs on host tissue are amplified by the significant local tissue damage that occurs during receipt of the conditioning regimen. Specifically, this local tissue damage induces the release of cytokines and creates an environment by which donor immune cells recognize and react against antigens in the host.
   - The risk of GVHD depends on many factors, including the degree of HLA compatibility, stem cell source, and conditioning regimen intensity; donor gender has even been reported to impact risk. Acute GVHD is estimated to occur in as many as 50% of patients undergoing an HLA-matched related stem cell transplant and up to 60% of patients undergoing an unrelated donor stem cell transplant. Chronic GVHD incidence varies in patients who undergo an allogeneic stem cell transplant, but occurs in the majority of patients who develop acute GVHD.

2. What are the organs affected in acute GVHD?

- Acute GVHD classically affects the skin, gastrointestinal (GI) tract, and the liver.
  - Skin involvement typically manifests as a maculopapular rash, which can be painful and pruritic and involve various surfaces, including the palms of the hands and upper trunk. In severe cases, the rash may even cover the whole body and be associated with bullae, vesicles, and desquamation.
  - GI GVHD can occur throughout the tract and is typically characterized by diarrhea, although abdominal pain, nausea, vomiting, or ileus may also be present.
  - Liver involvement is typically recognized by hyperbilirubinemia or elevated alkaline phosphatase levels. Isolated liver GVHD is uncommon.

3. How is acute GVHD quantified?

TABLE 27.1 ■ Staging Criteria for Cutaneous, Hepatic and Gastrointestinal/Luminal Graft-Versus-Host Disease (GVHD)

Stage	Skin	Liver–Bilirubin Level	Gastrointestinal Tract Stool Output/Day
0	No GVHD rash	<2 mg/dL	<500 mL/day
1	Maculopapular rash <25% BSA	2–3 mg/dL	500–999 mL/day *or* persistent nausea, vomiting, anorexia with a confirmatory upper GI tract biopsy
2	Maculopapular rash 25%–50%	3.1–6 mg/dL	1,000–1,500 mL/day
3	Maculopapular rash >50%	6.1–15 mg/dL	>1,500 mL/day
4	Generalized erythroderma (>50% BSA) *plus* bullous formation and desquamation >5% BSA	>15 mg/dL	Severe abdominal pain with or without ileus or grossly bloody stool, regardless of stool volume

BSA, body surface area; GI, gastrointestinal; GVHD, graft-versus-host disease.

- Overall clinical grade
  - Grade 0: no stage 1 to 4 GVHD of any organ
  - Grade I: stage 1 to 2 skin GVHD + no liver or GI involvement
  - Grade II: stage 3 skin, stage 1 liver, and/or stage 1 GI
  - Grade III: stage 0 to 3 skin with stage 2 to 3 liver and/or stage 2 to 3 GI
  - Grade IV: stage 4 skin, liver, and/or GI involvement

4. What organs are typically affected in chronic GVHD?

- Multiple organs may be affected, including the following:
  - Skin: Presentation varies but includes lichen planus or sclerosis-like changes, poikiloderma, and depigmentation. The hair or nails may be affected.
  - Eyes/mouth: Presentation includes lichen planus-like changes of the oropharynx, xerostomia, mucoceles and leukoplakia, manifesting as dry eye, and photophobia.
  - Liver: Presentation includes elevated total bilirubin, alkaline phosphatase, or alanine transaminase (ALT) >2x the upper limit of normal.

- Lungs: Bronchiolitis obliterans by biopsy. Patients with chronic disease may present with dyspnea or wheezing. Pulmonary function testing (PFTs) can reveal obstructive or restrictive changes.
- Musculoskeletal: Presentation includes localized sclerotic changes manifesting as fasciitis and/or joint contractures or stiffness.

5. How is chronic GVHD graded?

- Chronic GVHD is graded by the National Institutes of Health (NIH) grading system: Each organ is given a score of 0 to 3, with 0 being no GVHD and 3 representing the most severe GVHD manifestations for that tissue.
- Mild disease involves only one to two organs or sites, with no lung involvement, and a max score of 1 at each involved site.
- Moderate disease involves at least one site with a score of 2, or three or more organs with a score of 1. A score of 1 in the lungs is designated as moderate disease.
- Severe disease is when any organ or site is scored as 3 or ≥1 in the lungs.

6. What measures are used to prevent GVHD?

- Nonpharmacologic preventive measures include use of properly matched donors, T-cell depletion, and minimizing pretransplant end-organ damage.
- Medications used to prevent GVHD vary by transplant center, preparative regimen, and donor source, but commonly include cyclosporine, methotrexate, mycophenolate mofetil, sirolimus, and tacrolimus.

7. What medications are used to treat acute GVHD?

- First-line therapy for acute GVHD depends on the initial GVHD grade.
  - For grade I (skin stage 1–2), topical steroids are recommended.
  - For grades II to IV, topical therapy in addition to high-dose oral prednisone at 1 mg/kg/day is recommended. If unable to tolerate PO, intravenous methylprednisolone (2 mg/kg/day) is recommended.
- Although there is debate as to the definition of corticosteroid-refractory GVHD, a general convention is disease progressing after 3 days of therapy or that is not improving after 7 days. Should such refractory disease be present, alternative therapy should be offered.
- Ruxolitinib is Food and Drug Administration-approved and is commonly administered as second-line therapy. Other options include infliximab, ruxolitinib, antithymocyte globulin, etanercept, mycophenolate mofetil, sirolimus, alemtuzumab, and octreotide.

8. What medications are used to treat chronic GVHD?

- First-line therapy for chronic GVHD typically begins with prednisone (1 mg/kg/day) for moderate or severe disease.
- Steroid-refractory chronic GVHD (SR-cGVHD) is recognized when:
  - cGVHD progresses while patients are taking prednisone at ≥1 mg/kg/day for 1 to 2 weeks.
  - Stable cGVHD is still present after 4 to 8 weeks of sustained prednisone at ≥0.5 mg/kg/day.
  - Symptoms flare or patients remain steroid-dependent while tapering corticosteroids to <0.25 mg/kg/day.
- Alternative management should be offered for SR-cGVHD. There are no standard therapies, but second-line management include mycophenolate mofetil, ibrutinib, mTOR inhibitors (including everolimus, sirolimus), mycophenolate mofetil, rituximab, and extracorporeal photopheresis.

OPPORTUNISTIC INFECTIONS

1. What are the infectious risks associated with stem cell transplant?

- Infectious risks are distinct depending on the phase of transplant.
- Pre-engraftment period (approximately day 0 through 30 days posttransplant): The major risk is related to neutropenia and impaired innate immune response, alterations to both anatomic mucosal barriers (mucositis and diarrhea), and vascular structures. Accordingly, facultative bacterial organisms from skin, oral, and GI flora are the most common sources of infection. Invasive fungal infections and herpes simplex virus (HSV), typically reactivation, can be seen in this time period as well.
- Postengraftment period (approximately day 30 through day 100 posttransplant): Severe neutropenia has resolved and barrier defenses are healing. Patients, however, remain immunosuppressed due to impaired cell-mediated immunity (CD8+ T-cells), humoral immunity (antibody-producing B-cells), and decreased phagocyte function. If acute GVHD has occurred, impaired immune function can occur, leading to damaged immune barriers. Combining this process with the immunosuppressive effects of GVHD-directed therapies will amplify the patient's already-immunocompromised state. The types of infections follow the nature of impaired cell-mediated immunity, as bacterial infections become less prevalent and viral infections become more common during this period, including infections from cytomegalovirus (CMV), adenovirus, enterovirus, human herpes virus 6 (HHV-6), BK virus, and various community-acquired respiratory viruses. Invasive fungal infections can also continue to occur, especially in patients with GVHD, as well as parasitic infections with *Pneumocystis jirovecii*, necessitating the need for prophylaxis.
- Late posttransplantation period (>100 days posttransplant): Cellular-mediated and humoral immunity recovers and immunosuppressive therapy is slowly withdrawn. Infections are unusual during this period in the absence of GVHD. If chronic GVHD is present, however, there remain defects in both cellular and humoral immunity, as well as in the barrier function of the skin, oropharynx, and GI tract. Infections during this period, when present, tend to localize to the skin and both upper and lower respiratory tracts. Pathogens are predominantly viral, especially varicella zoster virus (VZV) and CMV, but bacterial infections may occur. Of note, patients with chronic GVHD commonly have functional asplenia and therefore are more susceptible to infections from encapsulated bacteria.

HEPATIC SINUSOIDAL OBSTRUCTION SYNDROME

1. What is hepatic sinusoidal obstruction syndrome (SOS)?

- SOS is characterized by painful hepatomegaly, ascites, jaundice, weight gain and, in severe cases, fulminant liver failure. SOS typically occurs 3 to 21 days posttransplant.
- The primary mechanism of injury is to the hepatic venous endothelium with progressive occlusion of the venules and sinusoids, ultimately leading to widespread hepatic venous outflow disruption and hemorrhagic necrosis. SOS is observed in patients undergoing hematopoietic cell transplantation (HCT) but is also possible in the following clinical scenarios:

- Ingestion of large quantities of herbal tea containing pyrrolizidine alkaloids
- High-dose radiation therapy administered to the liver without cytoreductive chemotherapy
- Receipt of a transplanted liver
■ Risk factors for the development of SOS following HSCT include the following:
  - Preexisting liver disease, due to baseline abnormalities in hepatic endothelial cells, rendering cells more susceptible to cytoreductive regimens
  - Viral hepatitis
  - Other risk enhancers including intensive conditioning therapy (use of ionizing radiation, specifically), advanced age at transplant, and poor baseline performance status
■ Diagnosis of SOS is often made clinically by history, examination, and with accompanying laboratory studies. Severe cases are often fatal.

2. **How is SOS prevented and treated?**
   ■ The risk of developing severe SOS is mitigated by the following:
     - Minimizing risk factors, including eliminating exposure to hepatotoxic agents (e.g., excessive use of alcohol, recreational drugs, or acetaminophen)
     - Utilizing a reduced-intensity conditioning regimen
     - Utilizing appropriate GVHD prophylaxis; in patients undergoing myeloablative allogeneic HCT, ursodeoxycholic acid (UDCA; 12 mg/kg daily, divided in two doses) can be used as prophylaxis prior to the preparative regimen and continued for 3 months posttransplant
   ■ Treatment of SOS depends on the severity of the disease. Mild to moderate cases may be treated with supportive care alone with maintenance of intravascular volume and forward renal perfusion. Severe cases may be treated with defibrotide (6.25 mg/kg every 6 hours for 21 days). Transjugular intrahepatic portosystemic stent-shunt has also been performed in a small number of patients with SOS.

MANAGEMENT OF RELAPSE

1. **What options are available after relapse?**
   ■ Relapse occurs in 40% to 75% of patients undergoing autologous HCT and 10% to 40% of those undergoing an allogeneic HCT.
   ■ Donor lymphocyte infusions (DLI), which allow expansion of an antileukemic cell population, can be used to treat relapse following an allogeneic HCT.
   ■ DLI efficacy depends on the underlying malignancy, the dose of infused lymphocytes, and the degree of host lymphodepletion. Best outcomes have been seen in patients with chronic-phase chronic myeloid leukemia (CML), followed by lymphoma, multiple myeloma, and acute myeloid leukemia.
   ■ Risks associated with DLI include emergence of GVHD and myelosuppression. Current investigative therapies include hypomethylating agents, immunotherapy, antigen-pulsed dendritic cells, and chimeric antigen receptor T-cells.

LATE EFFECTS

1. **What are some common complications seen in long-term survivors following HCT?**
   ■ Late relapse of primary disease and chronic GVHD are the most common causes of death after allogeneic HCT.

- Late infection in the absence of chronic GVHD also contributes to non–relapse-related death.
- Various end-organ toxicities may also be observed.
  - Cardiovascular: higher incidence of ischemic heart disease, cardiomyopathy, heart failure, and arrhythmia
  - Pulmonary: inflammatory pneumonitis and chronic respiratory failure
  - Kidney: renal dysfunction related to radiation injury and immunosuppressive therapies
  - Endocrine: type 2 diabetes mellitus, hypothyroidism, osteopenia, hypogonadism, infertility, and hypoadrenalism
- Treatment-related myelodysplasia and/or secondary leukemia may develop.
- Secondary solid tumors of the skin (e.g., melanoma), brain, liver, and buccal cavity may also be seen.

QUESTIONS

1. **A 45-year-old woman underwent a matched related full-intensity conditioning stem cell transplant 50 days ago for Philadelphia chromosome-positive acute lymphoblastic leukemia (ALL) in first complete remission. Her transplant course was uncomplicated and she was discharged home on day +20. She remains on full-dose tacrolimus for graft-versus-host disease (GVHD) prophylaxis and continues to take acyclovir, fluconazole, oral and intravenous magnesium, trimethoprim/ sulfamethoxazole, and ursodiol. Her tacrolimus level is therapeutic. However, over the past 2 days she has had loss of appetite, mild epigastric pain, and six to eight episodes of nonbloody diarrhea daily. What is the next step in management?**
   A. Increase tacrolimus dose.
   B. Start mycophenolate mofetil.
   C. Start extracorporeal photopheresis.
   D. Obtain both upper and lower endoscopies with biopsies.

Questions 2 and 3 both pertain to the following clinical vignette:
A 60-year-old man is post-120 days from a matched unrelated hematopoietic stem cell transplant for acute myeloid leukemia (AML). His early transplant course was complicated by gastrointestinal (GI) acute graft-versus-host disease (GVHD), which was treated with steroids with prompt improvement. He presents to the clinic complaining of blurry vision, skin changes on both of his arms, as well as muscle and joint tightness. His exam is notable for a mild weight loss (2 kg), irritation of the sclera bilaterally, and shiny, indurated skin on both of his arms. He has a moderate limited range of motion (ROM) of both his elbows but no muscle tenderness on exam. He remains on tacrolimus for GVHD prophylaxis, but his dosage has been tapered. In addition, he continues to take acyclovir, fluconazole, and trimethoprim/sulfamethoxazole for infectious disease prophylaxis.

2. **What is the most likely diagnosis?**
   A. Chronic GVHD
   B. Side effects from tacrolimus
   C. Infection with cytomegalovirus (CMV)
   D. Sjögren syndrome

3. **What is the next step in the management for this patient?**
   A. Stop tacrolimus.
   B. Start prednisone 1 mg/kg/day.
   C. Obtain skin biopsy.
   D. Start Ibrutinib

4. **A 57-year-old man with chronic myeloid leukemia (CML) intolerant to tyrosine kinase inhibitors (TKIs) underwent a matched unrelated transplant in the second chronic phase. Posttransplant course has been complicated by acute mild skin graft-versus-host disease (GVHD) that responded to corticosteroid treatment and an admission for pneumonia. He is currently taking tacrolimus for GVHD prophylaxis. He presents at 1-year follow-up with evidence of relapse. What is the best option?**
   A. Initiate tyrosine kinase inhibitor
   B. Donor lymphocyte infusion
   C. Reduce immunosuppression
   D. Both B and C

5. **A 55-year-old woman with hepatitis B and acute myeloid leukemia (AML) in first remission underwent a myeloablative transplantation conditioning with busulfan and cyclophosphamide, followed by infusion of matched unrelated peripheral blood stem cells 15 days ago. Graft-versus-host disease (GVHD) prophylaxis was initiated and consists of tacrolimus and methotrexate. She now presents with 7-kg weight gain over 2 days. She is noted to have tender hepatomegaly with ascites. Laboratory testing is notable for a total bilirubin of 5.0 mg/dL and transaminases that are five-fold above baseline. Which is the most likely explanation for her current condition?**
   A. Engraftment syndrome
   B. Hepatic sinusoidal obstruction syndrome (SOS)/hepatic veno-occlusive disease (VOD)
   C. Methotrexate toxicity
   D. Right heart failure

6. **Donor lymphocyte infusion (DLI) is a therapeutic option in patients with relapsed disease following allogeneic hematopoietic cell transplantation (HCT). For which of the following disease states has DLI been shown to have the greatest response?**
   A. Acute lymphoblastic leukemia (ALL)
   B. Acute myeloid leukemia (AML) without minimal residual disease (MRD) status
   C. Chronic-phase chronic myeloid leukemia (CML) in relapse following allogeneic hematopoietic stem cell transplantation (HSCT)
   D. Multiple myeloma

7. **A 45-year-old male with multiple-relapsed classic Hodgkin lymphoma underwent full human leukocyte antigen (HLA)-matched unrelated donor transplant. Posttransplant course has been complicated by mild skin graft-versus-host disease (GVHD) and he is currently receiving immunosuppressive methotrexate and cyclosporine. At 3 months (approximately 90 days) posttransplant, he develops gross hematuria**

with dysuria. His basic laboratory evaluation is normal apart from mild anemia (hemoglobin 11.1 g/dL) with unimpaired kidney and liver functions. BK virus is quantified at 100,000 copies/mL in the urine. What is the most appropriate next step in management?

A. Start cidofovir.
B. Check cytomegalovirus (CMV), adenovirus, and BK virus serum polymerase chain reaction (PCR).
C. Stop immunosuppression.
D. Start intravenous immunoglobulin (IVIG).

8. A 65-year-old woman presents 1 year after receiving a matched unrelated donor allogeneic stem cell transplantation for high molecular risk primary myelofibrosis. What vaccination(s) is/are appropriate at this time?

A. Hepatitis B, DTaP, *Haemophilus influenzae* type b (Hib)
B. Pneumococcal conjugate, pneumococcal polysaccharide, polio-live vaccine
C. Measles, mumps, and rubella
D. Varicella zoster virus (VZV)

ANSWERS

1. **D. Obtain both upper and lower endoscopies with biopsies.** This patient is developing symptoms concerning for acute GVHD at day +20 following allogeneic transplant, and endoscopies with biopsies should be obtained to confirm the diagnosis. Optimal first-line therapy for treating acute GVHD involving the gastrointestinal tract is oral prednisone, with intravenous methylprednisolone reserved for patients who cannot tolerate oral therapy. It is critical to recognize and initiate therapy promptly to minimize volume losses or progression to more severe GVHD of the gut. There is no role for increasing tacrolimus when levels are already therapeutic as there is significant risk for toxicity with limited increasing therapeutic effect. Photopheresis and mycophenolate can both be effective therapies for GVHD but are typically reserved for patients who are not responding to steroids.

2. **A. Chronic GVHD.** The patient's collective symptoms of blurry vision with skin tightness/induration and joint stiffness are characteristic symptoms of chronic GVHD. At day +120 posttransplant, this is also an appropriate time frame for chronic GVHD to begin, particularly given his risk factors of having a history of prior acute GVHD and having undergone unrelated donor transplant. Sjögren syndrome commonly presents with dry eyes and/or mouth due to immune-mediated inflammation of the salivary glands, but his skin findings are not consistent with this diagnosis. Viral infection with CMV can certainly manifest with visual impairment but again would not explain her skin changes. Tacrolimus does not induce dry eyes, mouth, or arthralgias. More commonly, it results in renal wasting of magnesium, and rarely microangiopathic hemolytic anemia, neurologic changes, and renal dysfunction. Clinically and perhaps most importantly in approaching this vignette, the patient's tacrolimus is being tapered, suggesting that his symptoms are related to the withdrawal of this immunosuppressant, that is, GVHD, and not to the tacrolimus itself.

3. **B. Start prednisone 1 mg/kg/day.** This patient has evidence of moderate chronic GVHD with three involved organs (eyes, skin, and joints), with two (eyes, skin) being mildly affected and one organ being moderately affected (limited ROM of the elbow joints). His physical exam findings are distinctive of chronic GVHD and a skin biopsy is not needed. For moderate disease, he requires systemic therapy with glucocorticoids. It is inappropriate to stop tacrolimus as this would further exacerbate his symptoms. Ibrutinib is currently approved for chronic GVHD after failure of one or more lines of systemic therapy.

4. **D. Both B and C.** This patient has completed allogeneic hematopoietic cell transplantation with evidence of relapse at 1 year. All patients with CML with relapse after transplant should be considered for treatment with a TKI, although the question indicates that he was intolerant to TKIs, so this would not be a safe option. Both reduction of immunosuppression and donor lymphocyte infusion should be incorporated into the initial management, unless there is concern for GVHD or intolerable myelosuppression.

5. **B. Hepatic sinusoidal obstruction syndrome (SOS)/hepatic veno-occlusive disease (VOD).** The patient's presentation is most suggestive of hepatic SOS/VOD as evidenced by her rapid weight gain with ascites, peripheral edema, tender hepatomegaly, and rise in liver function tests (LFTs). Her history of hepatitis B and myeloablative preparative regimen likely placed her at increased risk of developing SOS. This condition is most commonly observed 3 to 21 days after transplant, and while severe cases are almost universally fatal most patients with mild to moderate disease will recover with only supportive care. Engraftment syndrome typically presents with cytokine release-like symptoms, including fevers, chills, and headaches; LFT abnormalities would be uncommon. While methotrexate can induce LFT elevation, drug toxicity is not associated with tender hepatomegaly. Right heart failure may present with edema, weight gain, and ascites if severe, but would be unlikely in this patient with no baseline history of cardiac disease.

6. **C. Chronic-phase chronic myeloid leukemia (CML) in relapse following allogeneic HSCT.** Donor lymphocyte infusion has shown the greatest efficacy in patients with CML in chronic phase following relapse after transplant. Moderate responses have been observed in patients with multiple myeloma. The responses are also less robust in AML and lowest in ALL, largely due to the rapid proliferation of malignant cells in these acute leukemias. Clinical responses to DLI can take months.

7. **B. Check cytomegalovirus (CMV), adenovirus, and BK virus serum polymerase chain reaction (PCR).** This patient is presenting with symptoms concerning for hemorrhagic cystitis, which can be caused by BK virus or adenovirus in transplant recipients. It is essential, prior to starting treatment, to assess for concomitant infections as treatment for BK viral infection typically involves the use of IVIG, which itself has antibodies against BK virus, in addition to decreasing immunosuppression. Stopping immunosuppression abruptly at this time is not appropriate and will increase his risk for GVHD.

8. **A. Hepatitis B, DTaP, *Haemophilus influenzae* type b (Hib).** Following autologous and allogeneic stem cell transplants, patients are susceptible to infection with encapsulated organisms and certain viral infections. Vaccinations for hepatitis B, acellular tetanus and diphtheria, and Hib should be administered at 12, 14, and 24 months posttransplant. Pneumococcal pneumonia vaccination should also be administered at 12 and 24 months following transplantation and influenza at least 6 months posttransplant. Live vaccines, such as measles, mumps, and rubella, are administered at least 24 months after transplantation. VZV and live polio vaccines, at present, are not recommended in transplant recipients.

Cellular Therapy: CAR T-Cells

Marcus Geer and Monalisa Ghosh

1. **What are chimeric antigen receptor (CAR) T-cells?**
   - CAR T-cells are T lymphocytes genetically engineered to express receptors targeting cancer cell antigens.
   - Current products utilize autologous T lymphocytes, but study of allogeneic CAR T-cells is ongoing.

2. **What are the Food and Drug Administration (FDA)-approved indications for CAR T-cell products?**
   - CAR T-cell products have been FDA-approved in the relapsed and refractory setting for acute lymphoblastic lymphoma (pediatric and adult), diffuse large B-cell lymphoma (DLBCL) not otherwise specified (NOS), primary mediastinal large B-cell lymphoma, high-grade B-cell lymphoma, follicular lymphoma, mantle cell lymphoma, marginal zone lymphoma, multiple myeloma, and DLBCL transformed from follicular lymphoma.

3. **What are the structural components of a CAR?**
   - Antigen binding domain: extracellular component (Figure 28.1)
   - Hinge region: exists between antigen binding domain and the cell surface to reduce the spatial restrictions that might limit interaction between antigen and CAR T-cell
   - Transmembrane domain: serves as a cytoplasmic anchor that connects the hinge region to the costimulatory domain
   - Intracellular signaling domain: innate T-cell activation signals through CD3-zeta; CD3-zeta also used in the CAR construct but is insufficient by itself for persistent activation
   - Costimulatory domain: intracellular component that promotes persistent signaling after activation to trigger a more robust response; allows for activation and persistence independent of the tumor microenvironment; second-generation CARs utilize two different endodomains:
     - CD28 (used in the structure of axicabtagene ciloleucel): more robust signaling cascade, earlier expansion of CAR T-cells
     - 4-1BB (used in the structure of lisocabtagene maraleucel and tisagenlecleucel): associated with CAR T-cell persistence

4. **How are CAR T-cells engineered?**
   - For the manufacture of autologous CAR T-cells, the patient undergoes leukapheresis during which T lymphocytes are collected and then sent for manufacturing. Current manufacturing technology requires a period of 2 to 5 weeks. The CAR transgene is transferred into the patient's T lymphocytes through transfection with lentiviral vectors. The CAR T-cell product is expanded and passed through quality assurance mechanisms to ensure adequate cell dose and CAR expression prior to administration.

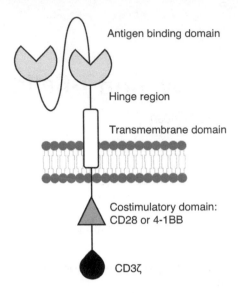

Antigen binding domain

Hinge region

Transmembrane domain

Costimulatory domain:
CD28 or 4-1BB

CD3ζ

FIGURE 28.1 ■ Second-generation chimeric antigen receptor structure.

5. What evaluation is necessary prior to CAR T-cell therapy?

■ Pretherapy evaluation typically consists of assessment of performance status and vital organ functions. Patient tolerance of lymphodepleting (LD) chemotherapy as well as the specific toxicities of CAR T-cell therapy must be considered when identifying eligible candidates.

6. Can chemotherapy be given before CAR T-cell administration?

■ Use of bridging therapies varied in the pivotal trials that have been completed thus far.

■ Use of lymphotoxic chemotherapy (e.g., bendamustine) within 3 to 4 weeks prior to leukapheresis could impact the number of the cells that can be collected for manufacturing.

■ Steroids should also generally not be administered within 7 days of leukapheresis due to the effect of steroids on absolute lymphocyte count and on the T-cell phenotype.

7. How are CAR T-cells administered?

■ LD chemotherapy is administered prior to infusing CAR T-cells. LD chemo must be completed at least 2 to 14 days prior to CAR T-cell infusion. LD chemo typically consists of a combination of fludarabine and cyclophosphamide. Bendamustine has also been used in some clinical situations. Proposed mechanisms to explain the benefit of LD chemotherapy include the following:

  ● Clearing endogenous lymphocytes which allows more opportunities for CAR T-cells to interact with endogenous cytokines and stimulate proliferation

  ● Clearing immune suppressive cells including regulatory T-cells and myeloid-derived suppressor cells that may suppress CAR T-cell activity and contribute to rejection of CAR T-cells

■ CAR T-cells are usually administered through a central venous catheter, but can be administered via a peripheral IV in some cases.

8. What are the common toxicities of CAR T-cell therapy?

- Cytokine release syndrome (CRS)
  - Acute systemic inflammatory reaction associated with T-cell activation, massive upregulation of proinflammatory cytokines, and recruitment of other immune mediators have been described.
  - CRS or similar syndromes have also been described in association with other disease states including use of bispecific antibodies, haploidentical hematopoietic stem cell transplants, and some viral infections (e.g., Covid-19).
  - Signs and symptoms must include fever. CRS may also be accompanied by malaise, hypotension, hypoxia, headache, rash, diarrhea, arthralgia, myalgia, vascular leakage, and organ dysfunction/failure.
  - Current American Society of Transplantation and Cellular Therapy (ASTCT) consensus grading criteria for CAR T-cell-related CRS is summarized in Table 28.1. The most severe symptom determines the grade and symptoms cannot be attributed other causes.
  - The typical timing and incidence of CRS is variable between CAR T-cell products. Most CRS starts between 1 and 14 days after CAR T-cell infusion and lasts for a median of 4 to 7 days.
  - Management of CRS:
    - Mild CRS (grade 1 and grade 2) is typically managed with primarily supportive measures: antipyretic, intravenous (IV) fluids, and supplemental oxygen.
    - Severe CRS (persistent grade 2, grade 3, and grade 4) is typically managed with the IL-6R antagonist tocilizumab ± high-dose glucocorticoids. Tocilizumab can be administered every 8 hours.
    - Persistent severe CRS sometimes warrants repeated tocilizumab dosing, usually with a maximum of three doses of tocilizumab within a 24-hour period.
    - If CRS does not improve or resolve with tocilizumab, corticosteroids are initiated.
    - More severe CRS frequently requires ICU level of care for monitoring and intensive intervention.
    - Use of alternative or additional agents such as the anti-IL-6 antibody siltuximab or JAK inhibitor, ruxolitinib, is primarily supported by small data sets and case series.

TABLE 28.1 ■ CRS Grading: ASTCT Consensus Grading Criteria

Grade 1	Fever (temperature ≥38.0°C)	and	No hypotension	and	No hypoxia
Grade 2	Fever (temperature ≥38.0°C)	and	Hypotension— fluid response	and/or	Hypoxia requiring ≤6 L/min nasal cannula
Grade 3	Fever (temperature ≥38.0°C)	and	Hypotension— requiring one presser[†]	and/or	Hypoxia requiring high flow O_2*
Grade 4	Fever (temperature ≥38.0°C)	and	Hypotension— requiring multiple pressers[†]	and/or	Hypoxia requiring positive pressure

*Includes nasal cannula (≥6 L/min), facemask, nonrebreather mask, or Venturi mask.

[†]Excluding vasopressin.

ASTCT, American Society of Transplantation and Cellular Therapy; CRS, cytokine release syndrome.

- Immune effector cell-associated neurotoxicity syndrome (ICANS)
  - Also known as neurotoxicity, the mechanism for ICANS is unclear. There is some component of endothelial cell activation and breakdown of the blood–brain barrier leading to infiltration of the central nervous system by CAR T-cells, other immune cell subsets, and inflammatory cytokines such as IL-6.
  - Signs and symptoms range widely and include change in level of consciousness, inattention, hallucinations, headaches, dysgraphia, apraxia, aphasia, seizures, cerebral edema, and death.
  - Current ASTCT consensus grading criteria for ICANS incorporates a 10-point immune effector cell-associated encephalopathy (ICE) assessment for level of consciousness, seizures, motor deficits, and increased intracranial pressure (Tables 28.2 and 28.3).
  - ICANS typically is preceded by CRS and tends to start 3 to 10 days after CAR T-cell infusion and lasts for a median of 5 to 7 days.
  - The CAR T-cell products targeting B-cell maturation antigen (BCMA), idecabtagene vicleucel and ciltacabtagene autoleucel, have a reported association with a unique neurotoxicity including parkinsonian dyskinesia.
  - Management of ICANS:
    - There are no FDA-approved therapies for ICANS.
    - Standard therapy typically consists of high-dose corticosteroids (e.g., dexamethasone 10 mg every 6 hours).
    - There are no approved second-line therapies for ICANS and data supporting the use of other agents are limited.
    - Severe or progressive symptoms frequently require ICU level of care for monitoring and intensive intervention.
    - Use of antiepileptic medications as prophylaxis is common, although the timing is controversial.
    - Some CAR T-cell constructs are associated with increased incidence of ICANS. This is generally the case with CAR T-cells that contain a CD28 costimulatory domain (e.g., axicabtagene ciloleucel or brexucabtagene autoleucel).
    - Use of additional or alternative therapies such as anakinra (IL-1 receptor antagonist), siltuximab (monoclonal antibody against IL-6), and intrathecal corticosteroids have been published in a few case reports.

TABLE 28.2 ■ ICANS Grading: ASTCT Consensus Grading Criteria

Grade	ICE Score	Level of Consciousness	Seizure	Motor Findings	Elevated ICP
Grade 1	7–9	Normal	None	None	None
Grade 2	3–6	Arousable to voice	None	None	None
Grade 3	0–2	Arousable to touch	Seizure spontaneously resolving	None	Focal edema on imaging
Grade 4	Unarousable/unable to assess	Unarousable, stuporous, comatose	Status epilepticus	Deep focal weakness	Diffuse cerebral edema/increased ICP on imaging or exam*

*Includes decerebrate or decorticate posturing, cranial nerve VI palsy, papilledema, or Cushing triad.

ASTCT, American Society of Transplantation and Cellular Therapy; ICANS, immune effector cell-associated neurotoxicity syndrome; ICE, immune effector cell-associated encephalopathy; ICP, intracranial pressure.

TABLE 28.3 ■ Immune Effector Cell-Associated Encephalopathy (ICE) Score

Orientation	Year, month, city, location	4 points
Naming	Name three objects	3 points
Following commands	Follow simple commands	1 point
Writing	Write a standard sentence	1 point
Attentiveness	Count backwards by 10 from 100	1 point

9. **What are the other common toxicities of CAR T-cell therapy?**
   - Cytopenia following LD chemotherapy and CAR T-cell infusion is common and multifactorial.
   - Hypogammaglobulinemia is commonly seen with prolonged B-cell aplasia.
   - The reported incidence of infection in the registration trials for tisagenlecleucel, axicabtagene ciloleucel, and lisocabtagene maraleucel is 12% to 55%. Mortality related to infection is low.

10. **What are the current indications for CD19-directed CAR T-cell therapy?**
    - B-cell acute lymphoblastic leukemia (B-ALL)
      - The CD19-directed CAR T-cell product, tisagenlecleucel, was first FDA-approved in 2017 for refractory or multiply relapsed B-ALL in pediatric patients up to age 25.
      - In the phase 2 ELIANA study for tisagenlecleucel in patients 3 to 21 years old, the overall response rate (ORR) was 81%, complete remission (CR) rate was 60%, and median overall survival (OS) was 19.1 months.
      - Brexucabtagene autoleucel was FDA-approved in 2021 for relapsed and refractory B-ALL in adults following the ZUMA-3 trial. The CR rate was 56%, with a median OS of >18 months. Severe CRS (grade 3–4) was reported in 24% and severe ICANS (grade 3–4) in 25% of subjects.
    - DLBCL
      - Three CAR T-cell products are FDA-approved for relapsed and refractory DLBCL.
        - In 2022, axicabtagene ciloleucel was FDA-approved for DLBCL that relapses within 12 months or is refractory to frontline chemoimmunotherapy based on the results of the ZUMA-7 trial. Axicabtagene ciloleucel was previously FDA-approved in 2017 for treatment of patients with DLBCL that relapsed after two or more lines of systemic therapy based on the phase 2, multicenter ZUMA-1 study. In the phase 3, multicenter, randomized ZUMA-7 study:
          - Median event-free survival (EFS) favored axicabtagene ciloleucel over standard of care (autologous stem cell transplant with EFS of 8.3 months in the CAR T-cell therapy arm vs. 2.0 months for standard of care autologous stem cell transplant arm). OS data remain immature.
          - The rate of severe CRS (grade 3–4) was 6% and severe ICANS (grade 3–4) was 21%, with no grade 5 toxicity.
          - FDA approval included primary mediastinal B-cell lymphoma, high-grade B-cell lymphoma, and DLBCL transformed from follicular lymphoma.

- Lisocabtagene maraleucel is also approved for DLBCL that relapses within 12 months or is refractory to frontline chemoimmunotherapy following the phase 3, multicenter, randomized TRANSFORM trial. Lisocabtagene ciloleucel was previously approved for DLBCL that was relapsed or refractory to greater than two lines of systemic therapy. In the TRANSFORM study:
  - Lisocabtagene ciloleucel demonstrated superior EFS compared with standard-of-care autologous stem cell transplant (10.1 vs. 2.3 months). OS was not yet reached.
  - The rate of grade 3 CRS was 1% and rate of grade 3 ICANS was 4%, with no grade 4 or 5 toxicity.
  - FDA approval included primary mediastinal B-cell lymphoma, high-grade B-cell lymphoma, and DLBCL transformed from follicular lymphoma.
- Tisagenlecleucel was FDA-approved for DLBCL after two or more lines of therapy following the phase 2, multicenter JULIET trial.
  - The ORR was 52%, with a 40% CR rate. The relapse-free survival (RFS) at 12 months was 79% for those reaching CR.
- Follicular lymphoma
  - Axicabtagene ciloleucel and tisagenlecleucel have both been given accelerated FDA approval for relapsed and refractory follicular lymphoma after two or more lines of therapy.
    - In the phase 2, multicenter ZUMA-5 trial, axicabtagene ciloleucel had an ORR of 94%, with 79% in CR. The median duration of response was not reached. At 18 months, the progression-free survival (PFS) was 73% and OS was 92%.
    - In the phase 2, multicenter ELARA trial, tisagenlecleucel showed an ORR of 86%, with 60% in CR. The median PFS at 12 months was 71% and duration of response was not reached.
- Mantle cell lymphoma
  - Brexucabtagene autoleucel was FDA-approved for mantle cell lymphoma following relapse after chemoimmunotherapy and a BTK inhibitor based on the results of the ZUMA-2 trial.
  - The reported ORR was 93% and CR was 67%. The PFS was 61% and OS was 83% at 12 months. The rates of severe CRS and ICANS (grade 3–4) were 15% and 31%, respectively.

11. What are the current indications for BCMA-directed CAR T-cell therapy?

- Multiple myeloma
  - Two products, idecabtagene vicleucel and ciltacabtagene autoleucel, are FDA-approved following four lines of systemic therapy, including an immunomodulatory agent, a proteasome inhibitor, and an anti-CD38 monoclonal antibody.
    - Ciltacabtagene autoleucel was FDA-approved in 2022 based on the phase 2, multicenter CARTITUDE-1 trial which showed an ORR of 98% and stringent CR rate of 82.5%. The median duration of response, PFS, and OS were not reached. At a median follow-up of 27 months, PFS was 54.9% and OS was 70.4% in a heavily pretreated population.
    - Idecabtagene vicleucel was FDA-approved in 2021 following the phase 2, multicenter, randomized KarMMA trial, which demonstrated an ORR of 73% and CR rate of 33%. The median PFS was 8.8 months and OS 19.4 months.

12. What is the mechanism of relapse following CAR T-cell therapy?
- Antigen loss: The CAR target antigen is no longer expressed or is down-regulated on malignant cells.
- T-cell dysfunction: There are multiple possible contributing factors, including poor expansion, inadequate persistence, and exhaustion due to prolonged activation.

QUESTIONS

1. A 64-year-old patient with immunoglobulin G (IgG) kappa multiple myeloma presents with right arm pain and evidence of new fluorodeoxyglucose (FDG)-avid lytic lesions involving the right humerus, sternum, and the seventh rib. The serum M-protein was previously undetectable in response to the most recent line of therapy but is now rising. She has previously been treated with combinations of lenalidomide, bortezomib, daratumumab, carfilzomib, dexamethasone, and the BCL2 inhibitor venetoclax as part of a clinical trial. What is the target antigen for the chimeric antigen receptor (CAR) T-cell products approved for this line of therapy?
   A. BCL2
   B. XPO1
   C. Cereblon
   D. B-cell maturation antigen

2. A 75-year-old patient is diagnosed with diffuse large B-cell lymphoma involving the mediastinal and axillary lymph nodes with fluorodeoxyglucose (FDG)-avid hypermetabolism in the spleen and bone marrow. Fluorescence in situ hybridization (FISH) testing is notable for rearrangements in the MYC and BCL2 genes. She receives treatment with chemoimmunotherapy for six cycles, with a complete response on end-of-treatment imaging. Two months later, she develops progressive abdominal pain, with a new abdominal soft tissue mass on imaging. Biopsy confirms relapse of high-grade B-cell lymphoma. Which chimeric antigen receptor T-cell product is approved in this clinical scenario?
   A. Brexucabtagene autoleucel
   B. Axicabtagene ciloleucel
   C. Idecabtagene vicleucel
   D. Sipuleucel-T

3. What advantage does the addition of a costimulatory domain to second-generation chimeric antigen receptor (CAR) T-cells offer?
   A. CAR T-cell excretion of proinflammatory cytokines
   B. Increased expansion and recruitment of both CAR-T and native immune cells
   C. Reduced incidence of severe neurotoxicity
   D. Limiting disease evasion by targeting multiple tumor antigens

4. A 42-year-old patient is diagnosed with mantle cell lymphoma following presentation with diffuse adenopathy, drenching night sweats, and progressive weight loss. He presents to the clinic to discuss the approved chimeric antigen receptor T-cell product for mantle cell lymphoma. Which of the following is true regarding brexucabtagene autoleucel?

A. Patients may experience prolonged cytopenias lasting >30 days follow-ing therapy.

B. Immune effector cell-associated neurotoxicity syndrome of any grade occurs in more than 80% of patients.

C. There may be an increased risk of infection due to prolonged hypogammaglobulinemia.

D. Brexucabtagene manufacturing is designed to limit T-cell exhaustion.

E. All of the above.

5. A 68-year-old patient is receiving chimeric antigen receptor (CAR) T-cell therapy for relapsed follicular lymphoma. Three days after receiving CAR T-cells, he develops fever to 39.0°C. His fever transiently improves with acetaminophen but the following day he develops progressive hypoxia requiring supplemental oxygen. He is transferred to the intensive care unit for monitoring. What is the target of the Food and Drug Administration (FDA)-approved therapy for cytokine release syndrome (CRS)?

A. Interleukin-6R

B. Granulocyte macrophage colony-stimulating factor

C. Interleukin-2

D. Tumor necrosis factor-alpha

6. A 70-year-old patient develops confusion and altered mental status 8 days following administration of tisagenlecleucel for relapsed diffuse large B-cell lymphoma. She is treated with corticosteroids with rapid improvement in her mentation. Which cell therapy product has been associated with risk of delayed neurotoxicity with parkinsonian features?

A. Axicabtagene ciloleucel

B. Tisagenlecleucel

C. Idecabtagene vicleucel

D. Lutetium 177 dotatate

7. Which of the following represents a barrier to broader use of cellular therapy products?

A. Toxicities requiring high levels of supportive care

B. Financial costs

C. Geographic limitations

D. Prolonged manufacturing time

E. All of the above

8. A 54-year-old patient with diffuse large B-cell lymphoma (DLBCL) presents for discussion of therapy for relapsed disease. He initially presented with extensive adenopathy above and below the diaphragm. He was treated with six cycles of R-CHOP therapy with a complete response on fluorodeoxyglucose (FDG)-PET. Three years later he presents with palpable adenopathy in the cervical nodes and biopsy is consistent with recurrent DLBCL. He is started on salvage chemotherapy with a near complete response after two cycles. What is the appropriate next step in management?

A. Referral for high-dose chemotherapy with stem cell rescue
B. Leukapheresis in anticipation of chimeric antigen receptor T-cell therapy
C. Continuation of salvage chemotherapy until progression or unacceptable toxicity
D. Observation

9. **A 72-year-old patient presents for consideration of chimeric antigen receptor (CAR) T-cell therapy for relapsed diffuse large B-cell lymphoma (DLBCL). He has active disease involving the mesentery root causing substantial abdominal pain. Which of the following therapies for relapsed DLBCL shares overlapping targets with the approved CAR T-cell products?**
A. Selinexor
B. Polatuzumab vedotin
C. Loncastuximab tesirine
D. Tafasitamab

10. **A 64-year-old patient with mantle cell lymphoma presents for consideration of chimeric antigen receptor (CAR) T-cell therapy. He was initially treated with combination chemotherapy followed by high-dose chemotherapy with stem cell rescue. He received rituximab maintenance followed by the BTK inhibitor ibrutinib after progression. He now has worsening adenopathy and cytopenias. Which of the following would most impact his ability to undergo successful CAR T-cell manufacturing?**
A. Bridging therapy with bendamustine prior to leukapheresis
B. Prior use of rituximab maintenance
C. A history of recurrent urinary tract infection
D. Inadequate peripheral venous access

ANSWERS

1. **D. B-cell maturation antigen.** Both approved CAR T-cell products for relapsed multiple myeloma, idecabtagene vicleucel and ciltacabtagene autoleucel, target B-cell maturation antigen (BCMA). BCMA is particularly expressed by plasma cells, both benign and malignant.

2. **B. Axicabtagene ciloleucel.** The ZUMA-7 trial established a progression-free survival advantage for axicabtagene ciloleucel over autologous stem cell transplant in patients with refractory disease or relapse within 1 year of primary chemoimmunotherapy. Patients with high-grade B-cell lymphoma were included in the ZUMA-7 trial and have historically inferior outcomes with salvage chemotherapy. Lisocabtagene maraleucel is also approved for this indication.

3. **B. Increased expansion and recruitment of both CAR-T and native immune cells.** The hallmark of second-generation CAR T-cell products is the addition of a costimulatory domain such as 4-1BB or CD28. Activation of these signaling pathways allows for more robust CAR T-cell expansion and persistence. This rapid proliferation contributes to increased rates of cytokine release syndrome and immune effector cell-associated neurotoxicity syndrome. CAR T-cell constructs that allow for cytokine secretion or targeting of multiple antigens are currently only available in the clinical trial setting.

4. **E. All of the above.** The manufacturing of brexucabtagene autoleucel removes malignant cells from the apheresis product to limit T-cell exhaustion before administration. Common CD19-directed CAR T-cell toxicities include prolonged B-cell aplasia resulting in hypogammaglobulinemia, prolonged neutropenia and thrombocytopenia, cytokine release syndrome (CRS) and neurotoxicity (ICANS).

5. **A. Interleukin-6R.** Tocilizumab is approved by the FDA for management of cytokine release syndrome and targets the interleukin (IL)-6 pathway by inhibiting both the soluble and membrane-bound IL-6 receptors. Tocilizumab has not been approved for the specific management of immune effector cell-associated neurotoxicity syndrome occurring without concurrent CRS.

6. **C. Idecabtagene vicleucel.** The chimeric antigen receptor T-cell products targeting B-cell maturation antigen (BCMA) carry Food and Drug Administration warnings for delayed neurotoxicity that presents with parkinsonian features. The reported incidence is very rare and may be related to expression of BCMA on cells in the central nervous system.

7. **E. All of the above.** Multiple barriers constrain the wider availability of chimeric antigen receptor (CAR) T-cells and other cellular therapies. CAR T-cell therapy is typically limited to high-volume centers with infrastructure in place to manage the complex logistics and toxicities. This may require patients to undertake significant travel and financial burdens to pursue therapy.

8. **A. Referral for high-dose chemotherapy with stem cell rescue.** This patient has had a significant interval of 3 years between initial chemoimmunotherapy and disease relapse. Chemosensitivity should be demonstrated with a platinum-based salvage regimen with consideration of autologous stem cell transplantation as consolidative therapy. In comparison, CAR T-cell therapy is considered in patients who relapse within 12 months of frontline therapy.

9. **D. Tafasitamab.** Tafasitamab targets the CD19 protein that is expressed near ubiquitously on B-cells. CD19 is also the primary target of the currently approved CAR T-cell products. There are very little data regarding the sequencing of CD19-directed therapies and what role antigen loss may play in disease progression.

10. **A. Bridging therapy with bendamustine prior to leukapheresis.** Bendamustine is a profoundly lymphotoxic therapy that may limit sufficient collection of healthy lymphocytes for CAR T-cell manufacturing. Bendamustine may be held from approved combination therapy regimens (bendamustine, polatuzumab, rituximab) prior to leukapheresis and then incorporated following confirmation of adequate collection. Rituximab will not interfere with T-cell collection. If peripheral access is not easily achieved, lymphocyte collection can be completed through a temporary central line.

Biostatistics

29

Christopher Su and Emily Bellile

BASIC CONCEPTS AND DEFINITIONS

TABLE 29.1 ■ Basic Biostatistical Concepts *p*-value

Term	Definition
P value	Assumes a **null hypothesis** (often that two measurements are equal) and describes probability that the observed difference is **due to chance or random variation alone**. **p-value <0.05 (5%) is usually sufficient to reject the null hypothesis** (i.e., difference between two datasets are NOT due to chance alone).
Prevalence	Number of **total cases** in a population at **a given point in time**.
Incidence	Number of **new cases** that occur over **a specific period of time.**
Incidence proportion	Number of **new cases** (during a period of time) divided by **total at risk** (at the beginning of this period). Also known as cumulative incidence.
Relative risk/ Risk ratio	Probability (incidence proportion) of an event in an exposed group (e.g. treatment) divided by probability (incidence proportion) of the same event in those not exposed. Used in **randomized controlled studies and cohort studies**.
Odds ratio	Odds (*probability*/[1 – *probability*]) of an event occurring in one group divided by the odds of the same event occurring in a different group. Summary measure in **logistic regressions to measure the strength of association between an outcome and predictors**. Used in **multivariable analysis** and **case-controlled studies.**
ARR/ Risk difference	**Change in incidence due to an exposure.** The proportion of patients who are spared the adverse outcome as a result of having received the experimental rather than the control therapy. Calculated by subtracting the incidence proportion of the exposed group from the incidence proportion of the control group over a period of time.
Number needed to treat	**Number of patients needed to be treated to prevent one event.** Inverse of the absolute risk reduction (1/ARR).

ARR, Absolute risk reduction.

EXAMPLE 29.1

There were 10 new cases in 100 subjects over a 1-year observation period. At the end of the observation period, there were 20 total cases (some had disease before the study).

Incidence proportion of disease is $10/100 = 10\%$ in this population over 1 year.

Prevalence of the disease at the end of the study is $20/100 = 20\%$ at the end of the study.

EXAMPLE 29.2:

Consider the following table.

TABLE 29.2 ■ Basic Concepts and Definitions

	Disease	No Disease	Total
Treated	5 (A)	45 (B)	50 (A+B)
Not treated	20 (C)	80 (D)	100 (C+D)
Total	25 (A+C)	125 (B+D)	150 (A+B+C+D)

Risk ratio = risk of disease in those treated / risk of disease in those not treated

$$RR = \frac{\dfrac{A}{A+B}}{\dfrac{C}{C+D}} = \frac{\dfrac{5}{50}}{\dfrac{20}{100}} = \frac{0.1}{0.2} = 0.5$$

Odds ratio = odds of disease in those treated / odds of disease in those not treated

$$OR = \frac{\dfrac{0.1}{1-.1}}{\dfrac{0.2}{1-0.2}} = \frac{\dfrac{1}{9}}{\dfrac{2}{8}} = \frac{4}{9} = 0.45$$

An easier way is (A*D) / (B*C) (odds ratio is also called the **cross-product ratio)** with the same result: (5*80) divided by (45*20) = 4/9 (0.45).

EXAMPLE 29.3

A new preventive treatment is introduced. Prior to the treatment, 10 people in 100 developed disease over a 1-year period. Now, only 5 people in 100 developed disease over the same period.

Absolute risk reduction is calculated: $5/100 = 5\%$ in the treated group subtracted from $10/100 = 10\%$ in the untreated group, so ARR is 5%.

Number needed to treat is 1 divided by ARR (0.05), which is 20 people.

DIAGNOSTIC TESTS

Test results		Condition or disease: Positive	Condition or disease: Negative	
	Positive	A	B	Positive predictive value = A/(A + B)
	Negative	C	D	Negative predictive value = D/(C + D)
		Sensitivity = A/(A+C)	Sensitivity = D/(B + D)	

FIGURE 29.1 ■ Sensitivity, specificity, positive predictive value, and negative predictive value.

TABLE 29.3 ■ Sensitivity, Specificity, Positive Predictive Value, Negative Predictive Value

Term	Definition
Sensitivity	# positive tests divided by # with disease. **How well the test detects disease in the population with disease – <u>screening</u> tests aim for high sensitivity (few false negatives).**
Specificity	# negative tests divided by # without disease. **How well the test confirms no disease in a population with no disease – <u>diagnostic</u> tests aim for high specificity (few false positives).**
Positive likelihood ratio (for positive tests)	Probability of an individual with disease testing positive divided by probability of an individual with NO disease testing positive. ***sensitivity/(1-specificity)*** **("how likely does an individual have the disease if they have a positive test?")** The more the likelihood ratio for a positive test (LR+) is greater than 1, the more likely the disease or outcome.
Negative likelihood ratio (for negative tests)	Probability of an individual with disease testing negative divided by probability of an individual with NO disease testing negative. ***(1-sensitivity)/specificity.*** **("how likely does an individual have the disease if they have a negative test?")** The more a likelihood ratio for a negative test is less than 1, the less likely the disease or outcome.
PPV	# positive tests in those that actually have disease divided by # of total positive tests. **High PPV is desirable for a screening test – although this is dependent on the prevalence of disease in the population** (i.e. a screening test can have high sensitivity and specificity, but have a low PPV if prevalence of disease is low in the studied population).
NPV	# negative tests in those that do NOT have the disease divided by # of total negative tests. **High NPV is also desirable for a screening test – similarly dependent on the overall population (see PPV above).**

NPV, negative predictive value; PPV, positive predictive value.

CLINICAL STUDY DESIGN BIASES

TABLE 29.4 ■ Selected Biases in Clinical Study Design

Term	Definition
Selection bias	Study population does not reflect the target population.
Referral/volunteer (response) bias	A type of **selection bias** where those who volunteer for medical studies may be more aware of their health, thereby biasing the study outcomes with a sample that is healthier than the population at large.
	A related bias is **centripetal bias** where patients may seek out certain medical centers or providers due to prestige (e.g. traveling from out-of-state), artificially inflating the number of observed cases at the institution/location.
Attrition bias	A type of **selection bias** where losses and withdrawals in the exposure and control groups are unequal. **Can be mitigated via intention-to-treat analysis in clinical trials.**
Classification (measurement) bias	Improper, inadequate, or ambiguous recording of exposure or outcome variables.
Recall bias	A type of **classification bias** where participants of different study subgroups may remember exposures differently (e.g. patients may recall exposures better than control).
Detection bias	A type of **classification bias** where the observations in one (often the treatment) group are followed-up more rigorously than those in the other (control) group. **Can be mitigated via study blinding.**
Observer (confirmation) bias	A type of **classification bias** where study personnel make subjective determinations of outcome, sometimes fitting observations to an existing belief/hypothesis. **Can be mitigated by study blinding and making outcomes objective rather than subjective.**
Confounding bias	Variable of interest is not directly associated with the outcome, but associated with a range of other variables that are also associated with the outcome. **Can be controlled for in analysis stage by statistically adjusting for confounders as long as they are properly identified.**
Lead time bias	**Artificial extension of perceived survival time by shifting forward the time of diagnosis** due to better detection/screening while the biological onset of disease remains unchanged. The earlier we diagnose a disease, the longer a patient appears to survive.
Length time bias	**Artificial inflation of the value of screening and survival time in slowly progressive disease over rapidly progressive disease, as screening is more likely to pick up slowly progressing disease** (i.e. the individuals with early-onset or rapidly progressive disease might be detected from symptoms prior to screening).

(continued)

TABLE 29.4 ■ Selected Biases in Clinical Study Design (*continued*)

Term	Definition
Reporting bias	Statistically significant results (and studies) are more likely to be reported over those which are insignificant.
Hawthorne effect	Study subjects who are aware that they are being observed behave differently from those who are not. **Can be controlled for by having a control group so all groups are under observation.**

CLINICAL STUDY BASICS

TABLE 29.5 ■ Selected Terms Used in Clinical Trial Design

Term	Definition
Confidence interval	Range of values **most likely to incorporate the true value** in a population following repeated sampling. Dependent on # of observation and variance in dataset – **confidence interval narrows with <u>increasing</u> observations and <u>decreasing</u> variance**. Often reported at 95% confidence interval (true value will fall within reported range 95% of the time).
Null hypothesis	**Claim that the study investigators want to disprove** (e.g. there is no difference between treated and untreated patients).
Type I error (alpha)	Probability of **rejecting the null hypothesis when it shouldn't be rejected** (false positive). **This is related to the *P* value** – if *P* value < alpha, we **reject** the null hypothesis. If *P* value > alpha, we **fail to reject** the null hypothesis.
Type II error (beta)	Probability of **failing to reject the null hypothesis when it should be rejected** (false negative). **Power** of study is related to **type II error (beta).**
Power	Probability of **rejecting the null hypothesis when it should be rejected** (true positive). **Defined as 1-beta, related to sample size, variance, defined significance level (alpha), and effect size.**
Cohort study	Type of **observational study** that compares two groups with **different exposures and following for outcome.** Can be prospective or retrospective. Helpful to **determine how common an outcome is, and what exposures are associated with the outcome of interest.** Measure of association between exposure and outcome can be **relative risk or odds ratio.**
Case-control study	Type of **observational study** that compares two groups with **different outcomes and examines prior exposures**. Retrospective. Helpful to **investigate exposures that lead to an outcome.** Measure of association between exposure and outcome is **odds ratio.**

(*continued*)

TABLE 29.5 ■ Selected Terms Used in Clinical Trial Design (*continued*)

Term	Definition
Randomized control trial (RTC)	"Gold standard" for clinical investigation – **randomly allocates subjects to control and treatment groups and follows for response.** Randomization helps control for confounders.
Intention-to-treat analysis	**Analyze study groups in a RTC according to randomization,** rather than adherence to treatment or the actual treatment received. This helps to reduce **attrition bias**.
Primary endpoint	**Goal of the study** – should ideally be clinically relevant, sensitive to intervention, practical and affordable to measure, ideally unbiased (e.g. objective measure like death), and interpretable within the context of study.
Composite endpoint	**Combination of several measures as a single endpoint** (e.g. death, stroke, and cardiac arrest as one endpoint in studying cardiovascular disease). Advantages include increasing the number of outcome events (thereby decreasing sample size needed to achieve sufficient power). Disadvantages include subjective determination of measures that form the composite endpoint and potentially unequal contribution of identified measures that form the composite endpoint.
Surrogate endpoint	**Selected measure that "stands-in" for a true clinical endpoint,** used usually when the true clinical endpoint takes a long time to achieve or is difficult to measure (e.g. the true clinical endpoint is rare or is the patient's death). **Progression-free survival** and **time to progression** are commonly assessed surrogate endpoints.
Phase 0	**First studies in humans** – very small sample sizes, focused on pharmacokinetics and pharmacodynamics. Not always done or required.
Phase I	**Safety and dose finding trials** – doses escalate in study groups until adverse events and desired treatment effects are seen. Often performed with patients of different cancer types.
Phase II	**Disease-specific/safety trials** – done in larger groups than Phase I on patients with the same type of cancer with tolerable doses found in Phase I studies. Target drugs may be combined with other existing drugs and treatment efficacy assessed.
Phase III	**"Which drug works better" trials** – large RTCs with treatment and control arms (often the standard-of-care drug or a placebo). Positive results for a study drug in Phase III trials usually lead to FDA application for approval.
Phase IV	**Post-marketing trials** – conducted to collect information on marketing data (cost effectiveness), long-lasting side effects, or other special considerations (drug-to-drug side effects, safety in special populations such as pregnant women).

RTC, randomized control trial.

QUESTIONS

1. **What is intention-to-treat (ITT) analysis?**
   A. All subjects randomized into a treatment group are included in the final analysis and analyzed according to the group they were randomized into, regardless of whether they took the trial drug.
   B. All subjects randomized into a treatment group are included in the final analysis and analyzed according to the group they were randomized into, only if they took the trial drug.
   C. Subjects are enrolled into treatment groups at the beginning of the study based on their intention or declination to take the trial drug.
   D. Subjects are only randomized into treatment groups if they intend to follow the results of randomization.

2. **Why are large randomized clinical trials often "double-blinded"?**
   A. It is required for intention-to-treat analysis.
   B. It reduces confounding.
   C. It reduces bias.
   D. It increases power.

3. **What determines whether a surrogate endpoint can be appropriately used in place of the primary clinical endpoint?**
   A. Allotted time and budget for the study.
   B. Demonstrated relationship between the surrogate endpoint and the primary clinical endpoint.
   C. Demonstrated improvement from the proposed intervention in both the surrogate and primary clinical endpoint in pilot studies.
   D. All of the above.

4. **A novel lymphoma treatment was developed. In the standard-of-care group, 60 out of 100 subjects experienced disease progression after 6 months. In the novel treatment group, only 10 out of 100 subjects experienced disease progression after 6 months. What is the number needed to treat?**
   A. 2
   B. 10
   C. 50
   D. 60

5. **You recently heard a colleague describe a clinical trial in which a first-in-class drug was tested across patients with different types of hematologic malignancies. All subjects received the drug; there was no placebo. The first enrolled patients received very low doses of the drug and were monitored for side effects. If the side effect profile was acceptable, the next patients enrolled received higher doses. The process was repeated until an anticipated therapeutic dosage had been reached and the side effect profile remained acceptable. Your colleague was most likely describing what type of clinical trial?**
   A. Phase 0
   B. Phase I
   C. Phase II
   D. Phase III

ANSWERS

1. **A. All subjects randomized into a treatment group are included in the final analysis and analyzed according to the group they were randomized into, regardless of whether they took the trial drug.** The advantage of intention-to-treat analysis is that it preserves randomization. In "per-protocol" analysis (choice B), in which subjects are analyzed according to the treatment they received, misleading results due to skewed treatment groups can occur. Intention-to-treat is an analytic method and does not determine how patients are enrolled into the trial (choices C and D).

2. **C. It reduces bias.** Blinding is a trial design component aimed at reducing observer bias due to awareness of group assignment by participants, investigators, or both. "Double-blinding" means that neither the participants nor the investigators are aware of treatment group assignment. Studies can even be "triple-blinded," in which the analysts who examine the outcomes are also unaware of group assignment. Blinding does not alter the existence of confounders, which must be recognized and adjusted for in statistical analysis. Blinding is unrelated to intention-to-treat analysis and statistical power.

3. **D. All of the above.** The advantage of utilizing a surrogate endpoint (biomarker or progression-free survival) in place of a primary clinical endpoint (diagnosis of cancer or overall survival) is that vast clinical trials with large sample sizes (aimed at increasing event rate) and prolonged observational periods may not be necessary. This helps with time or budget concerns (choice A). When designating a surrogate endpoint, the investigator should consider the demonstrated relationship of the surrogate to the primary endpoint. An improvement in the surrogate endpoint should be associated with an improvement in the primary endpoint. Furthermore, demonstrated relationship and improvement with the proposed intervention should be observed in both the surrogate and primary endpoints from pilot studies (choices B and C).

4. **A. 2.** To calculate the number needed to treat, the absolute risk reduction (ARR) must be derived. The novel treatment reduces the absolute risk from 0.6 (60/100) to 0.1 (10/100), yielding an ARR of 0.5. The number needed to treat is the reciprocal of the ARR, or 2. In other words, 2 patients need to be treated to prevent 1 patient progression.

5. **B. Phase I.** Phase 0 trials are designed to evaluate the pharmacokinetics and pharmacodynamics of a new drug. The sample size is small and there is no dose escalation. Phase I trials are safety and dose finding trials where doses vary in study groups until a therapeutic dosage with an acceptable side effect profile is reached. Phase I trials are often conducted with subjects with different types of cancer and there is no placebo group. Phase II trials build on the findings of Phase I trials by testing the tolerable dosages determined in Phase I trials on a patient population with the same malignancy. Often, the new therapeutic is combined with elements of existing therapy. Phase III trials are large randomized-controlled trials where the novel treatment regimen tested in the Phase II trials is compared against the standard-of-care ("gold standard") treatment to determine comparative treatment efficacy.

Index